W9-CNZ-656

Confronting AIDS

Directions for Public Health, Health Care, and Research

Institute of Medicine
National Academy of Sciences

NATIONAL ACADEMY PRESS
Washington, D.C. 1986

NATIONAL ACADEMY PRESS ● **2101 Constitution Ave., NW** ● **Washington, DC 20418**

NOTICE: The project that is the subject of this report was approved by the Governing Board of the National Research Council, whose members are drawn from the councils of the National Academy of Sciences, the National Academy of Engineering, and the Institute of Medicine. The members of the committee responsible for the report were chosen for their special competences and with regard for appropriate balance.

This report has been reviewed by a group other than the authors according to procedures approved by a Report Review Committee consisting of members of the National Academy of Sciences, the National Academy of Engineering, and the Institute of Medicine.

The National Academy of Sciences was established in 1863 by Act of Congress as a private, nonprofit, self-governing membership corporation for the furtherance of science and technology, required to advise the federal government upon request within its fields of competence. Under its corporate charter the Academy established the National Research Council in 1916 and the National Academy of Engineering in 1964.

The Institute of Medicine was chartered in 1970 by the National Academy of Sciences to enlist distinguished members of the appropriate professions in the examination of policy matters pertaining to the health of the public. In this, the Institute acts under both the Academy's 1863 congressional charter responsibility to be an adviser to the federal government and its own initiative in identifying issues of medical care, research, and education.

Support for this project was provided by the National Research Council (NRC) Fund, a pool of private, discretionary, nonfederal funds that is used to support a program of Academy-initiated studies of national issues in which science and technology figure significantly. The NRC Fund consists of contributions from several sources: a consortium of private foundations, including the Carnegie Corporation of New York, the Charles E. Culpeper Foundation, the William and Flora Hewlett Foundation, the John D. and Catherine T. MacArthur Foundation, the Andrew W. Mellon Foundation, the Rockefeller Foundation, and the Alfred P. Sloan Foundation; the Academy Industry Program, which seeks annual contributions from companies that are concerned with the health of U.S. science and technology and with public policy issues with technological content; and the National Academy of Sciences and the National Academy of Engineering endowments.

Library of Congress Cataloging-in-Publication Data

Institute of Medicine (U.S.).
  Confronting AIDS.

  Report prepared by the Committee on a National Strategy for AIDS of the Institute of Medicine.
  Includes bibliographies and index.
  1. AIDS (Disease)—Prevention—Government policy—United States. 2. AIDS (Disease)—United States—Prevention. 3. AIDS (Disease)—Research—Government policy—United States. 4. AIDS (Disease)—Research—United States. 5. AIDS (Disease)—Treatment—Government policy—United States. 6. AIDS (Disease)—Treatment—United States. I. Institute of Medicine (U.S.). Committee on a National Strategy for AIDS. II. Title. [DNLM: 1. Acquired Immunodeficiency Syndrome. 2. Health Policy—United States. WD 308 I59c]

RA644.A25I57   1986   362.1′9797′9200973   86-23779

ISBN 0-309-03699-2

First Printing, October 1986
Copyright © 1986 by the National Academy of Sciences   Second Printing, January 1987

Printed in the United States of America

Committee on a National Strategy for AIDS

STEERING COMMITTEE

DAVID BALTIMORE (*Cochair*), Whitehead Institute for Biomedical Research and Massachusetts Institute of Technology, Cambridge

SHELDON M. WOLFF (*Cochair*), Tufts University School of Medicine and New England Medical Center Hospital, Boston

JOHN J. BURNS, Roche Institute of Molecular Biology, Nutley, New Jersey

LEON EISENBERG, Harvard Medical School, Boston

BERNARD N. FIELDS, Harvard Medical School, Boston

HARVEY V. FINEBERG, Harvard School of Public Health, Boston

FRANK LILLY, Albert Einstein College of Medicine, Bronx

JUNE E. OSBORN, School of Public Health, University of Michigan, Ann Arbor

MARGERY W. SHAW, University of Texas Health Science Center, Houston

PAUL VOLBERDING, San Francisco General Hospital

IRVING WEISSMAN, Stanford University School of Medicine

HEALTH CARE AND PUBLIC HEALTH PANEL

SHELDON M. WOLFF (*Chair*), Tufts University School of Medicine and New England Medical Center Hospital, Boston

JAMES CHIN, California State Department of Health Services, Berkeley

WILLIAM J. CURRAN, Harvard School of Public Health, Boston

DAVID W. FRASER, Swarthmore College, Swarthmore, Pennsylvania

JEFFREY E. HARRIS, Massachusetts Institute of Technology, Cambridge

ARTHUR LIFSON, Equitable Life Assurance Society of the United States, New York City

DOROTHY NELKIN, Cornell University, Ithaca, New York

JUNE E. OSBORN, School of Public Health, University of Michigan, Ann Arbor

SAMUEL W. PERRY, Cornell University Medical Center, New York City

PAUL VOLBERDING, San Francisco General Hospital

LeROY WALTERS, Kennedy Institute of Ethics, Georgetown University, Washington, D.C.

RESEARCH PANEL

DAVID BALTIMORE (*Chair*), Whitehead Institute for Biomedical Research and Massachusetts Institute of Technology, Cambridge

LEON EISENBERG, Harvard Medical School, Boston

RESEARCH PANEL (Continued)

BERNARD N. FIELDS, Harvard Medical School, Boston
JEROME E. GROOPMAN, Harvard Medical School, Boston
MAURICE R. HILLEMAN, Merck Institute for Therapeutic Research, Merck Sharp & Dohme Research Labs, West Point, Pennsylvania
RICHARD T. JOHNSON, Johns Hopkins University School of Medicine, Baltimore, Maryland
ROBERT F. MURRAY, Jr., Howard University College of Medicine, Washington, D.C.
ROLAND K. ROBINS, Molecular Research Institute and ICN Pharmaceuticals, Costa Mesa, California
P. FREDERICK SPARLING, University of North Carolina School of Medicine, Chapel Hill
CLADD E. STEVENS, New York Blood Center, New York City
HOWARD M. TEMIN, University of Wisconsin School of Medicine, Madison
IRVING WEISSMAN, Stanford University School of Medicine

EPIDEMIOLOGY WORKING GROUP CHAIRMAN

J. THOMAS GRAYSTON, University of Washington, Seattle

STAFF

ROY WIDDUS, Project Director and Director, Division of International Health
DEBORAH COTTON, Deputy Project Director
MARK FEINBERG, Staff Officer
JEFF STRYKER, Staff Officer
JUDE PAYNE, Research Assistant
KAREN ZWEIG, Research Assistant
GAIL SPEARS, Administrative Secretary
STEVE OLSON, Project Editor
DOROTHY SAWICKI, Book Editor, National Academy Press
CAROL COFIELD, Secretary
CAREY O'BRIEN, Secretary
KATHLEEN ACHOR, Secretary

CONSULTANTS

PETER E. DANS, Johns Hopkins Medical Institutions, Baltimore, Maryland
JESSE GREEN, New York University Medical Center, New York City

iv

Preface

In October 1985 the Institute of Medicine devoted its annual meeting to the subject of acquired immune deficiency syndrome (AIDS). The information presented at that meeting has been summarized in a nontechnical volume entitled *Mobilizing Against AIDS: The Unfinished Story of a Virus* (Harvard University Press, 1986), which surveys knowledge on AIDS and the issues raised by the disease. That annual meeting was not intended to develop recommendations about the best course of action for dealing with the problems it surveyed, but the Institute of Medicine realized that recommendations were needed and that, to develop them, national leadership was essential. As a result, in early 1986 the presidents of the National Academy of Sciences (NAS) and the Institute of Medicine (IOM), with the approval of the councils of these organizations, decided to initiate a special effort to assess the extent of the problems arising from AIDS and to propose an appropriate national response. The congressional charter establishing the National Academy of Sciences, under which it and the Institute of Medicine operate, specifies that they shall undertake studies of issues of vital importance to the nation. This report results from such self-initiated activity.

The topics to be addressed in the study were specified as follows:

The committee shall assess the current understanding of the virus that causes acquired immune deficiency syndrome (AIDS), its transmission, the natural history of infection and associated disease, the epidemiology of conditions associated with the virus, and the likely trends in these.

v

The committee also shall review the nation's response to AIDS both in the public and private sector and the current planning in regard to:

- research necessary for prevention and treatment
- provision of care and its financing
- public health measures designed to control the disease.

The committee shall evaluate methods whereby the ultimate goals of controlling and combating the disease may be achieved. Questions to be addressed should include, but are not necessarily limited to, the following:

- Are there neglected research opportunities or needs with regard to the biology and epidemiology of the virus, the animal models of infection and disease, or the prospects for vaccines or antiviral agents?
- What are the impediments to the most expeditious pursuit of these opportunities and needs, and how can they be overcome? Specifically, what mechanisms should be instituted to achieve promotion of productive research, timely utilization of new knowledge, optimal communication among persons engaged in research and development (and with health care and public health professionals), integration and coordination of the R&D effort, recruitment of appropriate investigators, and the optimal involvement of industry?
- Is the care of AIDS and AIDS-related complex (ARC) patients (and seropositive persons) properly coordinated? What are the best approaches to the provision of care and what are the local, regional, and national implications of these models for the health care system?
- How are the costs of care being met? Are there ways in which these costs could be met in a more rational and/or equitable fashion?
- What public health measures (including educational programs) are desirable in light of present knowledge and circumstances? By whom should these be promoted, implemented, coordinated, and revised?
- What are the legal and ethical issues raised by the questions posed above; in particular, in the formulation of public health policy, how is a balance best achieved between the interests of the public and those of the individual?
- How should the United States address the international ramifications of the problem of AIDS? What will be its magnitude; what is the appropriate role for the United States; and what are its responsibilities?

The committee shall prepare a report outlining a strategy (or strategies) whereby these concerns can be addressed. The report shall contain recommendations for its implementation directed to the Executive Branch, the Congress, the research community, those who treat patients, state and local governments, corporate leadership, and the public. The report shall include a description of the basis for the committee's conclusions.

To prepare this report, a committee with an impressive breadth of credentials was established. To cover the broad range of issues raised in combating AIDS, two panels were constituted, one addressing issues in research, the other addressing issues in health care and public health. To integrate the activities of the panels, a steering group was formed, consisting of four members from each panel and four at-large members. Collectively, the panels and the steering committee comprised individuals with expertise in molecular biology, virology, immunology, epidemiology, neurology, psychiatry, infectious diseases, general medicine, health care, public health, economics, law, ethics, and other disciplines. They represented research experience in academia, several branches of the federal government, and industry, with substantial experience in managing research and development projects in all three of these areas. In addition, the panels and the steering committee included individuals with experience in developing and implementing public health programs at the national, state, and local levels, as well as those closely involved in the care of patients.

The councils of the National Academy of Sciences and the Institute of Medicine requested that a report be produced by the committee within six months of its initial meeting, reflecting the urgency with which they felt the problem should be addressed. In response, the committee undertook an intensive schedule of activities. Each panel held four meetings, which were attended by many of the at-large members of the steering committee. Also, two working groups were formed, one consisting of approximately 30 individuals who studied both the short- and long-term epidemiology of the disease, and the other a somewhat smaller group that met on two occasions to discuss issues in the financing of health care for AIDS patients.

The committee held two public meetings, one in San Francisco and one in New York City, where many individuals concerned with various problems raised by AIDS expressed their views. In addition to the public meetings, the committee invited a large number of individuals from the scientific, health care, and public health communities to contribute their thoughts. Many excellent papers were prepared at the committee's request and will be available upon request to the Institute of Medicine (see Appendix H). Many individuals involved in AIDS-related activities were also kind enough to submit prepublication data, greatly aiding the committee's awareness of ongoing research.

Committee and staff members participated in a workshop held by the Public Health Service at Coolfont, Berkeley Springs, West Virginia, June 4-6, 1986, to produce a plan for the prevention of AIDS and the control of the AIDS virus. A number of committee members and a representative of the staff also attended the Second International Conference on AIDS in Paris, June 22-25, 1986, where much new information was presented. In July 1986 the steering committee held its final meeting in Woods Hole, Massachusetts, to integrate the contributions from the panels and the working groups.

TERMINOLOGY

AIDS poses a number of problems related to terminology. First, the etiologic agent of AIDS has been given several different names, including lymphadenopathy-associated virus (LAV), human T-cell lymphotropic virus type III (HTLV-III), and AIDS-associated retrovirus (ARV). The committee followed the usual practice of NAS/IOM committees in using the name recommended by the appropriate international body charged with giving advice on nomenclature. In this case, the appropriate body is the International Committee on the Taxonomy of Viruses, a subcommittee of which has proposed that the virus be called human immunodeficiency virus (HIV). This designation for the virus is used throughout this report.

Terminology related to AIDS and other conditions related to HIV infection may also be confusing. The term AIDS itself was coined as a surveillance definition for epidemiologic purposes. It does not include the full spectrum of conditions now known to be associated with HIV infection.

Reference to the "AIDS epidemic" has become ubiquitous in discussions and publications on this topic. It must be understood, however, that the epidemic in its full extent includes not only individuals with AIDS but other infected individuals who have less severe manifestations of the disease or who are asymptomatic. (In some sense, the epidemic can even be said to encompass reactions such as fear of the disease and of the virus among the general public.) Indeed, because infection of humans with HIV is a relatively new phenomenon, the full spectrum of signs and symptoms that the virus may cause is yet to be known. Furthermore, the manifestations of HIV infections and immunodeficiency reflect, at least in part, the environmental pathogens to which individuals are exposed. Thus, these manifestations may appear to vary in different population groups in different parts of the world, but they still reflect the basic, underlying HIV infection. In general, the evolution of terminology related to HIV-associated conditions should be regarded as natural and desirable as our knowledge of the pathogen and its consequences increases.

There are other problems of terminology related to AIDS. Certain groups—for example, male homosexuals and intravenous drug users—have been designated as being at high risk of contracting the disease. However, the designation "at high risk" encompasses more people than is necessary, because not all members of these groups are at high risk of being infected with HIV. A more appropriate designation might be "persons who engage in high-risk behaviors," and references in this report to "high-risk groups" should be so interpreted. Furthermore, references to high-risk groups may lead persons outside of these groups to believe mistakenly that they are not susceptible to HIV infection even if they engage in high-risk activities. It may also lead individuals to consciously or unconsciously deny that they are at risk. For example, a man who has had infrequent homosexual contacts may regard himself as predominantly heterosexual and therefore not in danger of infection. This can lead to misconceptions about the desirability of taking action to avoid infection or about whether infection may have already occurred.

Identifying the risk of infection as being associated with certain "high-risk behaviors" is also not without problems. This is particularly so in the area of sexual transmission, where a multiplicity of sexual partners, homosexual or heterosexual, has been associated with a high risk of becoming infected. Unfortunately, some may interpret this to mean that many partners are required for a person to become infected. In fact, it merely represents a statistical phenomenon whereby the chances of having intercourse with an infected person increase as the number of partners increases.

The term "intravenous drug use" presents additional difficulties. In this report the term implies the intravenous administration of illicit drugs such as heroin for nonmedical purposes. Individuals who engage in this activity may or may not be addicted, and some may not regard their use of such drugs as abuse.

Care has been taken throughout the report to be as precise as possible. However, the reader should bear in mind potential problems of this nature when drawing conclusions from material presented here.

STRUCTURE OF THE REPORT

After a summary chapter that presents the report's major findings and recommendations, Chapter 2 lays out the present understanding of the disease and the current status of the AIDS epidemic, providing the essential background information upon which the committee based its conclusions and recommendations (which appear throughout succeeding chapters as well as in the summary chapter). Chapter 3 then projects the epidemic into the future, suggesting its most likely course and discussing the uncertainties that any such projections entail. It also includes a brief discussion of the resources that could be brought to bear on the problems the epidemic has generated. Chapter 4 examines the measures available now—e.g., education—that could alter the course of the epidemic. Chapter 5 discusses the implications of the epidemic's projections for the provision and financing of health care related to HIV infection and AIDS in the United States. Chapter 6 identifies areas of research that will be critical in the long term for devising better means of prevention and treatment. Chapter 7 looks at international aspects of HIV infection and AIDS and at the United States' contribution to solving those problems.

Given the complex nature of the problems and the time and resources available, the committee did not attempt to prepare a definitive monograph on AIDS or to make explicit recommendations on all of the problems related to the disease. Rather, it identified the most crucial problems and suggests, when necessary, mechanisms for addressing them. Some of these problems can be addressed by agencies that already exist; others may need new mechanisms or require the convening of disparate groups working together to solve them.

During the preparation of the report, the committee was continually reminded that it was assessing a "moving target," because the problem of HIV infection was evolving as it was being studied. Consequently, this report represents the committee's evaluation as of August 1986. The pace of developments in this field has also contributed to one of the committee's major recommendations—that the problem should be monitored on a continuing basis.

Limited time precluded the committee's addressing certain important areas as fully as would have been desirable. The areas needing further consideration are identified in the report. As discussed in Chapter 1, the committee hopes that a mechanism will be put in place to take up the important issues in more detail.

ACKNOWLEDGMENTS

The committee wishes to thank the many persons who took time from their activities to assess the current status of their fields for purposes of this report (see Appendix J). In addition, all committee members gave unstintingly of their time to this endeavor. As cochairmen, we thank them for their devotion to this important work. Finally, we wish to acknowledge the excellent substantive and organizational assistance provided to the committee by the staff of the IOM-NAS headed by Roy Widdus.

DAVID BALTIMORE
Director, Whitehead Institute for
Biomedical Research, and *Professor of
Biology*, Massachusetts Institute of
Technology

SHELDON M. WOLFF
Chairman, Department of Medicine, Tufts
University School of Medicine, and
Physician-in-Chief, New England Medical
Center Hospital

Contents

ABSTRACT 1

1 CONFRONTING AIDS:
   SUMMARY AND RECOMMENDATIONS 5
   Status of the Epidemic, 5
       Infection and Transmission, 6; Clinical Manifestations
       of the Disease, 7; Statistical Dimensions of the
       Epidemic, 7
   The Future Course of the Epidemic, 8
   Opportunities for Altering the Course of the Epidemic, 9
       Public Education, 9; Public Health Measures, 13;
       Funding for Education and Other Public Health
       Measures, 16; Discrimination and AIDS, 19
   Care of Persons Infected with HIV, 19
       Health Care Costs Resulting from HIV Infection, 21; The
       Financing of Health Care for HIV-Related Conditions, 22
   Future Research Needs, 23
       Basic Research, 23; The Natural History of HIV
       Infection, 23; Epidemiologic Approaches, 24; Animal
       Models, 25; Antiviral Agents, 25; Vaccines, 26; Social
       Science Research Needs, 27; Funding for Research on
       AIDS and HIV, 28

xi

International Aspects of AIDS and HIV Infection, 28
Rationale for U.S. International Involvement, 29;
Risks of Infection Outside the United States, 29;
International Research Opportunities, 30
Guidance for the Nation's Efforts, 31
What Is Needed?, 32; Establishment of the
Commission, 32
Major Recommendations, 33

2 **UNDERSTANDING OF THE DISEASE AND
DIMENSIONS OF THE EPIDEMIC** 37
The Causative Agent of AIDS, 38
Features of Retroviruses, 40; Related Viruses, 41
Pathogenesis of AIDS, 42
Natural History of the Disease, 44
Clinical Manifestations of HIV Infection, 46
Opportunistic Infections, 46; Kaposi's Sarcoma, 47;
Other Malignancies, 48; Neurologic Complications
Associated with HIV Infection, 49; Pediatric AIDS, 49
Modes of Transmission of HIV, 50
Sexual Transmission, 51; Parenteral Transmission, 52;
Maternal-Infant Transmission, 56
Population Groups at Increased Risk of HIV Infection, 57
Homosexual Men, 57; Intravenous Drug Users, 59;
Hemophiliacs, 60; Recipients of Blood Transfusions,
60; Heterosexual Contacts of HIV-Infected
Persons, 61; Infants and Children, 61; Health Care
Workers, 62
Epidemiologic Studies and Findings, 63
Surveillance, 63; National Disease Reporting, 63;
Epidemiologic Research, 65; Findings of
Epidemiologic Studies, 69
HIV Infection and AIDS Outside the United States, 73
African Countries, 74; Other Countries, 76
References, 77

3 **THE FUTURE COURSE OF THE EPIDEMIC AND
AVAILABLE NATIONAL RESOURCES** 85
Projections by the Public Health Service, 85
Problems in Making Projections, 86

The Epidemic Within and Beyond High-Risk
  Groups, 89
The Proportion of Seropositive Individuals Who Will
  Develop AIDS, 91
Long-Term Prospects, 91
National Resources for Dealing with AIDS and HIV, 92
    Impediments to Involvement, 92; Mechanisms for
    Coordinating Activities, 93
References, 94

**4 OPPORTUNITIES FOR ALTERING THE COURSE
    OF THE EPIDEMIC** 95
Public Education, 96
    What Should Be the Content of Public Education?, 97;
    What Are the Aims of Public Education?, 100; Who
    Needs Education?, 100; Who Should Do the
    Educating?, 103; Assessing Educational Interventions,
    104; A Special Case—Changing Behavior Among IV—
    Drug Users, 105; Recommendations, 110
Public Health Measures, 112
    Tests for Infection with HIV, 113; Blood Banking,
    115; Surveillance, 117; Reporting Schemes, 118;
    Contact Tracing and Notification, 119; Mandatory
    Screening, 120; Voluntary Testing, 122; Compulsory
    Measures, 126; Recommendations, 129
Funding for Education and Other Public Health
  Measures, 130
    Recommendation, 133
Discrimination and AIDS, 133
    Recommendations, 135
References, 135

5 CARE OF PERSONS INFECTED WITH HIV 139
Roles of Health Care Providers, 139
    Recommendations, 140
Health Care Settings for AIDS Patients, 141
    Hospital Care, 141; Outpatient Care, 142;
    Community-Based AIDS Care, 143;
    Recommendations, 145
Needs of Specific Patient Populations, 146

Psychiatric and Psychosocial Support, 148
Needs of Patients with AIDS, 148; Needs of Patients
with ARC, 149; Needs of Patients with Subclinical
HIV Infections, 150; Needs of Seronegative Persons,
151; Recommendations, 152
Ethical Aspects of Providing Care, 153
Costs of Health Care for HIV-Related Conditions, 155
Direct Costs of Care for AIDS Patients, 156; Costs
of Care for ARC Patients and Seropositive
Individuals, 158; Indirect Costs of HIV-Related
Conditions, 159; Cost Implications of Projected AIDS
Cases, 159; Projected Hospitalization Facilities, 160;
Conclusions and Recommendations, 161
Financing of Health Care for HIV-Related
Conditions, 162
Sources of Financing, 162; Improving the Coverage of
Health Care Costs, 165; Emerging Issues, 166; Policy
Issues, 171; Conclusions and Recommendations, 172
References, 173

6   FUTURE RESEARCH NEEDS 177
The Structure and Replication of HIV, 178
Retroviral Structure, 178; Retroviral Replication, 179;
Definition of the Structural and Functional
Constituents of HIV, 181; Determination of the
Structure of the HIV Virion, 182; Interrupting
Infection by HIV, 183; Conclusions and
Recommendations, 187
Natural History of HIV Infection, 189
Transmission of HIV, 189; The Immune System
Response to HIV Infection, 191; The Immunologic
Consequences of HIV Infection, 193;
Recommendations, 198
Epidemiologic Approaches to Understanding the
Transmission and Natural History of HIV
Infection, 199
Recommendations on Surveillance, 199;
Recommendations on Natural History of HIV
Infection, 200; Recommendations on Transmission of
HIV, 202; Recommendations on the Need for
Improved Serologic and Virologic Tests, 203

Animal Models, 204
    HIV Infection of Chimpanzees, 205; HIV-Related
    Viruses in Old World Primates, 205; Lentiviruses
    of Ungulates, 206; Conclusions and
    Recommendations, 207
Antiviral Agents, 209
    Drug Evaluation *in Vitro*, 212; Drug Evaluation in
    Humans, 212; Current Antiviral Agents Under Clinical
    Study, 213; New Antiviral Agents Against AIDS, 218;
    Conclusions and Recommendations, 219
Vaccines, 221
    Animal Retrovirus Vaccines, 222; Vaccines Against
    HIV, 225; Models of Vaccine Delivery, 226;
    Approaches to HIV Vaccine Development
    and Evaluation, 228; Conclusions and
    Recommendations, 229
Social Science Research Needs, 230
    Breaking the Chain of Transmission, 231; Reducing
    Public Fear and Its Effects, 234; Organizing Health
    and Social Services, 237; Conclusions and
    Recommendations, 238
Funding for Research Related to AIDS and HIV, 238
    Current Levels of and Mechanisms for Funding, 239;
    Current NIH Funding Mechanisms, 241; Distribution
    of Funds Among Agencies and to Specific Research
    Areas, 244; Assessing Desirable Levels of Research
    Support, 244; Recommendations, 248
References, 249

7   INTERNATIONAL ASPECTS OF AIDS AND
    HIV INFECTION 261
Projections of the Disease Outside the United States, 261
International Organizations, 263
Rationale for U.S. International Involvement, 264
    Foreign Policy Considerations, 264; Health Improvement
    Assistance, 265; International Spread of Diseases, 266;
    Opportunities for Mutually Beneficial Research, 266;
    Agencies and Organizations with International
    Responsibilities or Operations, 267; Importation, 268
Infection Risks Outside the United States, 268
    Sexual Exposure, 268; Exposure Through Blood

Transfusion, 269; IV Drug Use, 270; Use of Unsterile
Needles and Implements, 270; Lack of Evidence
for Transmission by Insect Vectors and Casual
Contact, 271; Conclusions, 271
International Research Opportunities, 272
The U.S. Contribution to International Efforts, 274
Conclusions and Recommendations, 276
References, 277

APPENDIXES

A. Clinical Manifestations of HIV Infection 281
B. Serologic and Virologic Testing 304
C. Risk of HIV Transmission from Blood Transfusion 309
D. U.S. Public and Private Sector Resources for Fighting
   AIDS. 314
E. The Centers for Disease Control's Surveillance
   Definition of AIDS 316
F. CDC Classification System for HIV Infections 320
G. PHS Plan for Prevention and Control of AIDS
   and the AIDS Virus 326
H. List of Background Papers. 334
I. List of Presentations at Public Meetings 336
J. Acknowledgments 339
K. Biographical Notes on Committee Members 343

   GLOSSARY 353

   INDEX 361

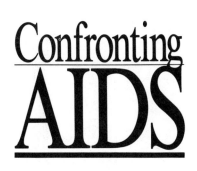

Confronting
AIDS

Abstract

Human immunodeficiency virus (HIV), the cause of acquired immune deficiency syndrome (AIDS), now infects more than a million people in the United States and millions more in other countries. The cases of AIDS reported thus far are only the beginning of the expected toll, because the damage the virus inflicts on the immune system—and the resulting inability of the victim to fight off infections and cancers—may not be apparent until years after initial infection. The epidemic is growing every day, partly because persons who may not know they are infected are spreading the virus. HIV is spread in only a few ways: transmission by anal or vaginal intercourse, by intravenous (IV) drug use, and from mother to fetus or newborn infant now predominate. Infection occurs mostly in young adults, usually the healthiest segment of the population.

A sizable proportion of those now infected will, in a few years, progress to severe disease and death. If the spread of the virus is not checked, the present epidemic could become a catastrophe. The Institute of Medicine-National Academy of Sciences Committee on a National Strategy for AIDS therefore proposes perhaps the most wide-ranging and intensive efforts ever made against an infectious disease. The situation demands both immediate action to stem the spread of infection and a long-term national commitment to produce a vaccine and therapeutic drugs.

A massive, continuing campaign should begin immediately to increase awareness of ways in which persons can protect themselves against infection, such as using condoms, avoiding anal intercourse, and not sharing drug injection equipment. The campaign should employ all the skills and tactics of education and media persuasion, and its message should be directed in language understandable to specific target groups, including homosexual men, intravenous drug users, sexually active heterosexuals (especially those who have had a number of partners), and adolescents. The committee estimates that by the end of the decade approximately $1 billion annually, much of it from federal sources, will be needed for education and other public health measures that it recommends, such as blood screening, voluntary confidential testing for infection, and increased efforts in the treatment and prevention of intravenous drug use.

The other arm of the attack on the epidemic is research. The committee believes that a vaccine is not likely to be developed for at least five years and probably longer. One drug has recently shown benefits in the treatment of AIDS, but agents that are acceptably safe for possible long-term treatment and that effectively halt or cure the disease may also not be available for at least five years. The committee calls for extensive basic and applied biomedical investigations to better understand the disease and increase the likelihood of producing a safe and effective drug or vaccine as soon as possible. This program must involve both private industry and the public sector working together. Within the overall research effort there is a need for extensive epidemiologic investigations to assess the spread of infection and the efforts to control it. Finally, there is a need for considerable research on sexual behavior and drug use and factors that influence them.

The committee believes that such a program of research will require at least $1 billion in public funds annually by 1990 and a continuing commitment over many years. These funds must be newly appropriated, not money taken from other research, because the nation's general health efforts as well as those directed against HIV need continuing progress in basic biomedical science on a broad front.

The increasing need for care of patients with AIDS and other HIV-associated conditions, including those with AIDS-related complex and HIV-related dementia, poses new and often difficult problems. These problems will spread widely in the next few years from the populations now affected. The $2- billion yearly expenditure proposed for responding to the epidemic is a small fraction of the billions of dollars for care that the epidemic is sure to cost, especially if it is not rapidly curbed. The optimal organization of care has only begun to be studied in a few cities with the heaviest case loads, but some evidence is emerging to support community-oriented care and minimal hospitalization. The provision of such care should be designed to guarantee equity of access, and the mechanisms for more appropriately financing this care need further evaluation immediately in light of various problems now apparent.

There are scientific and medical lessons to be learned about AIDS and HIV infection elsewhere in the world and compelling reasons for U.S.

involvement in efforts to control the disease worldwide. The committee believes that the United States should be a full participant in international efforts on the problem, both through the World Health Organization and through bilateral efforts.

Federal agencies, notably the Centers for Disease Control, the National Institutes of Health, and the Food and Drug Administration, have contributed enormously to the rapid acquisition of knowledge about AIDS and HIV or to techniques to help in its control. They should continue their efforts, but greater involvement of the academic and private sectors should be encouraged. Continuing evaluation of many matters will be needed, including the spread of HIV, directions for research and development, the effectiveness of various efforts to promote risk-reducing behavior, and the appropriate level of national effort. There is also a need to mobilize existing resources and encourage interaction of the public and private sectors. To fill these needs—and also for informing the American public, Congress, and the executive branch—the committee proposes a National Commission on AIDS, created either as a presidential or joint presidential and congressional entity. The commission should act in an advisory capacity, because the need for integration of the nation's efforts is not presently such as to require central control that supplants the existing administrative structures.

These and other of the committee's major recommendations are summarized at the conclusion of Chapter 1, with detailed recommendations appearing at the ends of major sections within later chapters.

1

Confronting AIDS: Summary and Recommendations

STATUS OF THE EPIDEMIC

The first cases of the disease now known as acquired immune deficiency syndrome (AIDS) were identified in 1981. Since then the disease has become an epidemic—as of September 1986 more than 24,500 cases had been reported in the United States, and between 1 million and 1.5 million people in the United States probably are infected with the virus that causes AIDS. In the same five years, great progress has been made in understanding AIDS. Much is known about the virus that causes it, about the ways in which the virus is transmitted, about the acute and chronic manifestations of infection, and about its impact on society. Although this knowledge is incomplete, it is extensive enough to permit projections of a likely 10-fold increase in AIDS cases over the next five years, to provide a basis for planning the provision of health care, to guide policy decisions on public health, and to envisage strategies for drug and vaccine development.

Early in the epidemic the diversity of diseases observed in patients was explained by the discovery that the common thread was damage to the patient's immune system. For this reason patients succumb to infections with usually harmless microorganisms or to unusual cancers that individuals with normal immune systems are able to ward off. The damage to the immune system results primarily from the destruction of certain crucially important white blood cells known as T lymphocytes. The death of these blood cells is a consequence of their infection with human immunodefi-

5

ciency virus (HIV), also known as lymphadenopathy-associated virus (LAV), human T-cell lymphotropic virus type III (HTLV-III), and AIDS-associated retrovirus (ARV). The geographic and biologic origins of HIV are not clear, but there is little doubt that this is the first time in modern history that it has spread widely in the human population.

Infection and Transmission

A test has been developed to detect the presence in a person's blood of antibodies that specifically recognize HIV and that serve as a marker for viral infection. The virus can be isolated from most persons who test positive for the presence of these antibodies. Anyone who has antibodies to the virus must be assumed to be infected and probably capable of transmitting the virus. Use of the test has greatly improved the safety of the banked blood supply by enabling elimination of donated blood that tests positive.

A person infected with HIV may not show any clinical symptoms for months or even years but apparently never becomes free of the virus. This long, often unrecognized period of asymptomatic infection, during which an infected person can infect others, complicates control of the spread of the virus.

The virus spreads from infected persons either by anal or vaginal intercourse or by the introduction of infected blood (or blood products) through the skin and into the bloodstream, which may occur in intravenous (IV) drug use, blood transfusion, or treatment of hemophilia. In addition, it can spread from an infected mother to her infant during pregnancy or at the time of birth. Studies show no evidence that the infection is transmitted by so-called casual contact—that is, contact that can be even quite close between persons in the course of daily activities. Thus, there is no evidence that the virus is transmitted in the air, by sneezing, by shaking hands, by sharing a drinking glass, by insect bites, or by living in the same household with an AIDS sufferer or an HIV-infected person. Male-to-male transmission of virus during anal intercourse and male-to-female and female-to-male transmission during vaginal intercourse have been well documented, but the relative efficiency of various types of sexual transmission is not known.

The risk of infection with HIV is directly related to the frequency of exposure to the virus. Groups now at highest risk of infection are homosexual men, IV drug users, persons likely to have heterosexual intercourse with an infected person, and the fetuses or newborn infants of infected mothers. The risk of infection to recipients of blood or blood products is now greatly reduced, although persons in this group already infected may progress to disease.

Clinical Manifestations of the Disease

HIV infection can result in a wide range of adverse immunologic and clinical conditions. The opportunistic infections (those caused by microorganisms that seldom cause disease in persons with normal defense mechanisms) and cancers resulting from immune deficiency are generally the most severe of these, but neurologic problems, such as dementia resulting from HIV infection of the brain, can also be disabling and ultimately fatal. Other clinical consequences of HIV infection include fevers, diarrhea, and swollen lymph nodes. Such cases, if not meeting the criteria for AIDS, are termed ARC (AIDS-related complex). It is not yet fully clear that asymptomatic HIV infection and ARC are stages of an irreversible progression to AIDS, but many investigators suspect this to be so.

The Public Health Service's Centers for Disease Control (CDC) has established a set of criteria to define cases of AIDS based on the presence of certain opportunistic infections and/or other conditions such as cancer. Opportunistic infections in AIDS patients are serious, difficult to treat, and often recurring. Among these infections, a type of pneumonia caused by a protozoan, *Pneumocystis carinii,* is the most common cause of death. Cures for any one of the host of opportunistic infections associated with AIDS, with the possible exception of *P. carinii* pneumonia, would not prolong survival much, because it is the HIV infection that causes the immune system damage and thus, ultimately, the death of AIDS patients. There have been no recorded cases of prolonged remissions of AIDS. Most patients die within two years of the appearance of clinical disease; few survive longer than three years.

Statistical Dimensions of the Epidemic

Because of the long symptom-free period between infection and clinical disease, HIV has spread unnoticed and widely in some population groups. Studies have shown that infection with the virus is far more common than is AIDS or ARC, and suggest that at least 25 to 50 percent of infected persons will progress to AIDS within 5 to 10 years of infection. The possibility that the percentage is higher cannot be ruled out.

As of September 1986, approximately 24,500 cases of AIDS had been reported to the Centers for Disease Control. The number of ARC cases—which is somewhat uncertain, depending on the definition adopted—is probably between 50,000 and 125,000. Among homosexual and bisexual men in some cities, as many as 70 percent may be infected. Substantial numbers of IV drug users also are infected, although precise figures are lacking.

HIV infection is a major and growing problem in some developed countries besides the United States, and it is nearing catastrophic proportions in certain developing countries, particularly in parts of sub-Saharan Africa. Worldwide, as many as 10 million persons may be infected.

There is no satisfactory treatment now for HIV infection. Prospects are not promising for at least five years and probably longer for a vaccine against HIV. One drug has recently shown benefits in the treatment of AIDS, but agents that are acceptably safe for possible long-term treatment and that effectively halt or cure the disease may also not be available for at least five years.

THE FUTURE COURSE OF THE EPIDEMIC

Estimates of the future course of the epidemic are important to the planning of health care, public health measures, and research. Following a June 1986 planning conference at Coolfont, Berkeley Springs, West Virginia, the Public Health Service (PHS) issued projections of the course of the epidemic through 1991. Among the most important PHS estimates are the following:

- By the end of 1991 there will have been a cumulative total of more than 270,000 cases of AIDS in the United States, with more than 74,000 of those occurring in 1991 alone.
- By the end of 1991 there will have been a cumulative total of more than 179,000 deaths from AIDS in the United States, with 54,000 of those occurring in 1991 alone.
- Because the typical time between infection with HIV and the development of clinical AIDS is four or more years, most of the persons who will develop AIDS between now and 1991 already are infected.
- The vast majority of AIDS cases will continue to come from the currently recognized high-risk groups.
- New AIDS cases in men and women acquired through heterosexual contact will increase from 1,100 in 1986 to almost 7,000 in 1991.
- Pediatric AIDS cases will increase almost 10-fold in the next five years, to more than 3,000 cumulative cases by the end of 1991.

Projections of the future incidence and prevalence of AIDS and HIV infection derived from empirical models such as those used by the PHS pose several difficulties, not the least of which is the assumption that past trends—such as the distribution of cases by age, sex, geographic location, and risk group—will not change with time.

Uncertainties notwithstanding, **the Institute of Medicine-National Academy of Sciences Committee on a National Strategy for AIDS believes** that the PHS estimates are reasonable, and the committee supports their use for planning purposes. This acceptance does not, however, obviate the need to acquire information that will facilitate the construction of better models that will lead to more reliable estimates. Data are needed on many aspects of the virus, its infectivity, the natural history and pathogenesis of disease, the size of the groups at risk, and the epidemiology of the epidemic.

The populations at highest risk for HIV infection in the near future will continue to be homosexual men and IV drug users. HIV infection will probably continue to spread in homosexual males, although possibly at a slower rate than in the past because of increased avoidance of anal intercourse and greater use of condoms. Continuing spread of HIV in IV drug users throughout the United States is also expected. Infected bisexual men and IV drug users of both sexes can transmit the virus to the broader heterosexual population where it can continue to spread, particularly among the most sexually active individuals. Although there is a broad spectrum of opinion on the likelihood of further spread of HIV infection in the heterosexual population, there is a strong consensus that the surveillance systems and studies presently in place have very limited ability to detect such spread. Better approaches to tracking this spread can be instituted, but general population surveys are probably neither practical nor ethical. **The committee believes** that over the next 5 to 10 years there will be substantially more cases of HIV infection in the heterosexual population and that these cases will occur predominantly among the population subgroups at risk for other sexually transmitted diseases.

In view of the numbers of people now infected, it is extremely unlikely that the rising incidence of AIDS will soon reverse itself. Disease and death resulting from HIV infection are likely to be increasing 5 to 10 years from now and probably into the next century. But the opportunity does exist to avert an increase in this burden by preventing the further spread of infection.

OPPORTUNITIES FOR ALTERING THE COURSE OF THE EPIDEMIC

Neither vaccines nor satisfactory drug therapies for HIV infection or AIDS are likely to be available in the near future, but actions can be taken now to reduce the further spread of HIV infection and thus to alter the course of the epidemic.

Public Education

For at least the next several years, the most effective measure for significantly reducing the spread of HIV infection is education of the public, especially those individuals at higher risk. (In fact, education will be a central preventive public health measure for this disease under any circumstances.) People must have information on ways to change their behavior and encouragement to protect themselves and others. "Education" in this context is not only the transfer of knowledge but has the added dimension of inducing, persuading, or otherwise motivating people to avoid the transmission of HIV. Education also is needed for those who are in a position to influence public opinion and for those who interact with infected persons. The present federal effort is woefully inadequate in terms of both the amount of educational material made available and its clear communication of intended messages. **The committee recommends** a major educational campaign to reduce the spread of HIV.

If an educational campaign is to change behavior that spreads HIV infection, its message must be as direct as possible. Educators must be prepared to specify that intercourse—anal or vaginal—with an infected or possibly-infected person and without the protection of a condom is very risky. They must be willing to use whatever vernacular is required for that message to be understood. Admonitions to avoid "intimate bodily contact" and the "exchange of bodily fluid" convey at best only a vague message.

In addition to knowing which sexual activities are risky, people also need reassurance that there are sexual practices that involve little or no risk. For example, unprotected sexual intercourse between individuals who have maintained a sexual relationship exclusively with each other for a period of years can be considered essentially free of risk for HIV transmission, assuming that other risk factors are absent. An integral aspect of an education campaign must be the wide dissemination of clear information about those behaviors that do not transmit the disease.

Condoms have been shown under laboratory conditions to obstruct passage of HIV. They should be much more widely available and more consistently used. Young people, early in their sexually active lives and thus less likely to have been infected with HIV, have the most protection to gain from the use of condoms.

Because in the United States the majority of AIDS patients are men, the implications of HIV infection in women have often been overlooked. Women need to know that if they are infected with HIV they may transmit the virus to their sexual partners and possibly to their future offspring. This message is particularly important for IV drug users and their sexual partners.

The most obvious targets for a campaign of education about AIDS are persons whose behavior puts them at special risk—for example, male homosexuals who practice anal intercourse without a condom. Education directed at this group could exploit the fact that although HIV infection prevalence higher than 50 percent occurs in male homosexuals in some urban centers, the much larger proportion of male homosexuals *not* infected outside these areas could protect themselves.

Many other groups, including health care professionals, public officials, and opinion makers, must receive education about AIDS. In addition, special educational efforts must be addressed to teenagers, who are often beginning sexual activity and also may experiment with illicit drugs. Sex education in the schools is no longer only advice about reproductive choice, but has now become advice about a life-or-death matter. Schools have an obligation to provide sex and health education, including facts about AIDS, in terms that teenagers can understand.

In planning the needed education programs for various groups, cultural traditions and practices should be taken into account, because blacks and Hispanics make up a disproportionately high percentage of AIDS cases. Because so many different groups must be educated in this campaign, its early activities must include the instruction of trainers suitable to each of the groups.

Not only must education about AIDS take many forms, but also it must have financial support from many sources. The most fundamental obligation for AIDS education rests with the federal government, which alone is in a position to develop and coordinate a massive campaign. **The committee recommends** consideration of the establishment of a new office or appointment that would be devoted exclusively to education for the prevention of HIV infection, possibly within the Office of the Assistant Secretary for Health. The office should be responsible for implementing and assessing a variety of innovative educational programs and for encouraging the involvement of state and local governments and private organizations.

The committee recognizes that the reluctance of governmental authorities to address issues of sexual behavior reflects a societal reticence regarding open discussions of these matters. However, the committee believes that governmental officials charged with protection of the public's health have a clear responsibility to provide leadership when the consequences of certain types of behavior have serious health outcomes.

If government agencies continue to be unable or unwilling to use direct, explicit terms in the detailed content of educational programs, contractual arrangements should be established with private organizations that are not subject to the same inhibitions.

A massive, coordinated educational program against HIV infection will not be cheap. Although there was an increase in funding by the federal government in Fiscal Year (FY) 1986 for such activities, many times the amount budgeted could be spent usefully.

The committee recommends that substantially increased educational and public awareness activities be supported not only by the government but also by foundations, by experts in advertising, by the information media, and by other private sector organizations that can effectively campaign for health. Legal and administrative barriers to the use of paid television for these educational purposes should be removed.

Preventing HIV Infection Among IV Drug Users

As a group, IV drug users have incurred the second-largest number of AIDS cases in the United States. IV drug users are also the primary source of heterosexual HIV transmission (via their sexual partners) and of perinatal transmission to newborn children. The large differences in the prevalence of HIV infection in IV drug users in different parts of the country is heartening, because it indicates an opportunity to halt the further spread of infection by changing behavior.

Preventing AIDS among the sexual partners of IV drug users may be a more difficult matter. The behavior changes required to prevent heterosexual and *in utero* transmission can entail disruption of sexual relationships and decisions to forgo having children. These behavior changes require intensive efforts with persons who are generally distrustful of authority and unlikely to be responsive to the mere dissemination of information. Sexual partners of IV drug users who do not themselves use drugs may also be difficult to reach, because they do not necessarily come in contact with treatment centers or with the criminal justice system.

There is no doubt that the best way of preventing HIV infection among IV drug users would be to stop the use of illicit IV drugs altogether. The United States' experience in curbing use of such drugs has not been wholly promising, however. The fear of AIDS will probably lead some IV drug users to seek treatment for their addictions. But in the United States as a whole, the availability of treatment for IV drug use was less than the demand even before the AIDS epidemic. Thus, a major possibility for reducing illicit IV drug use and the transmission of HIV is expansion of the system for treating IV drug use. Through treatment, users who have not been infected with HIV could greatly reduce their chances of being infected, and users who have already been infected would be less likely to infect others. At a purely economic level, treating AIDS costs from $50,000 to $150,000 per case, whereas drug abuse treatment costs as little as $3,000 per patient per year in nonresidential programs. **The committee believes** that more methadone and other treatment programs, detoxification programs, and testing and counseling services are needed.

In general, the life-styles and the frequent involvement of IV drug users in unlawful activity make it difficult to apply traditional public health measures in an effort to control the spread of infection in this population. It will not be possible to persuade all IV drug users to abandon drugs or to switch to noninjectable drugs. Many may wish to reduce their chances of exposure to HIV but will neither enter treatment nor refrain from all drug injection. Increasing the legal availability of hypodermic needles has received some support among public health officials but has generally been opposed by law enforcement officials, who predict that it would lead to greater IV drug use. However, if drugs are available and clean needles and syringes are not, IV drug users will probably use available unsterile equipment. **The committee concludes** that trials to provide easier access to sterile, disposable needles and syringes are warranted. Results of such trials should be measured both in incidence of HIV infection and in drug use.

Public Health Measures

The use of public health methods such as contact tracing is complicated in HIV infection by the frequently long lag between infection and identification of disease, the lack of satisfactory treatment for contacts, the impracticality of follow-up in some circumstances, and the potentially adverse social consequences for those identified (such as discrimination in housing or employment).

In 1983-1984, researchers discovered a way to culture the causative agent of AIDS and thus provided the basis for the HIV antibody test used to screen blood. Two years later, this test is used more than 20 million times a year, or about 80,000 times per working day. Although not 100 percent sensitive or specific, the test is at least as accurate as most serologic tests in routine use, and it has made the nation's blood supply much safer.

The use of the test remains controversial because of public perceptions about AIDS, the technical limitations of the test, and the sheer magnitude and diversity of the test's present and projected applications. Important questions about the use of the test relate to uncertainties over the long-term implications of positive results. As more data become available from longitudinal studies of the health of seropositive persons—those who test positive for HIV antibodies—the implications of a positive result will become clearer, and the significance of the test can be better explained to those tested.

Screening tests are of paramount importance in the context of blood, plasma, and tissue banking. The ability to screen blood rather than donors obviates some of the potential for discrimination arising with programs that depend on identifying individuals at risk. The small fraction of false-negative test results and the length of time between infection with the virus and the appearance of antibodies underscore the continuing need for those who have engaged in high-risk behaviors to refrain from donation. **The committee urges** that blood and plasma collection centers also establish administrative systems to further encourage self-deferral of donations and diversion of suspect blood to research while maintaining donor privacy.

Surveillance

Surveillance, which involves both the passive reporting and the active seeking of information, provides data on the prevalence, incidence, and distribution of disease or infection in the population. Such data can be used to monitor the spread of a disease, to shed light on the mechanisms of transmission of infectious agents, to help in designing public health measures to prevent the spread of a disease, to evaluate the effectiveness of interventions, and to guide planning for the provision of facilities. Data on HIV infection and related disease are critical to all aspects of coping with the epidemic.

All states require that AIDS cases be reported promptly to local and state health authorities, who then report the cases to the Centers for Disease Control. Unfortunately, anecdotal accounts suggest that the stigma associated with AIDS may have led to some underreporting of new cases and fatalities. Prompt reporting of individual AIDS cases, the disease's manifestations, the cause of death, and underlying risk factors is essential. **The committee supports** a vigorous program of early reporting of both AIDS and ARC cases (as soon as acceptable definitions for reporting ARC can be formulated) to local and state public health agencies under strict policies of confidentiality.

Surveillance of the general population for HIV infection presents ethical, logistic, and practical problems. Specific epidemiologic research is therefore needed to ascertain the spread of infection in certain populations, such as heterosexuals.

Mandatory Screening

Mandatory screening of the entire U.S. population for HIV infection would be impossible to justify now on either ethical or practical grounds. Mandatory screening of selected subgroups of the population—for example, homosexual males, IV drug users, prostitutes, prisoners, or pregnant women—raises serious problems of ethics and feasibility. People whose private behavior is illegal are not likely to comply with a mandatory screening program, even one backed by assurances of confidentiality. Mandatory screening based on sexual orientation would appear to discriminate against or to coerce entire groups without justification.

The committee is generally opposed to the mandatory screening now of population subgroups, but recognizes that arguments can be made for its application in the military.

Voluntary Testing

In the context of personal health services, the HIV antibody test enables a physician to identify an infected patient. But it should be the patient's decision to be tested, and only after being informed of the implications of a reaffirmed positive test and assured of strict confidentiality. The importance of confidentiality should perhaps be emphasized through the establishment of punitive measures against persons who make unauthorized disclosure of antibody test results.

Voluntary, confidential testing should be encouraged, because individual and aggregate antibody test results enable epidemiologists to assemble baseline data for longitudinal studies of the incidence, prevalence, and natural history of the disease. Such studies can be used to monitor the spread of the virus and to provide the data needed for changing control strategies.

Many persons in high-risk groups are already aware of the dangers their behavior poses to themselves or others. Yet screening programs possibly could identify many seropositive persons who had no reason to suspect they were at risk of infection—for instance, someone unaware of a sexual partner's infection or IV drug use. Persons who test positive in any circumstance have a right to know the results. No testing should be undertaken without adequate pre-test and post-test counseling. If situations arise in which the testing agency has no mandate to provide counseling—as by the military with applicants rejected because they test seropositive—counseling programs by third parties should be established.

The Role of Coercive Measures in Public Health Efforts

Proposals have been made to use coercive measures to control AIDS and HIV infection. Newspaper editorials and legislative bodies have discussed measures such as isolation and quarantine traditionally used to contain contagious disease. However, those diagnosed with AIDS do not usually pose great danger in the further spread of the epidemic. Rather, the greater danger lies with the hundreds of thousands of people who are already infected but asymptomatic. These individuals could not be identified without universal screening programs that would infringe on civil liberties in a manner unacceptable in this society.

The active voluntary cooperation of individuals who are at risk will be needed to curtail the epidemic. Coercive measures will not solicit this cooperation and could prevent it. Believing that coercive measures would not be effective in altering the course of the epidemic, **the committee recommends** that public health authorities use the least-restrictive measures commensurate with the goal of controlling the spread of infection.

Most state health authorities already have laws and regulations that could be applied in unusual situations, such as in the case of a seropositive person who refuses to obey reasonable public health directives. However, the public health statutes concerning infectious disease are outmoded in some states, may not afford civil rights protections adopted by the American courts, and should be reviewed accordingly.

Compulsory actions taken to deal with AIDS have largely affected closed populations, such as prisoners, psychiatric inpatients, and the institutionalized mentally retarded. The public authorities who administer these facilities have a legal obligation to care for residents by taking precautions to prevent the spread of diseases. However, although special precautions against the spread of HIV may be necessary in closed populations, coercive measures should be applied only as necessary for the protection of health. Such measures should not be regarded as models for compulsory programs among the general population.

Questions have previously arisen about admitting children with HIV infection to school classrooms. An accumulation of evidence about the transmission of the virus has now made it apparent that risk from contact with an infected child is negligible, and has made possible the establishment of guidelines for school attendance.

The committee recommends that, as a general policy, children with HIV infection be admitted to the same primary and secondary school classes they would attend if not infected. Guidelines published by the Centers for Disease Control are recommended for special circumstances.

Funding for Education and Other Public Health Measures

The committee did not attempt to work out in detail the cost of the education and other public health measures needed to stem the spread of HIV infection, but it estimated the general magnitude of the funds needed over the next few years. Resources are needed for education, serologic screening, surveillance, increased drug use treatment, and experiments designed to test the effects of greater availability of sterile needles and syringes to drug users. Present expenditures are inadequate.

Federal funds for AIDS education and other public health measures are appropriated to the Centers for Disease Control and also via that agency to states through a variety of arrangements, including cooperative agreements, contracts, and grants for activities such as establishing alternative serologic testing sites (independent of blood donation centers) and demonstration projects for risk-reduction education. The total funds allocated to the Centers for Disease Control for all AIDS education and public health measures are estimated to have been $64.9 million in FY 1986. The Public Health Service budget request to the U.S. Department of Health and Human Services for FY 1988 includes $68.8 million for all AIDS public health and education efforts within a total request of $471.1 million for AIDS-related activities.

Expenditures by states for AIDS-related prevention efforts have grown markedly in the last few years. For FY 1986-1987, a total of $65 million in state expenditures is projected. Five states (California, New York, Florida, New Jersey, and Massachusetts) account for 85 percent of the total spent since July 1, 1983 ($117.3 million), with California and New York jointly accounting for 66 percent.

If efforts to stop the spread of HIV infection are to be effective, they must start (or be expanded) immediately, not only in areas where there are reported AIDS cases but also in areas where there are few or no cases. Delaying such efforts until cases occur increases the likelihood that the problem of AIDS in those areas will subsequently be much greater. The opportunity to forestall the further spread of infection must not be lost.

Some examples illustrate the magnitude of funding needs:

• Testing at alternative test sites, including counseling, is estimated to cost $40 per person, and more than 10 million individuals may be candidates for testing.

• The most successful education programs to date (exemplified by the experience in San Francisco) have occurred within small geographic areas where there are educated homosexuals. Programs for other groups, such as IV drug users, will face more difficult problems of access and motivation; they will therefore probably require more resources per capita. In addition, large groups such as sexually active heterosexuals who have had a number of partners will need to be reached and motivated to adopt risk-reducing behaviors.

• Newspaper, radio, and particularly television advertising are influential means of communicating information, but the use of these media is expensive. One page of advertising in a major newspaper can cost around $25,000 per day, and a minute of national television time can cost between $60,000 and $400,000. Consequently, to influence the behaviors affecting HIV transmission, policymakers must begin to contemplate expenditures similar to those made by private sector companies to influence behaviors—for instance, $30 million to introduce a new camera, or $50 million to $60 million to advertise a new detergent. Furthermore, advertising campaigns are judged successful even when they produce relatively modest shifts in behavior. The efforts needed to influence the behaviors that spread HIV will have to be greater and more sustained.

California has moved earlier than most states to provide funds for AIDS prevention, undoubtedly because the need for such actions has been reinforced by the occurrence of large numbers of AIDS cases. (It is hoped that other states will not delay launching prevention efforts until they have the same stimulus.) Current annual state expenditures for AIDS prevention efforts in California average 65 cents per capita, and in San Francisco such expenditures approximate $5 per capita. Extrapolated on a population basis for the entire United States, these figures would amount to state expenditures nationwide of approximately $150 million and $1 billion, respectively. The committee believes that the desirable level of state expenditures probably falls between these two figures. It bases this conclusion on the fact that, although San Francisco has a sizable concentration of homosexual men, this group does not unduly bias the California population as a whole. In addition, the need for active prevention of spread among heterosexuals is only now becoming recognized, and efforts need to be directed to this group. The risk to heterosexuals is greater in areas of high prevalence, but prevention efforts will need to be relatively uniform nationwide.

The committee also believes that expenditures just from the states of the size mentioned above will be inadequate for a number of reasons. For one, the effectiveness of the educational message will be reinforced if it is delivered from a variety of agencies in a variety of settings. Thus, federal efforts should complement those of the states, which in turn should complement the local efforts of employers and private groups. Funds should be provided for these efforts at each level.

For these reasons, **the committee believes** that a necessary goal is a total national expenditure based on per capita prevention expenditures roughly similar to those made in San Francisco by the state of California. This suggests the need for approximately $1 billion annually for education and other public health expenditures by 1990. A major portion of this total should come from federal sources, because only national agencies are in position to launch coordinated efforts commensurate with the potential size of the problem.

The process of designing and implementing educational interventions to reduce the risk of HIV transmission, followed by evaluations of their effectiveness, will enable policymakers to evaluate over the next year or two the magnitude of effort needed to bring about a drastic reduction in the spread of HIV infection. It is possible that the amounts envisaged by the committee will not be sufficient to stem increases in the prevalence of infection, especially since some of the groups at risk are difficult to reach with conventional approaches and since, despite the expenditures noted above, the infection continues to spread in areas such as San Francisco, though at a reduced rate. More funding for prevention measures will be necessary if those projected here for 1990 do not prove sufficiently great to slow the epidemic.

Discrimination and AIDS

The stigma associated with AIDS has led to instances of discrimination in employment, housing, and access to social services. Sometimes AIDS or ARC sufferers are discriminated against by those who misunderstand the modes of transmission and fear infection from mere casual contact. Improved public awareness resulting from educational efforts may decrease this problem. In other instances, discrimination is rooted in prejudices against the behavior of those presently most at risk for AIDS or HIV infection.

The committee is of the opinion that discriminating against those with AIDS or HIV infection because of any health risk they may pose to others in the workplace or in housing is not justified and should not be tolerated. Laws prohibiting discrimination in employment and housing are encouraged and supported as formal expressions of public policy. Any form of discrimination against groups at high risk for AIDS should be prohibited by state legislation and, where appropriate, by federal laws and regulations. Participation by representatives of high-risk groups in policymaking bodies should be encouraged when appropriate and practicable, and the help of organizations representing high-risk groups should be enlisted for public service programs such as health education, personal counseling, and hospital and home treatment services.

CARE OF PERSONS INFECTED WITH HIV

The provision of care for persons with AIDS or other HIV-related conditions will place an increasing burden on the health care system of the United States for years to come. Based on experience to date, **the committee believes** that if the care of these patients is to be both comprehensive and cost-effective, it must be conducted as much as possible in the community, with hospitalization only when necessary. The various requirements for the care of patients with asymptomatic HIV infection, ARC, or AIDS (i.e., community-based care, outpatient care, hospitalization) should be carefully coordinated.

AIDS patients need an array of services that can prove difficult for hospitals to accommodate if they have not organized for the task. **The committee recommends** that, for provision of hospital inpatient care, AIDS units or teams should be established in high-incidence areas, with a nursing and psychosocial support staff trained in AIDS care and integrated with outpatient and community-based staff. Furthermore, for high-incidence areas, where HIV infection puts the greatest logistic and financial stress on health care systems, the development of multidisciplinary outpatient clinics dedicated to treating AIDS and other HIV-related conditions should be considered.

Systems of community-based care should be able to provide these patients with attendant or homemaking services up to 24 hours daily, as needed; nursing staff able to provide necessary specialized medical intervention; and social support, including small-group housing. The use of volunteer groups to assist in patient care and counseling should be encouraged. Also, representatives of existing agencies and health care providers should organize AIDS care groups to coordinate efforts toward community-based care.

Special systems of care may be required to meet the particular needs of certain AIDS patients, such as IV drug users.

All physicians should be alerted to the signs and symptoms of HIV infection; opportunities to train in the care of HIV-infected patients should be provided to physicians less familiar with the disease; and medical education programs should include academic and practical training related to HIV infection and disease.

Many AIDS patients, being young, have not previously considered the reality of severe illness and death. Therefore, it is important that psychiatric care and psychosocial support be provided to patients with AIDS and ARC, to individuals infected with HIV but asymptomatic, to members of risk groups, and to health care providers for these persons.

Various ethical issues pertain to HIV-related disease: society has an ethical obligation to provide an adequate level of health care to all of its members, and health professionals have an ethical obligation to care for all persons infected with HIV. Additionally, persons who may be infected have ethical obligations to protect others from possible infection. They may do this by avoiding unprotected sexual intercourse and by not sharing needles; by refraining from donating blood, sperm, or other tissues or organs; and by notifying care providers of their status so that recommended precautions against the spread of infection can be used during treatment.

Implicit in society's obligation to provide appropriate care for persons infected with HIV is the responsibility to ascertain and respect patients' wishes about terminal care. This obligation extends to the provision of a variety of settings such as hospices in which AIDS patients can spend their final days.

Health Care Costs Resulting from HIV Infection

The direct health care costs resulting from HIV infection include those for pre-test and post-test counseling associated with serologic testing, detection and confirmation of infection by serologic testing, monitoring of asymptomatic infected individuals, and treatment of the broad range of HIV-associated conditions.

Most studies to date have focused on the direct health care costs for AIDS patients arising from care in and out of the hospital. As estimated by these studies, the average total costs for inpatient care from the time of diagnosis until death range from about $50,000 to $150,000. The difference in the figures derives largely from differences in the numbers of hospital days used.

Several factors—including hospital readmission, length of stay, and type of care—have been identified as making the costs of treating AIDS patients higher than those for treating other patients. These costs also vary with the type of AIDS patient—IV drug user, homosexual male, infant—because the disease manifestations can differ accordingly.

The Public Health Service has estimated that the direct cost of care for the 174,000 AIDS patients projected to be alive during the year 1991 will be $8 billion to $16 billion in that year alone. Because this estimate does not include the care of ARC patients and seropositive individuals, and because it does not take into account the costs associated with experimental therapies or lengthened survival times, it significantly underestimates the total annual direct costs for HIV infection in that year.

The costs for care of ARC patients and seropositive persons—of whom there are many more than there are AIDS patients—also need consideration. These patients will incur costs for a longer period of time, and care for HIV-related conditions such as dementia is extremely costly. The committee found no attempts to estimate the future magnitude of the direct health care costs associated with ARC patients and seropositive individuals, but believes they will be substantial.

There are also large *indirect* costs associated with HIV-related conditions including AIDS. Some of these indirect costs are the loss of wages for sick persons, the loss of future earnings for persons who are permanently incapacitated or die because of illness, and the cost of infection control in the course of other health services, such as dental care.

For urban areas handling a large number of AIDS cases, the strain on available resources will be especially great. Large numbers of infected IV drug users in certain cities will seriously encumber their municipal hospital facilities. In New York City, AIDS patients who are IV drug users may occupy more than 10 percent of municipal hospital beds by 1991.

Having studied the projected course of the epidemic and its implications for health care costs, **the committee believes** that more information must be gathered on all aspects of the costs of care for persons with HIV-related conditions, especially AIDS. Such data should permit calculation of the direct lifetime health care costs resulting from HIV infection and the indirect costs associated with the disease. It is essential to determine which are the most cost-effective approaches to providing care for patients with AIDS and other HIV-related conditions. Thus, **the committee recommends** that all demonstration projects be designed to facilitate comparison of patients, their health outcomes (e.g., longevity, quality of life), the effectiveness of care, and the costs associated with its provision.

The Financing of Health Care for HIV-Related Conditions

The financing of care for patients with AIDS and other HIV-related illness now depends on the same variety of public and private plans that apply to patients with other diseases. Most of the public funds for care of AIDS patients come through the Medicaid program, which is estimated to cover about 40 percent of such patients. Medicare serves only a small percentage of AIDS patients, because its two-year time-to-eligibility for individuals below the age of 65 is longer than the remaining life of most AIDS victims (although this may change if survival increases). Private plans cover a substantial proportion of AIDS patient care, as would be expected from the fact that at least 85 percent of Americans have health insurance, much of it through their jobs.

Despite the fact that most Americans have health insurance, an estimated 80 million have inadequate coverage or none, mostly because they have no jobs, they have no fringe benefits in their jobs, or they are poor health risks. Their plight is indicative of many shortcomings in health care financing, most of which are underscored in the case of HIV-related conditions. In addition, AIDS poses such potentially large expenditures for care that some insurance companies and employers are already wary of offering coverage or employment to persons at high risk of exposure to HIV.

The committee believes that all persons with AIDS or other HIV-related conditions are entitled to adequate care and that mechanisms equitable both to recipients and to providers should be found for financing this care. It is preferable that solution of the problems arising from the financing of care for AIDS and other HIV-related conditions be achieved within a mechanism that ameliorates problems existing in general for the financing of care for other serious illnesses. Measures could include national health insurance for catastrophic illnesses or state-based pools for persons medically at high risk.

The Public Health Service has proposed the establishment of a commission to evaluate the problems of financing the costs of care associated with HIV-related conditions. Finding the optimal mechanism for financing the care of HIV-infected patients, especially those not now covered, should become the first order of business of such a commission.

FUTURE RESEARCH NEEDS

Basic Research

Since the identification of HIV as the cause of AIDS, analyses of the virus have characterized its entire genetic structure and have enabled the identification of many, if not all, of its genes. At the same time, increased knowledge of how the virus is transmitted has helped in the design of public health and education programs. Such insights, however, provide only the first milestone on what promises to be a long and difficult path toward effective therapy to minimize the effects of HIV infection and toward vaccines to limit the spread of the virus.

Developing an effective vaccine or acceptable drugs will depend on a better understanding of the basic biological processes and consequences of HIV infection. The characteristics of viral proteins and their interactions with cellular proteins and processes must be determined. And the design of strategies to prevent the clinical manifestations of HIV infection will require a greatly improved understanding of the normal functioning of the human immune system.

The same types of basic research that have generated the progress of the past few years can also be expected to yield valuable insights into ways to limit the establishment and progression of HIV infection. Thus, basic research in virology and immunology should be considered an important part of the AIDS research effort and should be fortified in the years ahead.

The Natural History of HIV Infection

Much remains to be learned about the natural history of HIV infection—how the virus establishes and maintains infection and how it leads to the immunologic deficits and pathologic consequences associated with ARC and AIDS. For instance, it is not known what factors activate the provirus; what influences the ability to isolate the virus from an infected person; whether the virus is transmitted as free virus, as cell-associated virus, or in both forms; or what proportion of infected individuals will become sick. In the study of HIV infections in human beings, there should be a greater emphasis on defining the introduction and spread of HIV *in vivo,* on identifying the *in vivo* reservoirs of infected cells, and on studying the effects of HIV on the immune and central nervous systems throughout the course of infection.

In addition, drug development efforts, epidemiologic studies, and public health measures all require more comprehensive immunologic and virologic analyses than are presently available. Such analyses could resolve questions about the efficiency with which infected persons infect others, the existence and extent of a virus-positive but antibody-negative population, the relevance of host or environmental cofactors in the development of AIDS, and the efficiency of heterosexual transmission.

Epidemiologic Approaches

Since AIDS was first identified in 1981, much has been learned from epidemiologic research about how HIV is transmitted and about how the virus affects people who are infected with it. But more must be discovered. For instance, epidemiologic studies could provide much of the information needed to fashion improved models of the future course of the epidemic.

Reporting of AIDS should be continued and augmented by the selective reporting of other stages of HIV infection. In addition, active surveillance is needed of groups of particular epidemiologic importance, such as heterosexuals and non-IV drug users in high-incidence areas, IV drug users and homosexual men in low-incidence cities, spouses of infected individuals, pregnant women, newborn children of infected mothers, prostitutes throughout the country, and recipients of blood products. Better information is also needed to quantify the number of persons infected with HIV.

Epidemiologic studies of the immunologic effects and pathologic manifestations of HIV infection can contribute to knowledge of the natural history of infection. Prospective cohort studies should be continued and expanded, and studies should be undertaken to determine differences in the characteristics of infection and disease among different populations.

Natural history and epidemiologic studies would be facilitated by better tests for antibodies to HIV and by simpler, quantitative ways of detecting virus. Tests for both virus antigen and infectious particles are necessary. In addition, viral isolation procedures need to be refined so that a standard is available for evaluating other techniques.

Animal Models

Animal models that reproduce or mimic the consequences of HIV infection in human beings can play a crucial role in improving the understanding of disease pathogenesis and in the development and testing of antiviral drugs and vaccines. However, no completely analogous animal model for HIV infection and disease is now available.

The most relevant and promising animal models are provided by nonhuman primates. Therefore, the nation's primate centers should be improved to permit the expansion of the primate populations available for AIDS-related research, the development of appropriate biocontainment facilities, and the education of appropriately trained investigators.

The committee believes that available supplies of test animals, especially chimpanzees, will be insufficient for future research needs, and that the plans for the conservation, expansion, and optimal use of these animals appear inadequate. Populations of primate models need to be expanded as rapidly as possible·to meet the future needs of research and testing. Furthermore, a national system should be set up to facilitate appropriate access to test animals for valid experimentation by qualified investigators, regardless of institutional affiliation.

Chimpanzees in particular must be treated as an endangered national resource that will be irreplaceable if squandered. Thus, mechanisms should be developed to ensure that AIDS-related experiments with chimpanzees proceed only if there is a broad consensus among the interested scientific community that the proposed experiment is critically important to the development of vaccines or antiviral agents and cannot be conducted in any other species or by any other means.

Antiviral Agents

The development of acceptably safe and effective antiviral agents for the treatment of HIV infection is likely to be a long, hard job with no certainty of success. The ideal AIDS drug must fulfill a number of requirements: it must be conveniently administered, preferably orally; it must be sufficiently nontoxic to be used for prolonged periods, perhaps for a lifetime; and it must be active not only in peripheral immune system cells but in the central nervous system, because HIV may infect the nervous system early in the disease process. Several drugs are under clinical evaluation, but thus far no drug meeting these criteria has been identified.

Until an agent effective against HIV and reasonably safe for prolonged administration is identified, the committee believes that the quickest, most efficient, and least-biased way to identify and validate the efficacy and safety of treatments for HIV infection is by means of randomized clinical trials in which control groups receive a placebo. When an effective and acceptably safe agent is found, newer candidate drugs should be compared against it.

Shortly before the publication of this report, data were released by the National Institutes of Health and the Burroughs Wellcome Company from a study of azidothymidine (AZT) administered for 20 weeks to a group of approximately 140 AIDS patients while a similar group received a placebo. The patients were selected for having had no more than one bout of *Pneumocystis carinii* pneumonia. There was 1 death in the AZT group compared with 16 deaths in the placebo group. Because of the time at which this information became available, the committee was not able to analyze the data from this study in enough detail to judge the risks and benefits of this drug. Further evaluation will be needed to fully determine the side effects of AZT treatment and its long-term efficacy and safety for various categories of patients.

Decisions on the design of studies to test new drugs for HIV infection must be made on a case-by-case basis. Such decisions should take into account the results of further studies on the efficacy and toxicity of AZT, the category of patients to whom the drug under consideration would be given, and preliminary information on the safety and efficacy of the drug.

It is essential that mechanisms for the efficient testing of candidate drugs be established. Efforts should be undertaken now to ensure that organizational and financial support will be sufficient to permit the expeditious evaluation of promising therapeutic agents for HIV infection.

Success in the development of antiviral agents will be much more likely if the expertise resident in the industrial, governmental, and academic research communities can be engaged and coordinated.

Vaccines

The development of a vaccine against viruses like HIV has never been seriously attempted, much less achieved. Except for a vaccine used in cats, no vaccine against such viruses is available. The properties of viruses related to HIV suggest that developing a vaccine will be difficult. It is also likely that a subunit vaccine, rather than a whole-virus vaccine, will be needed, and these have additional problems of efficacy. Moreover, even if the scientific obstacles were surmounted, legal, social, and ethical factors could delay or limit the availability of a vaccine. For these reasons, the committee does not believe that a vaccine is likely to be developed for at least five years and probably longer.

Because HIV attacks the immune system itself, a successful vaccine development program will require a greatly expanded knowledge base.

The urgency of the problem calls for the active and cooperative participation of scientists in government, academia, and industrial laboratories.

Much of the expertise in vaccine development is in the industrial sector. However, contributions of industry to the development of an HIV vaccine are inhibited by the substantial developmental costs in the absence of a significant probability of financial return and by apprehension over potential liability incurred in the course of vaccine distribution. Creative options for the governmental support of industrial research, guarantees of vaccine purchase, and the assumption of reasonable liability should, therefore, be actively explored and encouraged.

The committee finds that the federal coordination of vaccine development has been inadequate. The National Institutes of Health has recently reorganized its efforts on AIDS, and **the committee encourages** the appointment of strong leadership to the vaccine program with the authority and responsibility to develop a strategy for a broad-ranging vaccine development program.

Social Science Research Needs

Social science research can help develop effective education programs to encourage changes in behavior that will break the chain of HIV transmission. It can contribute to the design of policies that reduce the public's fear of AIDS and that help eliminate discriminatory practices toward AIDS patients. And it can shape the establishment of health care and social services for AIDS patients.

A major research need is for studies that will improve understanding of all aspects of sexual behavior and drug use and the factors that influence them. There has been little social science research specifically focusing on HIV infection and AIDS. Demographic features and social dynamics related to HIV infection should be thoroughly studied in order to develop effective means to reach people at risk, to delineate the obstacles to behavioral change, and to determine effective language and styles of communication among various population groups.

Different approaches to achieving behavioral change in the various groups at risk of HIV infection should be monitored. Wherever feasible, educational programs should have an evaluation component.

Treatment, social service programs, and hospital management practices should be assessed to determine which practices work best and are most cost-effective. Experiments based on different models of patient care should be evaluated with regard to their applicability to other areas, providing a foundation on which to build locally relevant programs.

Funding for Research on AIDS and HIV

Confronting the AIDS epidemic will require new and substantially increased financial support for basic biomedical and social science research activities. The rapid and effective application of the insights provided by basic research will also require the significant expansion of applied research activities. In addition, funds are needed to provide researchers with adequate equipment and facilities, to attract high-caliber individuals into the field, and to support the training of future investigators.

The Public Health Service's request to the U.S. Department of Health and Human Services for AIDS-related research in FY 1988 was $471 million. If appropriated, this budget would represent a doubling of funds from FY 1986 to FY 1988. The National Science Foundation spends just over $50 million annually on social science research, but presently a very small amount of this is on studies related to AIDS.

The committee believes that there are sufficient areas of need and opportunity to double research funding again by 1990, leading to an approximately $1 billion budget in that year. These funds must be new appropriations, not a reallocation of existing Public Health Service funds. Areas of clear need include high-containment facilities for primate research, better containment facilities for universities and research institutes, training funds, construction and renovation funds, equipment funds, social science and behavioral research funding, vaccine and drug development efforts, international studies, basic research efforts, and epidemiologic studies. In addition, funds diverted from NIH programs to support the AIDS effort should be returned.

In recent years there has been a steady decline in the proportion of NIH funds spent on grants for investigator-initiated research on AIDS and an increasing proportion expended on contracts for NIH-designed studies. A more balanced growth of support is desirable in coming funding cycles to promote the involvement of the nonfederal basic research community to a greater extent. The level of funding for investigator-initiated studies in all areas (including non-AIDS studies) must be adequate to continue to attract the most able younger scientists to clinical, social science, and basic biomedical research, or the quality and productivity of the scientific enterprise will suffer.

INTERNATIONAL ASPECTS OF AIDS AND HIV INFECTION

More than half the countries of the world have reported cases of AIDS. Although reporting may not be reliable in many countries, it has been estimated, based on studies in specific areas, on the number of identified cases, and on the U.S. ratio of cases to seropositive persons, that up to 10 million people worldwide may be infected with HIV. A substantial proportion of these are in sub-Saharan Africa, particularly central Africa.

It is likely that millions of infected adults will progress to AIDS in the next decade, and that tens of thousands of infants will contract the syndrome perinatally. In response to this situation, many developed and developing countries are initiating research and prevention programs, and the World Health Organization is initiating a global program for the control of AIDS.

Rationale for U.S. International Involvement

The United States has actively promoted the technological development of less developed countries for economic, altruistic, and political reasons. Because AIDS most often occurs in young adults, it imposes a particularly severe burden on development efforts in these nations by draining off intellectual and economic assets—namely, productive individuals.

U.S. technical assistance programs have often included major contributions to efforts in improving health through programs in immunization and nutrition. The burden of AIDS and other HIV-related conditions added to the lengthy existing agenda of health problems in developing countries may negate the hard-won gains made by these programs.

New knowledge critical to prevention and treatment of HIV infection may be more readily obtained outside of the United States. For instance, the extent of perinatal and heterosexual transmission in central Africa offers opportunities for U.S. research resources to complement local expertise in mutually beneficial investigations.

Certain federal agencies have special international responsibilities or may be able to make contributions to the global effort to control the AIDS epidemic through support of activities in the United States. These agencies include the Agency for International Development, the Food and Drug Administration, and the Centers for Disease Control. There is also need for U.S. involvement in AIDS internationally because the operations of many federal agencies and other organizations require that their personnel visit or live in countries where HIV infection may be relatively prevalent. Such personnel may be at risk of infection or need appropriate care.

Risks of Infection Outside the United States

Sexual transmission probably accounts for the largest proportion of transmission of HIV outside of the United States. Bidirectional heterosexual transmission is the dominant mode of HIV transmission in sub-Saharan Africa. HIV infection is also becoming a major problem among female prostitutes in many areas.

HIV transmission between homosexual men must be presumed to be possible wherever behavior involving risk of infection is practiced. Knowledge of the frequency with which homosexual behavior occurs in different countries and cultures is incomplete, however, and existing information may not be reliable.

Transfusion of blood poses a substantial risk of HIV infection in many countries of the world that have not adopted procedures necessary to prevent such transmission and that lack the laboratories, finances, or personnel needed to institute such measures.

Application of currently available serologic tests will be possible only in some situations. **The committee concludes** that simpler serologic tests that give sensitive and specific results rapidly and reliably are essential before widespread efforts to control HIV transmission via the blood supply in developing countries will be practicable.

Transmission of HIV through the sharing of needles and syringes used to inject IV drugs is well documented in countries where IV drug use is common. However, some evidence suggests that in Africa injections administered for medical purposes with unsterile needles and syringes may be a route of HIV transmission.

There is no evidence to support the hypothesis that HIV is transmitted through insect vectors or casual contact. Studies in Africa of household contacts of infected persons and the age distribution of AIDS and HIV infection suggest that transmission by casual contact is very infrequent or nonexistent. The relative ineffectiveness of needlestick transmission in health professionals and the age distribution of AIDS and HIV infection also suggest that mechanical transmission by insects is unlikely.

International Research Opportunities

The United States has contributed greatly to the understanding of AIDS and HIV infection through its investment in domestic research. The international efforts undertaken to date illustrate the reasons and opportunities for the United States to contribute to multinational and bilateral efforts.

As is appropriate, some of the United States' support for international efforts on AIDS and HIV is committed for use exclusively through the World Health Organization (WHO). The committee believes that additional bilateral or multinational activities involving the United States outside of the WHO program will be essential to enhancing the prospects for achieving rapid control over the disease.

The WHO program is in the early phases of organization, but the need for action in some countries is urgent. The focus of the WHO program is prevention and control of AIDS and HIV infection rather than research opportunities, and links of U.S. investigators or institutions with affected countries could provide a means of rapid response to their needs.

The committee recommends that the United States be a full participant in international efforts against AIDS and HIV infection. U.S. involvement should be both through support of WHO programs and through bilateral arrangements in response to the needs and opportunities in individual countries. These arrangements should be pursued in a fashion that is acceptable to host governments.

The magnitude of the problem internationally and the variety of reasons warranting U.S. participation in international efforts convince the committee that the United States should make clear its commitment to global prevention and control of AIDS and HIV infection.

The following are feasible goals: (1) the total amount of U.S. funding going to international efforts in AIDS-related research and prevention should reach $50 million per year by 1990 (this is approximately 2.5 percent of the amount recommended by the committee for use in the United States for these purposes); (2) increased funding should be provided to the WHO program on the basis of demonstrated capacity to use such funds productively; and (3) increased funds to bilateral research or technical assistance programs or projects abroad should be provided on the basis of review procedures involving persons familiar with the local conditions under which such projects are undertaken.

The committee found information to be lacking on the extent and kinds of work on HIV-related conditions by U.S. investigators in other countries or on their collaborations with foreign researchers. **The committee recommends** that an evaluation be initiated immediately to identify all work under way and to assess and coordinate the roles and responses of the various U.S. federal agencies, private voluntary groups, and foundations interested in international efforts on AIDS and HIV.

GUIDANCE FOR THE NATION'S EFFORTS

No single approach—whether education and other public health measures, vaccination, or therapy—is likely to be wholly successful in combating all the problems posed by HIV infection. Similarly, neither the public sector, the private sector, nor any particular agency, organization, or group can be expected by itself to provide the solution to the diverse problems posed by the disease. Federal agencies (notably the National Institutes of Health, the Centers for Disease Control, and the Food and Drug Administration) have contributed enormously to the rapid acquisition of knowledge about AIDS and HIV or to techniques to help in its control. They should continue their efforts, but greater involvement of the academic and private sectors should now be encouraged.

All of these approaches and entities must be organized in a national effort, integrated and coordinated so that participants are working toward common goals and are aware of each other's activities. Such coordination does not imply management by a centralized directorate. However, monitoring of the many activities in the effort is necessary to ensure that important matters are not overlooked and that periodic review can be conducted for the adjustment of priorities and general directions.

What Is Needed?

The committee found gaps in the efforts being directed against the AIDS epidemic and in the employment of the nation's resources. It also identified as a major concern a lack of cohesiveness and strategic planning throughout the national effort. A body is needed to identify necessary actions and to mobilize underused resources in meeting the challenge of the epidemic. Therefore, **the committee recommends** that a new entity—a National Commission on AIDS—be established to meet the need for guidance of the national efforts against HIV.

The commission would monitor the course of the epidemic; evaluate research, health care, and public health needs; encourage federal, state, philanthropic, industrial, and other entities to participate; stimulate the strongest possible involvement of the academic scientific community; encourage greater U.S. contribution to international efforts by relevant government agencies and other organizations; make recommendations for altering the directions or intensity of health care, public health, and research efforts as the problem evolves; monitor and advise on related legal and ethical issues; and report to the American public.

The commission should achieve its purposes by assuming an advisory role and by acting catalytically in bringing together disparate groups. It should not dispense funds but should be provided with sufficient resources to undertake its mission effectively.

Establishment of the Commission

To oversee and marshal the nation's resources effectively, the proposed commission should have certain attributes. It should be able to engage all of the diverse public and private resources that can be brought to bear on HIV-associated problems. It must be sufficiently independent to give critical advice to participants in these efforts. It should have sufficient national and international stature and credibility for its advice to command the attention of participants.

The advantages and disadvantages of various institutional locations for the commission were evaluated by the committee. The requirement for spanning both public and private sectors implies that it should not be created within the administrative structure of the federal executive branch. However, the desirability of affirming a national commitment to the control of AIDS and HIV suggests that the commission should be endorsed at the highest levels of government. Accordingly,

• **The committee recommends** that the proposed National Commission on AIDS be created as a presidential or joint presidential-congressional commission.

• **The committee recommends** that the President take a strong leadership role in the effort against AIDS and HIV, designating control of AIDS as a major national goal and ensuring that the financial, human, and institutional resources needed to combat HIV infection and to care for AIDS patients are provided.

• **The committee urges** all cabinet secretaries and other ranking executive branch officials to determine how AIDS and HIV relate to their responsibilities and to encourage the units within their purview to work collaboratively toward responding to the epidemic on a national and international level.

• **The committee recommends** that the U.S. Congress maintain its strong interest in the control of AIDS and HIV infection and increase research appropriations toward a level of $1 billion annually by 1990. In addition, it recommends that by 1990 there be significant federal contributions toward the $1 billion annually required for the total costs of education and public health measures.

MAJOR RECOMMENDATIONS

In summary, the committee recommends that two major actions be undertaken to confront the epidemic of HIV infection and AIDS. They are as follows:

1. Undertake a massive media, educational, and public health campaign to curb the spread of HIV infection.
2. Begin substantial, long-term, and comprehensive programs of research in the biomedical and social sciences intended to prevent HIV infection and to treat the diseases caused by it.

Within a few years these two major areas of action should each be supported with expenditures of $1 billion a year in newly available funds not taken from other health or research budgets. The federal government should bear the responsibility for the $1 billion in research funding and is also the only possible majority funding source for expenditures of the magnitude seen necessary for education and public health.

Furthermore, to promote and integrate public and private sector efforts against HIV infection, a National Commission on AIDS should be created. Such a commission would advise on needed actions and report to the American people.

Curbing the spread of HIV infection will entail many actions, including the following:

• Expand the availability of serologic testing, particularly among persons in high-risk groups. Encourage testing by keeping it voluntary and ensuring confidentiality.

• Expand treatment and prevention programs against IV drug use. Experiment with making clean needles and syringes more freely available to reduce sharing of contaminated equipment.

The care of HIV patients can be greatly improved by applying the results of health services research. In the meantime, the following actions should be taken:

• Begin planning and training now for an increasing case load of patients with HIV infection. Emphasize care in the community, keeping hospitalization at a minimum.

• Find the best ways to collect demographic, health, and cost data on patients to identify cost-effective approaches to care.

• Devise methods of financing care that will provide appropriate and adequate funding.

The recommended research efforts should include the following actions:

• Enhance the knowledge needed for vaccine and drug development through basic research in virology, immunology, and viral protein structure.

• Improve understanding of the natural history and pathogenesis of AIDS, and trace the spread of HIV infection by means of epidemiologic and clinical research.

• Study sexual behavior and IV drug use to find ways to reduce the risk of infection.

• Encourage participation of academic scientists in research against AIDS, in part by increasing the funding for investigator-initiated research proposals.

• Solicit participation of industry in collaboration with federal and academic research programs.

• Expand experimental animal resources, working especially to conserve chimpanzee stocks, and develop new animal models of HIV infection.

Because AIDS and HIV infection are major and mounting health problems worldwide:

• The United States should be a full participant in international efforts against the epidemic.
• United States involvement should include both support of World Health Organization programs and bilateral efforts.

NOTE: Reference documentation for material in this summary is presented in the respective chapters of the full report.

2

Understanding of the Disease and Dimensions of the Epidemic

In the middle of 1981, several outbreaks of *Pneumocystis carinii* pneumonia and Kaposi's sarcoma in previously healthy young male homosexuals were reported to the Centers for Disease Control (CDC), the division of the Public Health Service responsible for monitoring infectious diseases in the United States (Centers for Disease Control, 1981a,b). Before these reports, those diseases were essentially seen only in persons with recognized causes of immune system compromise, such as rare genetic diseases, immunosuppressive treatments for organ transplants, or cancer chemotherapy. Nevertheless, the sufferers of this novel and inexplicable syndrome demonstrated severely compromised immunologic defenses against a wide range of viral, bacterial, and parasitic infections.

Although the syndrome was first seen in homosexual men, soon other groups also were found to be "at risk" for the disease, including intravenous (IV) drug users, recent Haitian immigrants, hemophiliacs, recipients of blood transfusions, sexual partners of persons who had the disease or were at risk, and infants of mothers with the disease or at risk. As a result, the general term "acquired immune deficiency syndrome" (AIDS) gradually became accepted (Centers for Disease Control, 1982a).

By the end of 1982, the Centers for Disease Control had established a surveillance definition of AIDS that could enable its incidence in the United States to be monitored (Centers for Disease Control, 1982b). This definition described AIDS as "a reliably diagnosed disease process that is at least moderately predictive of a defect in cell-mediated immunity occurring in a person with no known cause for diminished resistance"

37

(see Appendix E). Initially, 11 opportunistic infections and diseases were considered specific enough to be diagnostic for AIDS. This definition was designed with more emphasis on specificity than on sensitivity and has permitted the collection of useful data because of its precision and uniform acceptance. It also resulted in a broader recognition of the syndrome's prevalence and in early concerted attempts to identify the causative agent. It has been used uniformly since 1982, with minor changes made in June 1985 (Centers for Disease Control, 1985).

Shortly after the recognition of AIDS, an array of other distinctive and pronounced clinical signs and symptoms were noted among homosexual men. These included persistent generalized lymphadenopathy (PGL) (Abrams et al., 1984; Metroka et al., 1983), fatigue, persistent fever, weight loss, diarrhea, and certain neurologic signs and symptoms. Some investigators suggested that these illnesses represented the early stages of AIDS, but at the time there was little understanding of whether all persons who manifested such symptoms would ultimately progress to clinical AIDS. Gradually the term AIDS-related complex (ARC) began to be employed to describe all of the clinical signs and symptoms that seemed to be related to AIDS but did not fully meet the CDC's criteria for the disease.

Developing and improving the definitions of AIDS, ARC, and PGL have been important in understanding the epidemic. However, like other definitions designed for epidemiologic investigation, they are meant to be specific and easy to apply. When used in individual clinical situations, they are somewhat arbitrary and do not fully reflect the morbidity caused by the illnesses associated with them. Some patients with ARC experience a rapidly fatal disease course, while a few people with an AIDS-related malignancy are in reasonably good health more than five years after diagnosis.

It has been extremely difficult to arrive at any consensus regarding the definitions of ARC and PGL. Many persons with lymphadenopathy are asymptomatic. Patients with ARC have varying clinical symptomatology, ranging from mild problems such as occasional fevers and night sweats to fulminant disease courses, including dementia and death. Definitions of HIV-related conditions must therefore be applied cautiously. Nevertheless, they are helpful in monitoring the progression of the epidemic in various groups of people.

THE CAUSATIVE AGENT OF AIDS

Because AIDS was first recognized in male homosexuals, initial hypotheses of the cause of the disease focused on exposures common to this group. Suggested causes included the use of amyl and butyl nitrites (known as poppers) to heighten sexual pleasure, autoimmune reactions due to repeated exposure to sperm, "immune overload" due to repeated and varied infections, or an infectious agent.

The appearance of AIDS in population groups other than homosexual males lent strong support to the hypothesis that the disease was caused by an infectious agent rather than by an exposure specific to some homosexuals. In particular, the early epidemiologic analysis of AIDS delineated a pattern of spread very reminiscent of hepatitis B. This pattern strongly suggested a transmissible infectious agent in the blood or body fluids of affected individuals. However, the search for such an agent was frustrated by the large number of other infections commonly found in AIDS patients. Well-known and prevalent viruses such as Epstein-Barr virus and cytomegalovirus were advanced as possible etiologic agents, yet none could account for the novel character of AIDS or for its appearance in diverse populations.

Meanwhile, several contingents of medical scientists began exploring the possibility that the cause of AIDS might be a member of a family of viruses known as retroviruses. Such viruses are prevalent in certain species of animals but had only recently been described in human beings. In 1983, research efforts yielded very suggestive evidence for the involvement of a novel human retrovirus in AIDS. Shortly thereafter, the isolation and characterization of a previously unknown retrovirus variously known as LAV (lymphadenopathy-associated virus), HTLV-III (human T-cell lymphotropic virus type III), or ARV (AIDS-associated retrovirus) led to its definitive identification as the cause of AIDS (Barre-Sinoussi et al., 1983; Gallo et al., 1984; Levy et al., 1984). These early isolates of immunosuppressive retroviruses were later recognized to be closely related, and a generic name—human immunodeficiency virus (HIV)—has been proposed for them and for subsequently isolated and related viruses (Barre-Sinoussi et al., 1983; Gallo et al., 1984; Levy et al., 1984).

Initial attempts to isolate novel retroviruses from persons with AIDS were stymied by an inability to grow the cells in which human retroviruses proliferate—a type of white blood cell known as a T lymphocyte. Rather than continuing to proliferate, T lymphocytes derived from AIDS patients showed short-term growth and then extensive cell death. However, these T-lymphocyte cultures revealed the presence of viral particles resembling retroviruses and an enzymatic activity known as reverse transcriptase that is a marker for retrovirus production (Barre-Sinoussi et al., 1983; Gallo et al., 1984). The viability of T lymphocytes markedly deteriorated soon after these still-uncharacterized retroviruses were produced, an observation consistent with the expected effects of an "AIDS virus" (Klatzmann et al., 1984a; Popovic et al., 1984). Furthermore, the retroviruses derived from lymphocyte cultures of individuals with AIDS or associated conditions could easily be transferred to cultures of normal lymphocytes, where they would reproduce the pronounced cytopathic effects seen in the original culture. The finding that the target for viral infection *in vitro* is a vitally important subset of lymphocytes fits well with the profound depletion of these cells seen in persons with AIDS (Dalgleish et al., 1984; Klatzmann et al., 1984b; see section on "Pathogenesis of AIDS," below).

The next advance came in the identification of an immortal T-cell leukemia line that could be used to propagate the novel retroviruses without demonstrable cytopathic consequences (Popovic et al., 1984). It allowed the viruses to be produced on a large scale and characterized in detail. Furthermore, critical reagents could be prepared for use in epidemiologic studies and for delineating the modes of transmission of the virus.

Testing of sera from AIDS patients and persons with AIDS-associated conditions disclosed the presence of antibodies reactive with the protein constituents of HIV in almost all instances, whereas sera from individuals not in "at risk" groups were uniformly negative (Brun-Vezinet et al., 1984; Safai et al., 1984; Sarngadharan et al., 1984). Serum samples from individuals in groups at risk for the development of AIDS demonstrated a prevalence of antibodies to HIV that correlated well with the time of appearance, extent, and geographic clustering of cases of AIDS and ARC. HIV can be isolated from lymphocytes from the majority of persons, including most AIDS and ARC patients, demonstrating serologic reactivity with the virus (Salahuddin et al., 1985). (The failure to isolate the virus from all infected persons is most likely due to technical limitations in the lymphocyte culture methods and to the depletion of target cells in advanced stages of the disease.) The etiologic role of HIV in AIDS was further demonstrated by the study of AIDS cases associated with blood transfusions, which clearly showed that the virus could be transmitted to a previously uninfected person who could then develop AIDS (Feorino et al., 1985; Jaffe et al., 1985b). Because HIV can be isolated from most people with antibodies to it, all persons having antibodies to HIV must be assumed to be infected and, for practical purposes, capable of transmitting the virus.

Features of Retroviruses

The pathogenic features of the infectious agents that later became known as retroviruses were first described at the beginning of the twentieth century, when they were identified as the causative agents of certain leukemias and sarcomas in chickens. Since then, retroviruses have been identified as the causes of many other malignant and nonmalignant diseases in a wide variety of animals. Some of these animal diseases appear analogous to certain malignant or degenerative conditions in human beings, a similarity that caused many attempts to demonstrate the relevance of retroviruses to the pathogenesis of human diseases. But it was not until 1980 that a retrovirus was definitively isolated in a human disease, an unusual type of T-cell leukemia (Poiesz et al., 1980). This retrovirus, human T-cell lymphotropic virus type I (HTLV-I), is the cause of an aggressive form of leukemia known as adult T-cell leukemia that is common in certain parts of the world. A related but clearly distinct retrovirus known as HTLV-II was subsequently isolated from a person with a less aggressive type of leukemia (Kalyanaraman et al., 1982). HIV (also known as HTLV-III) is the third type of human retrovirus to be isolated.

The genetic information of retroviruses is transmitted as single-strand molecules of RNA (ribonucleic acid) in the virus particle. To be replicated and expressed in the cells that retroviruses infect, the information in these single-strand RNA molecules must be transferred into double-strand DNA (deoxyribonucleic acid), which is the form that can become integrated into the chromosomes of the infected cell (Varmus and Swanstrom, 1984). The backward, or "retro," flow of information from RNA to DNA—the reverse of most genetic message movement—gives the virus its family name. The retro movement is made possible by an enzyme, reverse transcriptase, encoded by the virus.

Related Viruses

The taxonomic family Retrovirinae is composed of three subfamilies: Oncovirinae, Lentivirinae, and Spumivirinae (Teich, 1984). The oncoviruses (oncogenic, or cancer-causing, viruses) include the causative agents of a number of naturally occurring leukemias and lymphomas in cats, wild mice, birds, cows, and gibbons. HTLV-I and HTLV-II most closely resemble members of this subfamily, though they have a number of distinctive structural and functional attributes.

Lentiviruses cause a number of naturally occurring, progressive, nonmalignant disorders in animals. They are responsible for a variety of protracted neurologic, musculoskeletal, hematologic, and respiratory diseases of hoofed mammals that generally arise after a long incubation period. HIV shares a number of genetic, structural, and biologic similarities with members of this group, although none of the previously described lentiviruses is known to directly affect the immune systems of infected hosts (Gonda et al., 1985; Sonigo et al., 1985). As discussed in Chapter 6, this classification of HIV as a lentivirus has a number of important implications for the analysis of the pathogenic mechanisms of

AIDS and for the development of potential interventions to prevent the effects of HIV infection.

Spumiviruses include bovine and feline syncytial viruses and simian and human foamy viruses. They persist in animals despite a host immune response and are not known to be involved in any disease processes.

Following the identification of HIV, a syndrome of acquired immunodeficiency that closely resembled AIDS was described in certain species of monkeys (Daniel et al., 1985; Kanki et al., 1985a; Letvin et al., 1985). Retroviruses isolated from the affected animals shared many biologic and immunologic characteristics with HIV. These related viruses have been named STLV-III (for simian T-cell lymphotropic virus type III) or SIV (for simian immunodeficiency virus). Although infection with this virus produces profound immunosuppression in certain species of monkeys, it results in no untoward effects in other species (Kanki et al., 1985b; Letvin et al., 1985). These related simian lentiretroviruses may provide extremely useful models for HIV infection in humans.

Very recently, analysis of newly discovered types of human retroviruses termed HTLV-IV and LAV-2 has shown that they are more closely related to the simian viruses than to HIV. The relationship of HTLV-IV and LAV-2 to each other is presently unclear, because infection with HTLV-IV reportedly results in no apparent immunodeficiency, while LAV-2 has been isolated from individuals suffering from immunologic abnormalities typical of AIDS.

PATHOGENESIS OF AIDS

AIDS is primarily a disease of the body's immune system. The consequences of HIV infection are such that infected persons exhibit in an apparently progressive manner a spectrum of immunologic compromise. In its most extreme manifestation, this immunologic compromise results in an inability to counter many infections with an effective immune response. HIV infection may also result in symptoms such as neurologic damage (see Appendix A).

The primary function of the immune system is to identify, isolate, and eliminate foreign (predominantly microbial) invaders of the body (Weissman, 1986). The human immune system is composed of a wide variety of differentiated cells that interact in an exceedingly complex and as yet poorly understood manner to provide protection against infectious diseases. Much of the future understanding of the pathogenesis of AIDS will derive from increasingly sophisticated insights into the human immune system.

Most of the *in vivo* measures of immune function are markedly depressed in patients with AIDS. Similarly, immunodeficiency is apparent in analyses of many of the *in vitro* measures of immune reactivity. Shortly after AIDS was first recognized, patients suffering from the syndrome were found to have reduced numbers of a subset of white blood cells known as T lymphocytes that expressed on their cell surfaces a molecule known as CD4 (such cells are also known as T4 cells). Such lymphocytes, most of which are included in what is functionally defined as the helper/inducer subset, constitute the major population of mature T cells. Another major subset of T cells express the CD8 molecule on their cell surfaces (such cells are also known as T8 cells). Most of these are classified as suppressor/cytotoxic cells. Normally, the CD4-to-CD8 ratio in humans is 1.5 to 2.0. In AIDS patients, however, this ratio is inverted, so that it is less than 1.0. Generally, this inversion has been found to be due to a decrease in the absolute numbers of CD4 cells, with the normal numbers of CD8 cells usually being preserved.

Given the enormous complexity of the human immune system, the simple distinction between CD4 and CD8 cells is bound to be an oversimplification. But measurement of the CD4-to-CD8 ratio was the earliest marker for immunologic impairment in AIDS, and it has proved to be a reasonably sensitive measure.

CD4 cells perform a multitude of essential functions in the immune system. They specifically recognize and proliferate in response to antigens (foreign molecules) that they encounter in the body, at the same time releasing a variety of proteins known as lymphokines that regulate other immune system cells. Upon signaling by CD4 cells, cells known as B lymphocytes, recognizing antigens, secrete specific antibodies to neutralize or eliminate antigenic bacteria and viruses as they travel through body fluids between cells. Similarly, following recognition of antigens and signaling from CD4 cells, some CD8 cells called cytotoxic T cells become activated to kill cells infected with intracellular pathogens; others called suppressor T cells dampen an ongoing immune response. Furthermore, CD4 cells are known to modulate the activities of immune system cells known as natural killer cells and macrophages, which are involved in responses to infection and perhaps to incipient malignancies.

The mechanisms by which CD4 cells might be depleted by HIV have remained mysterious (see Chapter 6). Once HIV was isolated, it was found *in vitro* to specifically infect a subset of CD4 cells and to initiate events leading to the depletion of most CD4 cells in the culture, accurately mirroring the depletion of CD4 cells *in vivo* (Klatzmann et al., 1984a; Popovic et al., 1984). This led investigators to test whether and subsequently to prove that the CD4 molecule is the receptor used by HIV to initiate viral infection of these cells (Dalgleish et al., 1984; Klatzmann et al., 1984b). The CD4 molecule at the cell surface thus appears to distinguish potential target cells for HIV and to act as the receptor molecule that binds the virus and allows infection and subsequent viral replication. Recent experimental evidence has also suggested that the interaction between HIV and the CD4 molecule contributes to the cytopathic consequences of viral infection (Lifson et al., 1986; Sodroski et al., 1986).

The immunodeficiency of AIDS clearly demonstrates the importance of CD4 T lymphocytes. Because of the loss of these cells, the remaining T lymphocytes from AIDS patients have diminished or absent responses to antigens, to certain chemicals known as mitogens that make T cells divide, and to blood cells from nonidentical individuals. In addition, T lymphocytes from AIDS patients show subnormal production of essential immunoregulatory factors, and due to their decreased numbers and functional capacity they are unable to fulfill their necessary role in providing direction for the maturation of B cells and cytotoxic T cells. The ability of AIDS patients to mount antibody reactions to new antigens is severely compromised, though paradoxically high levels of antibodies to previously encountered antigens, including HIV, are often present in patients' sera.

NATURAL HISTORY OF THE DISEASE

Since the initial recognition of the AIDS epidemic, much information has accumulated regarding the natural history of the disease. Prior to the identification of HIV as the causative agent of AIDS and the development of serologic testing to detect the presence of antibodies (and thus infection) in asymptomatic persons, information on the cause of the disease was limited to data on those who developed clinical dysfunction.

Since the virus was isolated, however, it has become increasingly feasible to study HIV-infected individuals prospectively for development of laboratory abnormalities as well as disease manifestations. The earliest markers now known to indicate that HIV has been transmitted to an individual are either the isolation of HIV from that person or the detection of antibodies to the virus in the person's blood. The appearance of antibodies directed against HIV in the serum of exposed persons—which is known as seroconversion—appears to predate any detectable immunologic defects.

Recent data suggest that seroconversion is accompanied within a five-year period by evidence of immunologic defects in more than 90 percent of individuals, including those who remain clinically asymptomatic (Melbye et al., 1986). Furthermore, the development of characteristic abnormalities, as revealed by certain laboratory measures of the immune system, often occurs very rapidly after the appearance of antibodies. The long-term health significance of these early alterations in immune functioning are not yet fully appreciated, but they must be regarded as a cause for concern.

The typical time between transmission of the virus and seroconversion has been estimated to be six to eight weeks, based on observation of cases in which an isolated exposure to the virus was known to have occurred (Melbye, 1986). This period is highly variable, however, with reported instances of seroconversion occurring up to eight months after an isolated exposure to HIV. Isolated and unusual cases have been reported in which individuals remained seronegative for long periods of time although they were infected, as evidenced by cultivation of virus from the blood (Groopman et al., 1985; Salahuddin et al., 1984). This possibility has implications for blood donation, as discussed in Chapter 4.

The number of viral particles needed to initiate infection, the form in which they are transmitted, and the relationship of these factors to possible routes of entry are not known (see Chapter 6). Also, the earliest events of the infection process and the sites of replication of the virus in the body are not well defined. One hypothesis for the initial events is that HIV enters the blood directly. If this is the case, the virus might appear in the plasma, where presumably it could bind to CD4 lymphocytes and initiate infection. Other possibilities for the initial route of viral entry or site of infection include macrophages or other local antigen-presenting cells that populate the surface epithelial cell lining of the vaginal, urogenital, or gastrointestinal tracts, or other specialized cells of the immune system located near the site of viral entry. HIV is known to multiply in lymphocytes and macrophages, but there is no evidence that it can multiply in other cells, such as neurons. Involvement of disseminated sites (including the central nervous system) during AIDS may be due to the migration of infected cells, such as macrophages, into the sites, or to infection of these cells *in situ*.

It is not known what proportion of individuals who are seropositive for HIV antibodies will ultimately develop clinical AIDS (see Chapter 3). In one recent study in San Francisco of 33 homosexual men known to have been seropositive since 1978-1980 and followed for an average of 68.2 months, 15 percent have developed AIDS, 27 percent lymphadenopathy, and 24 percent only hematologic abnormalities; 39 percent have no abnormal clinical findings (Rutherford et al., 1986).

Another major question has been whether cofactors in the form of environmental agents, genetic influences, or coexisting infectious diseases might increase the likelihood of HIV infection or the presence of clinical disease. The existence of such cofactors is often suggested, but there are no data to support the concept, with the possible exception in Africa of genital ulcers. Furthermore, some recent data fail to support the previously proposed association between either nitrite use or elevated cytomegalovirus titers and the development of clinical AIDS (Polk et al., 1986).

Another area of great concern is whether PGL and ARC will in most cases advance to AIDS. Some investigators had suggested soon after the early description of AIDS and its associated conditions that these conditions might reflect containment or repression of HIV infection by the immune system. However, although many cases of AIDS have been preceded by some manifestations of these symptoms, PGL, ARC, and AIDS cannot be considered simply as stages of an orderly progression in the spectrum of HIV infection. It is not now known to what extent PGL or ARC may predict the eventual development of frank AIDS (Abrams et al., 1985). This important question has yet to be clearly resolved.

There are no recorded cases of the spontaneous remission of AIDS, of related clinical conditions, or of immune defects in HIV-infected persons, and only anecdotal reports of reversion from seropositive to seronegative status (Burger et al., 1985).

CLINICAL MANIFESTATIONS OF HIV INFECTION

Of the many clinical conditions associated with HIV infection, most are the consequences of immunologic damage and not the direct result of HIV infection itself. These conditions range from those that are annoying but not in themselves life threatening to some of the most serious and uniformly fatal infections and tumors known. The significance of these manifestations lies in their role as a common cause of or contributing factor to death from HIV infection, in their importance for tracking the epidemiology of the disease, in their further elucidation of the pathogenesis of disease, and in their implications for determining future health care needs and costs. (See Appendix A for a more detailed discussion of the presentation, diagnosis, and treatment of the clinical manifestations of HIV infection.)

The current CDC definition of AIDS reflects those opportunistic infections and cancers observed in the United States. The most common manifestations of HIV infection are not the same in all parts of the world; they differ, for instance, between the United States and Africa. With longer experience, additional manifestations—opportunistic infections, cancers, or direct consequences of HIV infection—may need to be added to those described below.

Opportunistic Infections

Opportunistic infections are caused by microorganisms that take advantage of the opportunity offered by lowered immunity but would seldom cause disease in persons with normal defense mechanisms. The occurrence of opportunistic infections in AIDS has been of central interest for at least two reasons. First, their unusual appearance in young, otherwise healthy men was one of the first indications that a new disease syndrome was emerging. Second, they are among the most common causes of death in AIDS patients. Opportunistic infections that have assumed a major role in the epidemic include *Pneumocystis carinii* pneumonia; toxoplasmosis; tuberculosis; viral infections due to herpes simplex, herpes zoster, and cytomegalovirus; cryptococcal disease (especially meningitis); oral and esophageal candidiasis (thrush); and cryptosporidiosis (see Appendix A).

As a group, these infections are the most common presenting clinical manifestations that ultimately lead to a diagnosis of AIDS. Traditionally, opportunistic infections have been associated with impaired immunity. However, therapy for these infections has been more successful in other immunocompromised populations, such as cancer patients and transplant recipients, than in patients with AIDS. Probably because the immune deficit is so profound, in AIDS patients these infections are characterized by an aggressive clinical course, resistance to therapy, a high rate of relapse, and a high incidence of drug toxicity during treatment.

It is not known whether improved therapy for opportunistic infections would significantly lengthen the overall survival of patients with AIDS. Given the number of characteristic infections seen and the underlying immune defects of these patients, it seems unlikely that cure of any single infection would significantly change the ultimate outcome of the disease. However, an effective treatment for *Pneumocystis carinii* pneumonia might prolong average survival somewhat, since a high proportion of AIDS patients succumb to this infection.

Kaposi's Sarcoma

Kaposi's sarcoma is a cancer originating from the cells that comprise the lining of blood vessel walls. It was one of the earliest recognized manifestations of AIDS, and because it produces lesions of the skin and other body surfaces it remains the most visible (and often disfiguring) indication of AIDS, leading to severe social as well as medical problems. While it can directly cause death when it results in respiratory failure, its diagnostic significance is as a readily detectable indication of underlying immune deficiency. Patients with Kaposi's sarcoma are also often less severely immunocompromised than are other groups of AIDS patients, making this population the focus of several clinical therapy trials for the malignancy itself.

For reasons as yet unclear, Kaposi's sarcoma is much more frequent in homosexual men than in other AIDS patients (Cohn and Judson, 1984;

Des Jarlais et al., 1984), although its incidence in this population is said to be decreasing, also for unknown reasons. Both cytomegalovirus infection (Drew et al., 1982) and the use of inhaled nitrites (Marmor et al., 1982) have been suggested as possible cofactors responsible for the increased incidence of Kaposi's sarcoma in homosexuals, but data to support these hypotheses are lacking at this time.

Kaposi's sarcoma can be readily recognized clinically by experienced physicians. Recently there have been anecdotal reports of a decline in the use of biopsies to confirm diagnoses (as required to meet the CDC definition of AIDS). The contribution of this trend to underreporting of AIDS cannot be determined at this time, but it illustrates the conflicts that can arise between clinical practice for individual patients and the need for accurate surveillance data on AIDS.

Other Malignancies

Since 1982, clinically aggressive (high-grade) non-Hodgkin's lymphomas have been seen with increased frequency in patients at risk for AIDS (Ioachim et al., 1985; Kalter et al., 1985). In 1985 this observation led the CDC to add this disease, when accompanied by a positive serologic test for HIV antibodies, to the surveillance definition of AIDS. Non-Hodgkin's lymphoma related to HIV infection occurs at unusual sites for that disease—e.g., the central nervous system, the rectum, and gastrointestinal sites. Many affected patients have a marked generalized lymphadenopathy that precedes by several years the diagnosis of lymphoma.

Despite dramatic advances in the treatment of non-Hodgkin's lymphoma in the general population in the last decade, the prognosis for the disease among individuals infected with HIV is poor. Even with aggressive treatment these patients have a low response rate, a high incidence of associated opportunistic infections, and high relapse and mortality rates.

People with HIV infection have also been reported to be at increased risk for the development of Hodgkin's disease (Schoeppel et al., 1985). While the disease appears to respond in a conventional manner to standard chemotherapy, treatment is more frequently accompanied by secondary opportunistic infections and is complicated by therapy-induced persistent and severe bone marrow failure.

Several other cancers have been reported to occur with increased incidence in people with HIV infection, including squamous cell cancers, malignant melanoma, testicular cancer, and primary hepatocellular carcinoma. These cancers are statistically associated with HIV infection, but there is no evidence of a direct causal relationship with HIV. HIV cannot be isolated from at least one malignancy in this group (Groopman et al., 1986), suggesting it is not the direct cause of the malignancy.

Neurologic Complications Associated with HIV Infection

Neurologic complications are becoming increasingly recognized as an important cause of the morbidity and mortality associated with HIV infection. As many as 90 percent of patients dying from HIV-related conditions have histopathologic abnormalities of the nervous system at postmortem examination, and the majority of patients have some clinical manifestation of neurologic disease during their lifetime. Neurologic complaints are the initially evident symptom in about 10 percent of patients. Of the HIV-related neurologic complications, dementia is among the most severe and disabling.

A wide variety of central and peripheral nervous system diseases are seen in AIDS patients (Appendix A). About 30 percent of these patients develop opportunistic infections of the central nervous system (CNS), including toxoplasmosis, cryptococcal meningitis, and disseminated herpes infection. Some 2 to 5 percent develop CNS neoplasms, particularly primary CNS lymphomas but also secondary lymphomas and metastatic Kaposi's sarcoma. Of patients with neurologic involvement, at least two-thirds develop a subacute encephalitis (mild brain inflammation) (Britton and Miller, 1984; Krupp et al., 1985), and 20 percent develop a myelopathy (Petito et al., 1985), both of which are thought to be related to primary infections of the central nervous system with HIV. In addition, peripheral neuropathies develop in approximately 25 percent of patients.

Central nervous system involvement of HIV may lead to neurologic deficits that mimic many psychological problems, posing difficulties in diagnosis, and it may have a chronic course. The occurrence of severely debilitating neurologic disease, especially dementia, will place a major strain on the health care system and on society as a whole in caring for affected patients (see Chapter 5).

There are many unanswered questions surrounding infection of the central nervous system by HIV. They include the timing and frequency of infection, the amount of time that may elapse between involvement of the central nervous system and the development of subacute encephalitis with dementia, and the primary site of infection in the central nervous system. The answers to these questions will have major implications for the design of future therapeutic agents, which will have to cross the blood-brain barrier; for social, ethical, and legal issues involving AIDS; and for the planning of future health care for AIDS patients.

Pediatric AIDS

The clinical manifestations of AIDS in children are significantly different from those in adults. In contrast to the most common diseases associated with adult AIDS—*Pneumocystis carinii* pneumonia and Kaposi's sarcoma—the most common clinical manifestations of pediatric AIDS are recurrent bacterial (Bernstein et al., 1985), viral, and candidal infection; failure to thrive; lymphocytic interstitial pneumonitis; and encephalitis. Because there are so many different clinical findings in pediatric AIDS and because the diseases associated with AIDS in this population are similar to those seen in general pediatric populations, testing for HIV antibodies assumes more importance in children suspected of having AIDS than in adult populations.

Some investigators believe that an attempt to fit observations from children into definitions for adult patients is unwise due to the broad and different presentations of AIDS in children (Parks and Scott, 1986). (See Appendix A for a detailed description of pediatric AIDS.)

MODES OF TRANSMISSION OF HIV

Transmission of an infectious agent requires five basic elements: (1) an infected source, (2) a vehicle or mechanism of spread, (3) a susceptible host, (4) an appropriate site of exit from the source, and (5) an appropriate site of entry into the susceptible host. Given these basic elements, infectivity will be related to such factors as the levels of the infectious agent present or the efficiency of possible mechanisms of transmission (see Chapter 6).

Knowledge of the routes of transmission of infectious agents in human populations is derived primarily from epidemiologic data. Direct evidence related to the efficiency of specific routes of HIV transmission cannot be derived experimentally, because it is unethical to deliberately infect a human being. However, chimpanzees and other animals susceptible to HIV or related viruses may in the future be used as models in experimental transmission studies. Isolation of an infectious agent such as HIV from certain secretions, body fluids, or tissues may suggest possible routes of transmission. But such findings do not imply that transmission by that route occurs, and the interpretation must be tempered by other evidence of transmission.

Epidemiologic data indicate that transmission of HIV is limited to sexual, parenteral, and maternal-infant (possibly including *in utero*) routes. It has been postulated, but not proved, that adult infection may require direct blood exposure and may be enhanced by coincident damage to skin or mucous membranes to facilitate viral entry.

There is no evidence for other routes of HIV transmission. In fact, there is now substantial evidence against transmission through so-called casual contact, including regular close contact (such as that occurring in sharing accommodations, eating utensils, or even toothbrushes), that does not involve parenteral or sexual exposure, despite the fact that HIV has been reported to have been occasionally isolated from saliva and tears in small amounts (Friedland et al., 1986).

Sexual Transmission

Numerous case-control studies have identified receptive anal intercourse (with ejaculation of semen) and having a number of sexual partners as the primary risk factors for HIV infection in homosexual men. Among men who practice receptive anal intercourse, rectal douching appears to further increase the risk, probably through trauma to the rectal mucosa or damage to normal protective barriers (W. Winkelstein, University of California, personal communication, 1986). Other factors associated with an increased risk of infection in homosexual men include manual-rectal intercourse ("fisting"), a history of sexually transmitted disease, recreational drug use (especially the use of amyl or butyl nitrites, known as poppers), IV drug use, and sexual contact with partners from bathhouses or from areas with a high prevalence of AIDS. These factors are frequently associated with the presence of HIV infection in potential partners or with the practice of anal intercourse and rectal douching; they are not regarded as independent primary risk factors for HIV transmission.

The capacity of available studies to define precisely the risk of HIV infection associated with oral intercourse (including ingestion of semen) or the risk to the insertive partner in anal intercourse is limited by the small number of individuals available for study who practice only these behaviors. A risk of infection to those who practice only these behaviors cannot be ruled out, but it is probably lower than the risk from receptive anal intercourse (Winkelstein et al., 1986).

Studies of homosexual men have identified couples with long-term, exclusive relationships in which one partner was infected with HIV and the other has remained uninfected over a considerable period, despite the seronegative partner's continued practice of receptive anal intercourse. Questions of possible individual variability in viral shedding and/or susceptibility need to be investigated further.

Although the virus has been isolated from semen and saliva, numerous studies have found no evidence that HIV is transmitted between homosexual men through kissing, oral-genital sex, oral-rectal sex, or mutual masturbation. HIV may be transmitted by these routes, but at relatively low efficiency.

HIV can also be transmitted during heterosexual intercourse. Saltzman and co-workers (1986) reported that 21 of 57 (37 percent) of persons who were long-term heterosexual partners of AIDS or ARC patients but had no other AIDS risk factors had confirmed antibodies to HIV; this included

17 of 48 (35 percent) female partners and 4 of 9 (44 percent) male partners. Redfield and co-workers (1986a) also reported approximately equal proportions of heterosexual partners with no other AIDS risk factors becoming infected in long-term sexual relationships with infected persons; 6 of 18 female and 2 of 6 male spouses became infected. In another study the Centers for Disease Control found 1 seropositive man among 20 husbands of women with transfusion-associated AIDS (T. A. Peterman, Centers for Disease Control, personal communication, 1986), as compared with 8 seropositive women among 50 wives of men with transfusion-associated AIDS. All of these studies suggested that vaginal intercourse was a route of transmission. Such findings document the existence of male-to-female and female-to-male transmission.

The committee concludes that data are not presently adequate to assess the relative efficiency of male-to-male, male-to-female, or female-to-male virus transmission during anal or vaginal intercourse. Even if a particular direction (male to female or female to male) and mode of transmission are relatively inefficient, repeated exposure to infected single or multiple partners may result in a significant risk of infection.

The high and nearly equal prevalence of seropositivity among men and women in central Africa and an age distribution of infected persons suggesting sexual transmission are other indications of female-to-male transmission (see section on "HIV Infection and AIDS Outside the United States," later in this chapter). The situation in Africa is complicated, however, by widespread heterosexual promiscuity among some groups and by the use of unsterile needles and syringes in some medical settings.

It is not clear whether tissue trauma leading to breaks in genital mucous membranes is necessary for and/or enhances sexual transmission of HIV. However, the increased risk attributable to rectal douching for men who practice receptive anal intercourse suggests that this may be the case. Furthermore, one study in Africa detected an increased risk, independent of the numbers of sexual contacts, among men who have a history of genital ulcers, suggesting that the virus may have gained entry when normal skin or mucous membrane barriers were disrupted (K. K. Holmes, University of Seattle, personal communication, 1986).

Parenteral Transmission

Epidemiologic data have indicated parenteral HIV transmission in a number of populations, including IV drug users, hemophiliacs, and blood transfusion recipients.

IV drug users commonly share injection paraphernalia (syringes and needles) and thereby transmit HIV through residues of blood. HIV can disseminate very rapidly if there is sharing of injection equipment outside of small, closed circles of IV drug users—for example, through the sharing of equipment with strangers that occurs in "shooting galleries" (places common in New York City where IV drug users can rent previously used injection equipment).

Transfusion-associated HIV infections occurred primarily from the late 1970s until about mid-1985, when screening of the blood supply for HIV antibodies began (see Appendix B). The available studies demonstrate that many blood components or products can transmit HIV, including packed red cells, frozen plasma, clotting factors, whole blood, and platelets. Albumin has not been implicated in the transmission of HIV, probably because it is routinely heated during preparation, a process known to destroy the infectivity of HIV. Nor has gamma globulin been implicated, at least when prepared by cold ethanol fractionation, as is the case in preparations for intramuscular use.

Follow-up of blood donors implicated in cases of transfusion-associated HIV infections has nearly always identified at least one donor who was a member of a high-risk group. More recently, studies have followed the recipients of units of blood that were found in retrospect to be seropositive. In the majority of cases, the recipient of a positive unit was later also found to be seropositive.

Self-exclusion of donors who are members of high-risk groups (i.e., their refraining from donating blood) began in 1983 and no doubt reduced the risk of exposure to HIV among transfusion recipients. Screening donors for HIV antibodies has further reduced the risk related to transfusion or the provision of blood products. (As discussed in Appendix C, the introduction of antibody testing has reduced the risk of HIV transmission to blood recipients by more than 95 percent.) However, even screening cannot guarantee absolute safety of the blood supply, because transmission can occur when the virus is present (viremia) but before the appearance of HIV antibodies and because the sensitivity of the test for detecting antibodies (and hence infection) is less than 100 percent (see Appendix B).

The current risk of HIV transmission from a blood product to a recipient depends on a number of factors. These include (1) the sensitivity of the screening test(s) in detecting antibody, (2) the prevalence and duration of viremia prior to the appearance of antibody in the donor population, (3) the likelihood of donation during the phase of infection that precedes the development of antibodies, and (4) the number of units of blood or blood products the recipient receives.

Of greatest concern to the general public is the risk of HIV transmission from packed red blood cells, which are the blood component most frequently transfused (although the much smaller number of patients who receive other nonsterile blood components or products are also at risk). Each donated unit of blood produces one unit of packed red blood cells. In the United States, approximately 10 million units of blood or blood components are transfused each year into approximately 3.5 million recipients. Thus, the average recipient is exposed to blood from three donors.

The risk of HIV exposure for an average recipient of packed red blood cells is estimated, on the basis of reasonable assumptions, to be fewer than 1 in 34,000 (see Appendix C). Under slightly more optimistic assumptions, the risk should fall to fewer than 1 in 140,000. Under slightly more pessimistic assumptions, the risk rises to approximately 1 in 11,000.

With the risk of HIV transmission to blood recipients reduced by more than 95 percent through antibody testing, instead of 4,000 infected units out of 10 million used, the baseline calculations presented in Appendix C project the transfusion of about 100 infected units each year. Since approximately half of transfusion recipients die of other causes relatively soon after receiving blood, the number of infections directly resulting from transfusion would be smaller.

Most of the current risk in blood transfusion relates to the possibility of blood donation during the preantibody phase of HIV infection. These considerations reinforce the importance of continued self-selection by potential donors to exclude those who have engaged in high-risk behaviors.

Transmission of HIV to persons receiving blood-derived clotting factors has also been demonstrated. In particular, hemophiliacs lack one of several blood proteins required for normal clotting and as a consequence are likely, without interventions, to endure severe and prolonged bleeding. Injected clotting factors (VIII for hemophilia A or IX for hemophilia B) concentrated from human plasma can alleviate this problem. Until recently, the procedures used to manufacture these concentrates, involving plasma pooled from many donors, allowed HIV to be transmitted from an infected plasma donor to recipients. Since late 1984, however, most manufacturers have heat-treated concentrates in such a way as to inactivate HIV, and such products no longer pose a risk of infection.

Exposures through accidental needlesticks have resulted in few infections. A CDC study of nearly 1,000 health care workers with accidental needlesticks showed no clinical AIDS and only two seroconversions (McCray, 1986). In only one of these cases were there adequate data to clearly implicate transmission by the needlestick. There are isolated instances of seroconversion after needlestick, including a case report of HIV transmission by needlestick from an African AIDS patient reported from England (*Lancet*, 1984). In this instance, whole blood was thought to have been injected at the time of the needlestick.

The greater risk of infection from transfusions as compared with that from accidental needlesticks suggests that the dose of virus is probably an important factor in parenteral transmission. This could also explain the apparently greater risk among IV drug users than that following needlesticks (IV drug users commonly draw blood into the syringe, and blood residues are injected when equipment sharing occurs). The frequency and direct IV route of exposure could also contribute to this difference.

Hemodialysis units are potential sources of parenteral exposure to infectious agents, as is seen with hepatitis B virus (HBV) infections (Peterman et al., 1986). However, the extensive use of disposable equipment has greatly reduced the risk of HBV and other infections in this setting in recent years. HIV could easily be introduced into dialysis units either through prior blood transfusions or through other dialysis patients who are seropositive. Seropositive dialysis patients have, in fact, been identified. However, available data have not demonstrated transmission between dialysis patients, and it seems unlikely, given the current standards of hygiene practiced within most units.

Questions have been raised about the possibility of HIV transmission from two other blood products: immune globulins and plasma-derived hepatitis B vaccines. The Centers for Disease Control actively monitors reported AIDS cases for evidence of an association with immune globulin. Thus far, none has been detected (Centers for Disease Control, 1984). Prospective evaluation of immune globulin recipients, including some who have received hepatitis B immune globulin containing detectable HIV antibodies, has demonstrated no transmission of the virus. Furthermore, the cold-ethanol treatment used to prepare immune globulin for intramuscular injection has been found experimentally to inactivate HIV. Thus, in the absence of flawed or altered manufacturing techniques, there is no reason to believe that intramuscular immune globulin can transmit HIV.

A recent case report of HIV infection in a long-term recipient of intravenous immune globulin suggested the possibility that the virus was transmitted from this material, although other sources were not completely excluded. The production steps for intravenous immune globulin would not be expected to inactivate virus with the same degree of certainty as those used for intramuscular preparations, and their ability to inactivate HIV has not yet been evaluated.

Follow-up of recipients of the American and French plasma-based hepatitis B vaccines has shown no evidence of HIV transmission from these products, even though some of the plasma used in their manufacture is known to have contained antibodies reactive with HIV. Moreover, each of the three inactivation steps used for the American vaccine has been shown experimentally to inactivate HIV. These hepatitis B vaccines have therefore been convincingly demonstrated to be safe with regard to HIV transmission.

An unusual case of apparent transmission from a child to his mother has been reported (Centers for Disease Control, 1986a). The child was born with congenital abnormalities and became infected with HIV as a result of a blood transfusion. The child required extensive hospital and home medical care, and the mother acted as nurse but did not adopt routine procedures—such as the wearing of gloves—appropriate to health care providers in such a situation. She was frequently and extensively exposed to bloody fecal material from the infant. This strongly suggests that the route of transmission would have been parenteral, with infection resulting from percutaneous exposure through microscopic (or unrecalled macroscopic) breaks in her skin.

Maternal-Infant Transmission

Transmission of HIV from an infected mother to her infant probably occurs during pregnancy and/or delivery rather than postnatally, although the issue of transmission through breast-feeding is yet to be resolved. Some investigators suspect that HIV is transmitted *in utero,* because the time to development of AIDS in some infants is relatively short. Recently a series of cases has been reported in which HIV-infected infants were described who exhibited a distinctive dysmorphic appearance, which supports the possibility of early *in utero* transmission (Marion et al., 1986). Sprecher and co-workers (1986) have reported HIV transmission as early as the fifteenth week of gestation. Transmission *in utero* would preclude, at least for those cases, the possibility of providing immunoprophylaxis to infants at high risk if effective means became available in the future. It is also important to determine precisely when (and how) transmission can occur in order to assess the usefulness of procedures such as caesarean delivery (Chido et al., 1986; Lifson and Rogers, 1986).

One case of HIV transmission to an infant via breast milk has recently been reported, suggesting the possibility that the virus could be transmitted orally to infants through breast-feeding (Ziegler et al., 1985). This issue would be of special importance in the developing countries of central Africa, where breast-feeding is otherwise extremely desirable.

The rate of maternal-infant transmission is unknown. In one study of 20 infants born to infected mothers who had already delivered 1 infant with AIDS, 13 infants (65 percent) had evidence of HIV infection several months after birth (Scott et al., 1985). This study may overestimate the average risk of transmission for all infected pregnant women, however, because the women were known to have previously transmitted the virus.

It appears that perinatal transmission is not inevitable; other studies have found transmission rates ranging from 0 to 22 percent (Centers for Disease Control, 1986b). Attempts are being made to screen women in high-risk categories for HIV antibodies and then to follow their infants prospectively (W. P. Parks, University of Miami, personal communication, 1986). This approach should define the risk of maternal-infant transmission and clarify the factors related to that risk.

It appears that pregnancy may increase the risk of developing AIDS or ARC for HIV-infected women. The Centers for Disease Control (1986b) has reviewed information on maternal-infant transmission and has made recommendations for assisting in the prevention of perinatal transmission of HIV.

POPULATION GROUPS AT INCREASED RISK OF HIV INFECTION

In the United States, homosexual males, IV drug users, neonates born to infected mothers, and persons such as hemophiliacs who received pooled blood products, including clotting factor, before testing for HIV antibodies have the highest risk of acquiring HIV infection. These groups have the most cases of AIDS and the highest prevalence of seropositivity. Homosexuals and IV drug users have a higher risk of infection because their behaviors and the prevalence of infection in those with whom they share these behaviors increase the likelihood of their being exposed to an infected person. However, individuals within all of the "high-risk behavioral groups" noted above have varying risks of infection depending on the extent of their exposure.

Within the rest of the population, which is generally at lower risk of infection, there also exists a spectrum of risk largely dependent on behavior. Instances of infection with HIV and of AIDS have been documented in this low-risk population and have been attributed to heterosexual transmission of the virus. HIV transmission from men to women has made up the majority of AIDS cases thus far attributed to heterosexual spread of the virus. These cases include spread to sexual partners of infected hemophiliac men, of IV drug users, and of bisexual men. There have also been some cases, cited as examples, of heterosexual spread to men from prostitutes (Redfield et al., 1985), but so far the number of such cases has been small.

Homosexual Men

The homosexual male population (which in this report is defined to include bisexual men) is probably the largest group in the United States at high risk of AIDS, but accurate demographic data on this population are extremely limited. There has not been a national estimate of the homosexual population in the United States since the Kinsey study, published in 1948 (Kinsey et al., 1948). The Kinsey report, which was based on a study of 5,300 white men between 1938 and 1948, estimated that 10 percent of males are more or less exclusively homosexual for at least three years between the ages of 16 and 55, and that 4 percent are exclusively homosexual throughout their lifetime. Extrapolations of the Kinsey data based on recent population figures give a rather wide range of estimates of the number of homosexual men, ranging from a low of 2 million or 3 million to a high of about 10 million in the United States.

The Kinsey survey was a pioneering effort in the study of human sexual behavior. However, it was not based on either random or stratified sampling of the U.S. population; those interviewed were all volunteers. Because Kinsey and his colleagues deliberately oversampled some populations (such as criminal and delinquent males), Gagnon and Simon (1973) reanalyzed the Kinsey data for the 1,900 males in the sample who were under the age of 30 and attending college. They found 3 percent with exclusively homosexual histories and another 3 percent with bisexual histories, rates lower than the Kinsey projections. There have been other surveys of self-reported responses of sexual behavior among males (Hite, 1981) and females (Hite, 1976), but they are not representative of the population at large.

The occasional demographic studies on this subject done since the Kinsey era seem to show that the percentage of male homosexuals has remained a stable percentage of the population (Bell and Weinberg, 1978). Yet with the advent of the gay liberation movement in the 1960s and 1970s, homosexual men and women have become more visible. This is especially true in the urban areas, such as San Francisco and New York City, to which they have gravitated. Homosexual men constitute a sizable proportion of the population over age 15 in a number of major American urban areas, although exact figures are not available. One study estimates that from 70,000 to 100,000 homosexual men reside in San Francisco, nearly a quarter of all of that city's male population aged 15 and over. Los Angeles, New York City, and Chicago probably have even larger numbers of homosexual men.

In the 1960s and 1970s many homosexuals asserted their claim to tolerance of their sexual orientation. At the same time they established a subculture where they could live openly—in common parlance "come out of the closet" and hence into the public consciousness. The taboo against homosexuality was challenged in a number of quarters; homosexuals began in greater numbers to live openly as homosexuals, being frank about their sexual orientation with business associates, family, and friends.

One component of the sexual liberation of the 1960s and 1970s was a proliferation of bars and bathhouses that fostered frequent, sometimes anonymous sexual liaisons among a certain proportion of homosexual men (FitzGerald, 1986). (Lesbians have tended to have more exclusive relationships.) Some homosexual men reported hundreds or even thousands of sexual partners during their lifetime. A consequence of this sexual freedom was a dramatic rise in the rates of syphilis, gonorrhea, amoebic dysentery, hepatitis, and other sexually transmitted diseases.

While the danger of sexual contact with large numbers of anonymous partners had been established with regard to sexually transmitted diseases other than AIDS, those diseases were largely regarded as treatable. With AIDS, sexually transmitted disease became a more serious matter, and sexual practices came under intense scrutiny. Often, descriptions of sexual activity implicated in the acquisition of HIV infection and AIDS seemed to imply a condemnation of those engaging in that behavior.

AIDS and the fear of AIDS may reveal just how tenuous are the tolerance and acceptance of homosexuals. In writing about AIDS, some have invoked explanations entailing divine retribution. There have also been calls for the incarceration of homosexuals and for eliminating future tax dollars for AIDS research. Though such recommendations remain extreme, there is still considerable institutionalized discrimination against homosexuals. In about half of the states, private consensual sexual activity between adults of the same sex remains a criminal offense. The U.S. Supreme Court upheld the right of states to pass such sodomy laws in an opinion issued in July 1986.

Intravenous Drug Users

The second-largest risk group for AIDS in the United States is IV drug users. According to the Centers for Disease Control, 17 percent of reported AIDS cases currently occur in people whose only known risk factor is IV drug use. As with homosexual men, accurate demographic data on IV drug users are very limited. However, experts in this field estimate that 750,000 Americans inject heroin or other drugs intravenously at least once a week, while at least an additional 750,000 inject drugs less often (D. C. Des Jarlais, New York State Division of Substance Abuse Services, personal communication, 1986).

Demographic data on IV and non-IV drug users who enter treatment programs are readily available, but data on IV drug users who do not seek treatment are scant. Within the former population, the median age is 28 years, and approximately 75 percent are men. There is a recognized urban concentration of "hard core" IV drug users who are mostly from lower socioeconomic strata. Typically, members of such groups have low-paying jobs or are unemployed and have received far fewer years of education than the average. Blacks, who make up approximately 13 percent of the nation's population, are nearly 40 percent of the IV-drug-using population (Ginzburg and Weiss, 1986).

In prison populations, IV drug users are known to be overrepresented, because IV drug use is an important factor predisposing to crime and incarceration. A national study of 12,000 state prison inmates in 1979 indicated that 30 percent of the inmates had used heroin at some time and that 12 percent had used heroin in the month prior to the crime for which they were imprisoned (U.S. Department of Justice, 1983).

Hemophiliacs

Hemophilia is a lifelong, hereditary blood-clotting disorder that affects males almost exclusively. The development of federally supported regional treatment centers and the introduction of clotting-factor concentrates in the 1970s markedly increased the life expectancy of hemophiliacs. The median age of persons with hemophilia rose from 11.5 years in 1972 to 20.0 years in 1982. As of 1986, more than 9,500 severe hemophiliacs (close to half of the total hemophiliac population in the United States) were being served by these centers.

Because of the pooling of plasma from numerous donors for the production of clotting-factor concentrates, a person with severe hemophilia may be exposed to as many as 100,000 blood donors per year. This exposure led to extensive, initially unrecognized transmission of HIV through these plasma concentrates beginning as early as 1980. The first cases of AIDS in hemophiliacs were diagnosed in 1982 (Evatt et al., 1984). Since 1984, the risk of transmission of HIV from these plasma products has been very markedly reduced by virus inactivation steps in their production, but a large proportion of hemophiliacs (including 60 to 80 percent of severely affected hemophiliacs) now test positive for HIV antibodies (Johnson et al., 1985).

Recipients of Blood Transfusions

In early 1983, with the growing realization that the etiologic agent of AIDS might be a virus that could be bloodborne, national guidelines were developed to have persons in the recognized AIDS risk groups refrain from blood donation. How many transfusion recipients received HIV-infected blood or blood components from the late 1970s until the routine adoption of this national policy is difficult to estimate, but it is likely to have been many thousands. Thus far, nearly 400 AIDS cases have been reported to the Centers for Disease Control among the recipients of whole blood, packed red blood cells, or platelets.

By March 1985, tests capable of detecting HIV antibodies had been developed and licensed; they allowed blood from most persons potentially capable of transmitting the virus to be identified. With donor screening in this manner and self-exclusion from blood donation by members of high-risk groups, the current risk of HIV transmission via transfusion is exceedingly small (see section on "Modes of Transmission of HIV," above, and Appendix C).

Heterosexual Contacts of HIV-Infected Persons

The heterosexual contacts of persons infected with HIV include heterosexual partners of IV drug users, female sex partners of bisexual men, sexual partners of infected hemophiliacs or of persons infected through transfusions, clients of infected prostitutes, and the heterosexual partners of other infected individuals. Accurate estimates of the numbers and characteristics of the spouses of infected hemophiliacs and persons infected through transfusions are either available or could be obtained. However, such data are only recently becoming available for the heterosexual contacts of IV drug users, of bisexual men, and of female prostitutes and other persons infected by HIV. These groups are potentially large, and they constitute the major threat for increasing transmission of HIV to the heterosexually active population, especially to those individuals who are currently at some risk of contracting a sexually transmitted disease (Winkelstein et al., 1986).

Infants and Children

Infants and children infected with HIV have been placed in a separate category for national surveillance because their clinical manifestations differ in many respects from those of adults (see Appendix A).

Pediatric AIDS was first recognized in 1980-1981, and since then the number of reported cases has been rising rapidly—to a total of 348 cases in children under 13 years of age as of September 8, 1986. This number represents approximately 1.5 percent of all reported AIDS cases in the United States. Half of these cases have occurred in children under one year of age. Of the children with AIDS, 60 percent have been black, and 21 percent Hispanic; 55 percent have been male; and 59 percent have died. About three-fourths of the AIDS cases in children have occurred in four states: New York (38 percent of the total in the four states), California (34 percent), Florida (14 percent), and New Jersey (14 percent).

The proportion of reported AIDS patients who are children under 13 years of age has not changed greatly over time. Of all the pediatric cases, approximately 54 percent have been children of IV drug users. An additional 10 percent have been children of parents who have AIDS or who are in other AIDS risk groups. About 15 percent of pediatric AIDS patients have received blood transfusions, while 4 percent have hemophilia. Thirteen percent are children of Haitian-born parents. Information on risk factors is incomplete or missing for the remaining 4 percent of cases.

Infants who acquire their infection from an infected mother are generally the offspring of female IV drug users, female sexual contacts of male IV drug users, female sexual partners of bisexual males, and women from Haiti or central Africa. As HIV infection continues to spread within the general heterosexual population, it would be expected that more children infected with HIV will be born to women with multiple sexual partners or to women whose male sexual partners have had contact with multiple sexual partners. Thus, pediatric AIDS may serve as an important marker of the heterosexual spread of HIV infection. In addition, it is theoretically possible that some children infected with HIV may survive to sexually active adulthood, thereby constituting a continuing reservoir of potential infection.

Health Care Workers

Health care workers comprise a significant segment of the labor force in the United States, accounting for about 6.3 million (5.3 percent) of the approximately 117 million persons employed in the United States. These workers have a wide range of earning levels and of educational and racial backgrounds.

Many health care workers are considered at increased risk for infections such as hepatitis B because of their occupational exposure to infected blood, primarily though needlestick-type exposures or abrasions of the skin (e.g., in dentistry). Because HIV can be readily transmitted between IV drug users by the sharing of needles and syringes, its potential for transmission by occupational exposure among health care workers has been studied. The CDC recently conducted a prospective study of 938 health care workers who had a reported parenteral or mucous membrane exposure to blood and other bodily fluids from AIDS patients. Of 451 of these workers tested, 2 (0.44 percent) were found to have developed HIV antibodies (McCray, 1986). In a comparable study of persons exposed to patients testing positive for hepatitis B surface antigen, about 26 percent developed infection.

Other studies have also reported a low risk of HIV infection among health care workers following occupational exposure (Henderson et al.,

1986). However, there have been a few reports of health care workers who have seroconverted after accidental needlestick injuries, which underscores the need for attention to safety precautions when caring for AIDS and HIV-infected patients or when handling blood in laboratories (Stricof and Morse, 1986).

As of early 1986, about 4 percent, or almost 800, of the more than 20,000 reported AIDS cases in the United States had occurred among health care workers. This percentage is similar to the proportion of the population employed in health care. In all cases fully investigated, risk factors other than being a health care worker were identified.

EPIDEMIOLOGIC STUDIES AND FINDINGS

Surveillance

Since the initial recognition of AIDS in 1981, public health surveillance of the epidemic has collected data essential to the understanding of the epidemiology of this disease. By September 1982, the Centers for Disease Control was using a case definition of AIDS designed for epidemiologic investigation (see Appendix E), and a CDC-organized national surveillance system was in place. Reporting of AIDS to public health officials has been required in most states since 1983. The CDC definition of AIDS was designed for precision, consistent interpretation, and specificity. Though modified slightly in June 1985, its primary purpose is still for epidemiologic rather than diagnostic use (i.e., to help track the disease rather than facilitate treatment of individuals).

The national surveillance system has been responsible for charting the growing magnitude of the AIDS epidemic, for delineating the occurrence of AIDS in the major risk groups, and for monitoring geographic patterns and trends in the occurrence of the disease. These surveillance efforts have been an overall success, but a method of case reporting designed for surveillance purposes cannot always be expected to yield data useful in answering research questions concerning disease pathogenesis, transmission, or outcomes.

National Disease Reporting

In the United States infectious disease surveillance is carried out primarily through a so-called "passive" reporting system by which physicians or hospitals send case reports to local and/or state health departments. State laws and regulations for the reporting of infectious diseases vary. In most states the list of reportable diseases consists of 40 to 60 infectious diseases, which generally include most of the diseases that the CDC requests be reported nationwide. Reporting by states to the CDC is voluntary; the CDC can request reports but cannot require states to report. However, states routinely comply with such requests.

Because of the severity of AIDS, the medical and media attention it has received, and the measures used to supplement the normal reporting procedures, the reporting of AIDS cases meeting the CDC surveillance definition (Appendix E) has been relatively complete. Studies of this issue in several cities have shown the reporting of hospitalized cases to be higher than 90 percent (Chamberland et al., 1985). Underreporting from hospitals probably does not obscure a large number of AIDS cases, because the majority of large city health departments visit hospitals and laboratories where most AIDS cases would be diagnosed. More under-reporting may occur with nonhospitalized cases, partly because of physicians' concern for maintaining confidentiality. Such concerns un-doubtedly lead to underreporting on death certificates, but this would have a more negative effect on research projects using death certificates than on national surveillance data.

With the increasing availability of the HIV antibody test to assist in determining infection status, there have been anecdotal reports that skin biopsies to diagnose Kaposi's sarcoma definitively and bronchoscopy to diagnose *Pneumocystis carinii* pneumonia are being obtained less fre-quently. This may be contributing to a gradual decline in verified diagnoses meeting the CDC surveillance criteria for AIDS even though such diagnoses would be made if appropriate diagnostic studies were performed. In some areas, particularly in nonurban areas, clinical inex-perience in the diagnosis of AIDS, plus the general lack of appropriate laboratory testing, may also have resulted in missing some AIDS cases. Finally, some illnesses due to HIV infection that are very severe and life threatening do not fit the CDC definition even if all of the appropriate laboratory tests are done.

In May 1986 the CDC introduced a clinical classification system for HIV infections (Appendix F). This classification system is intended primarily for public health purposes and was not designed or intended to be useful as a research classification or as a means of staging or classifying the clinical severity of symptoms or of making prognoses. Others have developed a clinical staging system (Redfield et al., 1986b). According to the CDC, its new classification system does not imply any change in its surveillance definition of AIDS for national reporting. However, the CDC is developing criteria for a "presumptive" diagnosis of AIDS that can be considered for national reporting.

The original CDC surveillance definition of AIDS was tailored to fit adult cases and was not particularly useful or sensitive for pediatric cases, because the types of conditions and clinical presentations in infants and children are significantly different from those in adults. Definitions for pediatric use have recently been developed by the Centers for Disease Control.

All cases of AIDS in which no risk factor is identified are referred for further investigation to local health departments. Of those cases for which additional information is obtained, most are reclassified into one of the known risk groups. Of the remainder, most stay in this "no identified risk" category because of incomplete information.

Because the CDC has not requested national reporting of ARC, no data on it are currently available from this source. Such reporting has not been requested for two main reasons. First, homosexuals have expressed concern that public health agencies will not maintain absolute confidentiality for such data. (However, no personal identifiers are transmitted to the CDC.) Second, there is no nationally accepted definition of ARC, and operational definitions can range from very mild signs and symptoms to severe illness and death.

The new CDC classification system for clinical manifestations of HIV infection should eventually lead to a better definition of ARC. In time it may contribute to an accepted national definition of ARC that for practical reasons, if not for prognostic reasons, could be subdivided into categories ranging from mild to severe.

As with ARC, the CDC has not requested national reporting of asymptomatic HIV infections. Nevertheless, a few states have followed Colorado in requiring the reporting of persons who have tested positive for HIV antibodies. Many public health epidemiologists believe that the data collected from mandatory reporting of laboratory results are incomplete and of little use. In addition, such mandatory reporting runs counter to current PHS recommendations that all persons at increased risk for HIV infection seek antibody testing on a strictly voluntary, confidential, and, if requested, anonymous basis (see Appendix G and Chapter 4). The confidential reporting of seropositive individuals *is* desirable at blood banks.

Epidemiologic Research

Epidemiologic research, in contrast to surveillance, usually involves more detailed study of a population selected for characteristics of interest. In AIDS, such populations have usually consisted of high-risk groups, such as homosexual men or transfusion recipients. With the isolation of HIV and the general availability of antibody tests, epidemiologic studies began to measure the prevalence and to some extent the incidence of infection among various population groups.

Epidemiologic research in AIDS has been centered largely in the National Institutes of Health's intramural and extramural programs, in ... and state departments of public health, and at the

...tain-

Shortly after the recognition of AIDS, many case-control studies of AIDS patients were carried out to supplement data collected from the initial clinical and laboratory studies. Case-control studies are generally not expensive to carry out, but they require personnel and resources that are not overly abundant in most local or state health departments today.

Case-control studies carried out during the past few years have provided valuable information on specific risk factors associated with AIDS in different population groups. In one of these studies the CDC compared male homosexual AIDS patients to healthy homosexual men selected from outpatient clinics and the practices of private physicians (Jaffe et al., 1983). The most important variables differentiating AIDS cases from controls were measures of homosexual activity. AIDS patients had a larger number of male sexual partners per year, began having sex at an earlier age, and were more likely than controls to have had syphilis and some form of hepatitis.

Another case-control study, carried out in New York City, compared men with Kaposi's sarcoma to homosexual controls from a private physician's practice (Marmor et al., 1984). This study also found that the number of male sexual partners in the year prior to diagnosis was significantly higher for AIDS patients than for controls. Other important variables identified included receptive anal intercourse and other traumatic sexual practices. Other studies have since borne out the findings implicating sexual transmission and receptive anal intercourse.

A case-control study conducted in New York and Miami showed significant differences between Haitian men with AIDS and Haitian men who acted as controls (Castro et al., 1985). The men with AIDS were more likely to report a history of gonorrhea and sexual contacts with female prostitutes. Among female Haitian AIDS patients, the variable most significantly associated with disease was having been offered money for sexual acts. This case-control study strongly implicated heterosexual contact as the predominant route of transmission in this population group.

Prospective Cohort Studies

The need for comprehensive longitudinal investigation of the natural history of AIDS was recognized early in the epidemic. The systematic and uniform collection of epidemiologically well-characterized biologic specimens was also needed as new test methods were developed. Several cohorts of homosexual men were enrolled in New York City, San Francisco, and other cities beginning in the late 1970s to participate in hepatitis B vaccine field trials. Study of these cohorts has continued, but the emphasis has shifted primarily to the retrospective and prospective study of risk factors associated with HIV infection and disease.

To supplement those studies, the National Institutes of Health provided funding in 1983 for collaborative prospective cohort studies of homosexual men in five cities. During 1984 and 1985, the centers that conducted these studies enrolled more than 5,000 volunteers (R. A. Kaslow, National Institutes of Health, personal communication, 1986).

In contrast to the cohorts from the other four cities, the San Francisco cohort was recruited from a probability sample and thus can be considered representative of the census tracts from which it was drawn. The other cohorts were recruited mostly from sexually transmitted disease clinics and from advertisements directed to homosexual populations. These groups must therefore be considered to represent a different population than the San Francisco cohort.

Participants in all of these cohorts are now being followed at least semiannually to collect social and sexual histories and biologic specimens or until they reach designated clinical milestones, such as ARC or AIDS.

Serologic Surveys

With the increased use of the HIV antibody test, public health surveillance of the AIDS problem will increasingly shift to serologic surveillance. The surveillance of the clinical manifestations of HIV infection will still be important, but such illnesses reflect infections that occurred an average of several years before the onset of signs or symptoms. Serologic studies of cohorts of homosexual men or periodic cross-sectional serologic surveys can provide valuable information on the current prevalence of HIV infection. Also, when compared with prior surveys, they can give some indication of the incidence of infection.

Serologic studies can accurately document the continuing spread of HIV infection in the known high-risk groups. They can also monitor the potential spread of HIV to heterosexuals. In addition, antibody studies can help evaluate the effectiveness of education and prevention measures or other programs designed to limit the spread of the virus.

Routine serologic testing is currently being done in the United States in the following situations:

1. About 12 million blood donors are being screened per year. Although there is some geographic variation (e.g., positive results are more common in high-incidence areas like New York City), early data indicated that an average of about 4 donors per 10,000 donors were antibody positive (with confirmatory testing) (Schorr et al., 1985).

2. All applicants for entry into the military services and all active-duty military personnel are being screened. These programs have just started, but preliminary data indicate that the seropositivity of recruit applicants averages 1.6 per 1,000 applicants nationally but can be as high as 2 percent in census tracts where the reported AIDS rate is highest (Burke et al., 1986).

3. Beginning in 1985, alternative test sites—which are physically separated from blood banks—were established to provide testing for persons who might be at some risk for HIV infection. Without alternative test sites it was felt that these persons might consider donating blood at a blood bank in order to be tested. The availability of such alternative test sites varies considerably throughout the country. The data obtained from these sites will be of limited value, because most of them provide testing on an anonymous basis and because repeat testing may be frequent.

The difficulty of fostering confidence in provisions to ensure confidentiality of test results continues to be a major obstacle to the full public health use of the HIV antibody test. Because of concerns over this issue, some jurisdictions have passed very strict consent and disclosure laws to prevent potential misuse of these tests. Thus, the routine testing of persons attending public sexually transmitted disease clinics cannot be carried out in many areas without the specific, written consent of the person to be tested. Such restrictions make it difficult but not impossible to carry out epidemiologic surveillance.

Except for contact notification (discussed in Chapter 4), public health use of information related to test results generally does not in itself appear to require identification of individuals. Various population groups are being routinely tested by unlinking personal identification information from the collected blood specimen. General demographic data are obtained in such unlinked testing, but the result of any test cannot be connected to any individual. The CDC is planning to carry out a national serologic study on a selected sample of hospital patients throughout the country on an unlinked basis to monitor the possible spread of HIV infection to other population groups.

Findings of Epidemiologic Studies

The Prevalence of HIV Infection

Epidemiologic and surveillance efforts have demonstrated that HIV infection is far more common than is AIDS, and that HIV infection causes a wide spectrum of illnesses. To put the current magnitude of the AIDS problem in perspective, the prevalence of HIV infection must first be estimated.

Most of the studies of HIV infection published to date have been based on individuals who may not be representative of the risk groups to which they belong. Most of the studies carried out in homosexual men have been based on patients from sexually transmitted disease clinics and on patients visiting private physicians for an illness. These men are likely to be among the most sexually active in a given population and are therefore more likely to have been exposed to HIV. In addition, many are already ill, possibly as a result of having AIDS or ARC.

Results from such studies indicate that the estimated prevalence of seropositivity among homosexual and bisexual men during 1985 ranged from 44 percent in a cohort from Washington, D.C., to 68 percent for men in San Francisco (Jaffe et al., 1985a). Data from a different cohort of homosexual men in San Francisco drawn from a probability sample indicate that in 1985 about 50 percent of these men were infected. Some limited survey data from nonurban areas of California and from other U.S. cities where the prevalence of reported AIDS in 1985 was low indicate the prevalence of seropositivity among homosexual men in these areas to be about 20 percent in 1985.

Most studies of HIV infection conducted among IV drug users are also potentially biased, since the majority of these patients are recruited from methadone treatment or detoxification programs. Published estimates of infection range from a low of 9 percent in San Francisco to a high of 64 percent in New York City. These large differences are believed to reflect in part that HIV infection was introduced into IV drug communities earlier on the East Coast than on the West Coast. Other factors related to patterns and practices of IV drug use in these areas may also be involved.

From studies of HIV infection among homosexual men and IV drug users, it is clear that a large number of persons in the two largest AIDS risk groups have been infected. Using estimated prevalence of infection and estimates of the size of these risk groups, estimates of the total number of infected persons in the United States can be derived. Using this method, the Public Health Service estimated as of mid-1986 that this number is somewhere between 1 million and 1.5 million (Appendix G). The estimate corresponds reasonably well with the estimate (approximately 1.25 million) derived using an infected-to-AIDS-case ratio of 50 to 1 (Curran et al., 1985). Morgan (Centers for Disease Control, personal communication, 1986) has estimated that there are between 50,000 and 125,000 cases of ARC in the United States, although this number is uncertain and depends on the definition adopted.

AIDS Cases By Risk Group

Because of the long incubation time for AIDS, disease trends will lag several years behind trends in infections. Between June 1, 1981, and September 8, 1986, the CDC received reports of 24,576 patients (24,228 adults and 348 children under 13 years of age) meeting its surveillance definition of AIDS (Centers for Disease Control, 1986c). While the number of reported AIDS cases has increased steadily, the increase has not been exponential. The doubling time for AIDS cases has increased from about four months in 1981 to almost one year in 1985-1986.

A total of 23,426 of the adult AIDS patients have been identified as being in one of the known HIV transmission categories: homosexual men with a history of drug abuse (8 percent); homosexual men who are not known IV drug users (65 percent); heterosexual IV drug users (17 percent); persons with hemophilia (1 percent); heterosexual cases (4 percent)—i.e., sexual partners of persons with AIDS, HIV infection, or at risk for AIDS (413 cases) and persons with no other identified risks who were born in countries where heterosexual transmission is believed to play a major role even though precise means of transmission have not yet been fully defined (525 cases); and recipients of transfused blood or blood components (2 percent). Cases with more than one risk factor other than the combinations listed above are tabulated in the first category only.

About 55 percent of the heterosexual cases are persons born outside the United States—e.g., in Haiti or central Africa. It is believed that most of the remaining 762 cases that fall in no identified transmission category could be assigned to a risk group if additional information were obtained either from the patient or from family members and friends. In a recent follow-up study of those cases initially not found to be in an identified risk group, 40 percent had a history of some other sexually transmitted disease such as gonorrhea or syphilis, suggesting that sexual contact may account for a significant number of these cases (Lifson et al., 1986).

The relative proportion of reported cases among the largest AIDS risk groups has remained remarkably stable over time. In the smaller risk groups, slight but statistically significant changes have occurred. AIDS cases among people born outside the United States, primarily in Haiti, have become proportionately less. Haitians accounted for 4.5 percent of total U.S. cases before 1984 but only 1.5 percent in 1986. The reason for this may be that the early cases were in Haitians who migrated to the United States from 1978 to 1981 and who were infected prior to their entry into this country.

The proportion of cases associated with blood transfusions has increased slightly, from 1.1 percent in 1983 to 1.9 percent in 1986, though the absolute number remains small. This increase represents additional cases among persons infected before an effective mechanism for donor screening was available. It may also represent increased recognition of the disease among transfusion recipients. With the long incubation period of AIDS, more cases are to be expected from the prescreening era. But with the institution of routine donor screening, the number of transfusion-associated AIDS cases should begin to decline as a proportion of total cases before the end of this decade.

The proportion of AIDS cases in the heterosexual contact risk group has also increased significantly over time, rising from 1 percent in 1983 to 1.4 percent in 1985 to a projected 2 percent in 1986, though the total number of such cases is still small (cumulatively totaling 413 cases as of September 8, 1986). However, in addition to those cases identified as caused by heterosexual exposure, it is likely that an undefined proportion of the cases among persons in no known risk group (totaling 762 cases) was caused by heterosexual transmission.

AIDS Case Trends by Geographic Area

The distribution of reported AIDS cases by geographic region has changed markedly over time. Relative to the New York City Standard Metropolitan Statistical Area (SMSA) and the San Francisco SMSA, the proportion of cases from the rest of the United States has increased significantly. This proportional change is greatest relative to New York City. It is primarily among homosexual men, but it is also seen among IV drug users and in the remaining risk groups. The most recent doubling time of reported AIDS cases was 14 months in New York City, 13 months in San Francisco, and 10 months in the rest of the country.

At least three hypotheses may account for the observed changes in the geographic distribution of AIDS cases. First, because the virus was introduced in New York City and San Francisco earlier than in the rest of the country, there has been more time for those persons who engage in high-risk activities to become infected. Second, in these cities the groups at highest risk are probably becoming relatively saturated with HIV infection and thus the incidence of new infections is slowing. Third, the intensive educational programs instituted in these cities may also have resulted in a marked reduction of unsafe sexual activities (see Chapter 4).

Additionally, changes in the methods of diagnosis or the consistency of reporting could at least in part account for these trends.

The national surveillance data can easily mask trends that differ within particular geographic areas. The overall proportion of reported cases by risk factor has changed little over time, but substantial and significant changes have occurred in individual areas. In New York City the proportion of AIDS cases in IV drug users (irrespective of sexual preference) has increased slightly—from 35 percent to 38 percent. In Newark, New Jersey, the proportion of cases in IV drug users has declined over time—from 67 percent to 61 percent.

AIDS Case Trends by Sex, Race, and Age

The distribution of AIDS cases by sex and race has not changed significantly over time, although there has been a slight increase in the average age of cases. Ninety-three percent of the reported cases in the United States are men. By race, 60 percent are white, 25 percent are black, and 14 percent are Hispanic. Less than 1 percent of the nonpediatric AIDS patients in the United States are between 13 and 19 years of age. About 90 percent of adult AIDS patients are between 20 and 49, with almost 50 percent between 30 and 39 years of age.

There are differences in the age, sex, and race distribution of cases by geographic region, but these are primarily because of differences in the patient risk groups. For example, in San Francisco the majority of AIDS cases are among homosexual men, and fewer than 1 percent of cases have been reported in women. By contrast, in New York City, which has a higher percentage of cases involving IV drug use and heterosexual contact, 10 percent of reported cases are in women. The slight increase in the age of AIDS patients does not necessarily indicate an increasing rate of new infection among older persons.

AIDS Case Trends in Disease Presentation and Mortality

Pneumocystis carinii pneumonia (PCP), the most common disease seen in AIDS patients, has been diagnosed in 64 percent of reported cases. Kaposi's sarcoma (KS), the second most common disease, has been diagnosed in 23 percent of cases (Centers for Disease Control, 1986c). PCP is common in all adult patient groups, while the vast majority (95 percent) of patients with KS are homosexual men.

The distribution of these two diseases is changing over time. PCP is accounting for an increasing proportion of AIDS-associated disease diagnoses, while KS is accounting for relatively fewer. Of the opportunistic diseases diagnosed before December 1984, PCP accounted for 34 percent and KS for 20 percent. Since then, PCP has accounted for 45 percent and KS for 14 percent. The decline in the proportion of KS and the increase in PCP can be seen in all adult risk groups. The trends are statistically significant in cases in New York City, San Francisco, and some other areas of the United States.

The reasons for this apparent shift in disease presentation are unclear, but at least three explanations have been hypothesized: (1) the occurrence of KS is associated with some cofactor, such as a second infection (e.g., cytomegalovirus) or the use of toxic substances (e.g., butyl and amyl nitrites), and the incidence of the cofactor is decreasing; (2) there is less reporting of KS, a condition somewhat more likely to be diagnosed and managed on an outpatient basis without biopsy-confirmed diagnosis; (3) there are relative differences in the distribution of incubation times for KS and PCP.

After PCP and KS, *Candida* esophagitis is the most common opportunistic disease, being seen in 14 percent of AIDS cases. This is followed by cytomegalovirus disease (7 percent), cryptococcosis (7 percent), chronic herpes simplex (4 percent), cryptosporidiosis (4 percent), toxoplasmosis (3 percent), and other opportunistic infections (3 percent). These percentages underestimate the number of diseases diagnosed in a given group of patients because health care providers frequently do not provide follow-up information on diseases that occur after a case has been reported initially.

Approximately 55 percent of all AIDS patients reported to the CDC are known to have died. The reported one-year mortality is 48 percent and increases to approximately 75 percent two years after the initial diagnosis is made (Centers for Disease Control, 1986c). These values, particularly the two-year estimate, are low because of underreporting of deaths.

The type of opportunistic illness initially diagnosed in AIDS patients relates significantly to short-term mortality. In one follow-up study of more than 1,000 AIDS cases, the median survival time after diagnosis for those with PCP was only 8 months, compared with a median survival of 30 months for those with KS alone.

HIV INFECTION AND AIDS OUTSIDE THE UNITED STATES

The fact that there are cases of AIDS in more than 80 countries has clearly demonstrated that HIV infection and its resulting diseases are a growing international problem. In an era of intercontinental travel, HIV has spread rapidly, and all countries share interests in finding and implementing effective control measures. Furthermore, analysis of the differences in the epidemiology of HIV infection from country to country can offer important clues to the biology of the virus and new opportunities, through international cooperation, to exploit those clues for control purposes.

African Countries

Infection with HIV appears to be widespread in central Africa and rapidly increasing in prevalence in eastern and southern Africa. Most available data are from central Africa. In Kinshasa, Zaire, the annual incidence of AIDS in adults as of February 1985 was estimated to be 38 per 100,000, up from 24 per 100,000 the previous July (Mann et al., 1986a). In October 1983 the estimated annual incidence in Kigali, Rwanda, was 80 per 100,000 (Van de Perre et al., 1984). AIDS has been seen in epidemic form in Zambia and Uganda since 1982, and subsequently in Tanzania (Biggar, 1986). High rates of infection, at that time without much disease, were noted in Nairobi in 1985, with some evidence of transmission from central Africa (Kreiss et al., 1986). Seropositivity has also been found in some areas of western Africa. Whether this reflects infection with HIV or with a related retrovirus is unknown. By December 1985 AIDS had been diagnosed in citizens of at least 23 African countries.

The presence of simian retroviruses with considerable genetic and immunologic homology to HIV raises the possibility that the virus arose in Africa and recently passed from monkey to human populations, although it could also have recently spread from an isolated human population to urban centers. The recent recognition that infection by retroviruses distinct from HIV and more closely resembling these simian retroviruses is also widespread in Africa has significant implications for public health measures and the improved understanding of the pathogenesis of HIV infection (see Chapter 6). Preliminary indications suggest that this spectrum of related viruses may cause varying degrees of immunosuppression and disease.

AIDS seems to have been rare and perhaps nonexistent in Africa before the mid-1970s. Cases consistent with AIDS occurred in a European visitor to Zaire in 1976 and in a Zairian citizen in Europe in 1977 (Bygbjerg, 1983; Vandepitte et al., 1983). Until the 1980s, however, cases were not seen with sufficient frequency to attract attention. The vast majority of reports of high rates of seropositivity in sera collected in the 1960s and 1970s are questionable, in view of an apparent lack of specificity in the initial antibody tests.

Clinically, AIDS cases in Africa differ from those in North America and Europe. There is a paucity of instances of documented *Pneumocystis carinii* infections in Africa, and a high frequency of oral candidiasis and tuberculosis, especially extrapulmonary (Biggar, 1986; Mann et al., in press). *Salmonella*, *Pseudomonas*, disseminated strongylosis, and

Entamoeba infections have also been noted in African AIDS patients. "Enteropathic AIDS," or "slim disease," is a syndrome seen in Africa and characterized by wasting, recurrent fever, and diarrhea. Endemic Kaposi's sarcoma was more common in Africa than in the developed world before the AIDS epidemic and does not appear to be associated with AIDS, but an increasing number of aggressive Kaposi's sarcoma cases are. As in the United States, these cases typically involve the lymph nodes and viscera, produce plaques on the trunk and face, and are rapidly fatal.

Several lines of evidence suggest that transmission of HIV in Africa is largely through heterosexual activity. The majority of cases are in adults. Unlike the situation in the United States, where the ratio of cases in men to those in women is greater than 10, in most African populations studied the ratio is approximately unity. In Kinshasa, the risk in men relative to women has been estimated to rise from 0.4 in those 20 to 29 years old to 4.0 in those 50 to 59 years old (Mann et al., 1986a). Striking clusters of AIDS cases among heterosexual partners have been anecdotally reported (Piot et al., 1984). Men with AIDS report an average 10-fold more heterosexual contacts than do controls (Clumeck et al., 1985), and up to half of the women with AIDS in some series are reported to be prostitutes (Van de Perre et al., 1984). Furthermore, seropositivity has been found in 31 to 66 percent of Nairobi women who are prostitutes and in 8 percent of men attending a Nairobi clinic for sexually transmitted diseases, in contrast to 2 percent of medical personnel (Kreiss et al., 1986). A survey of seropositivity in household contacts of AIDS patients and controls in Kinshasa showed a statistically significant increase in the seropositivity rate in spouses (61 percent in cases versus 4 percent in controls) but not in other contacts (4.8 percent in case households versus 1.6 percent in control households) (Mann et al., 1986b).

Little information exists on the particular sexual activities that transmit HIV or on the relative efficiency of transmission from women to men and men to women. Practices of scarification and "female circumcision" (genital mutilation) in some African societies have led some to wonder whether anal intercourse or trauma during vaginal intercourse might contribute to heterosexual transmission of HIV in Africa. However, the distribution of AIDS cases in Africa does not correspond closely with the practice of female circumcision, and anal intercourse is reported to be rare. Among Nairobi prostitutes, seropositivity was greatest (66 percent) in the lower socioeconomic class, whose clients were mainly Kenyan. In this group, only vaginal intercourse was reported to be practiced, but the average number of sexual encounters was 963 per year. Among higher-priced prostitutes, whose clients were mainly African and non-African tourists and businessmen, seropositivity was 31 percent, receptive oral sex (but not anal sex) was practiced by about 25 percent, and the average number of encounters was 124 per year. The risk of seropositivity seemed more closely linked in this study to the number of sexual encounters than to a particular sexual practice.

The importance of parenteral transmission of HIV in Africa is unknown but potentially great. Frequency of injections has been shown to be a risk factor for HIV infection there, a finding that might have been predicted from the practice in many medical clinics of reusing needles without sterilization. One of the common occasions for intramuscular injections in urban areas is treatment of sexually transmitted diseases, so it has been difficult to separate the role of the injection from that of the sexual encounter itself in contributing to transmission. The issue is confounded further by the observed statistical association of genital ulcers with seropositivity (K. K. Holmes, University of Seattle, personal communication, 1986). Interpretation of this association is difficult; the ulcers might be sites of inoculation of the virus, or they could have been a reason for attendance at a sexually transmitted disease clinic, where the virus might have been transmitted through unsterile needles or syringes.

Other Countries

The problem of AIDS in Haiti was recognized early, because initially some 40 percent of U.S. cases in which no known risk factor was found were in Haitians. Epidemiologic studies in Haiti have shown a ratio of cases in males to those in females of 4, which is intermediate between the ratios in the United States and Africa. Cases continue to increase rapidly and seem to be concentrated in urban centers.

Several lines of evidence point to both heterosexual and homosexual transmission of HIV in Haiti. Half of the men among recent cases are bisexual. Also, women with AIDS are much more likely to be sexually promiscuous than are their sisters, female friends, or the female sexual partners of men with AIDS (Pape et al., 1986).

A striking association has been observed in Haiti between AIDS and the receipt of an intramuscular injection in the preceding five years (Pape et al., 1986). As in Africa, the use in Haiti of unsterile needles and syringes is common. In one series, 7 of 34 cases, including 4 of 8 women, gave a history of a blood transfusion in the preceding five years. However, the overall degree of risk associated with blood transfusions in Haiti has not been determined.

The pattern of AIDS in Europe largely mirrors that in the United States. A large proportion of cases occur in homosexual men and IV drug users, with small numbers in heterosexual partners of people in high-risk groups, recipients of blood products, and travelers from countries with high rates of HIV infection. Particularly high rates of seropositivity have been reported among drug users in Italy and Spain, indicating a potential for rapid spread in this group. In Scotland a crackdown on the availability of hypodermic needles that coincided with the introduction of HIV may have contributed to the high (50 percent) seropositivity rate in IV drug users.

In southeast Asia, cases of AIDS have appeared in homosexual and heterosexual prostitutes in cities, despite the absence of much IV drug use in those groups. If HIV infection acts like other sexually transmitted diseases, the opportunity for amplification in that setting is worrisome.

REFERENCES

Abrams, D. I., B. J. Lewis, J. H. Beckstead, C. A. Casavant, and W. L. Drew. 1984. Persistent diffuse lymphadenopathy in homosexual men: Endpoint or prodrome? Ann. Intern. Med. 100:801-808.

Abrams, D. I., T. Mess, and P. A. Volberding. 1985. Lymphadenopathy: End-point prodrome? Update of a 36-month prospective study. Adv. Exp. Med. Biol. 187:73-84.

Barre-Sinoussi, F., J. C. Chermann, F. Rey, M. T. Nugeyre, S. Chamaret, J. Gruest, C. Dauguet, C. Axler-Blin, F. Vezinet-Brun, C. Rouzioux, W. Rozenbaum, and L. Montagnier. 1983. Isolation of a T-lymphotropic retrovirus from a patient at risk for acquired immune deficiency syndrome (AIDS). Science 220:868-871.

Bell, A. P., and M. S. Weinberg. 1978. Homosexualities: A Study of Diversity Among Men and Women. New York: Simon and Schuster.

Bernstein, L. J., B. Z. Krieger, B. Novick, M. J. Siddick, and A. Rubinstein. 1985. Bacterial infection in the acquired immunodeficiency syndrome of children. Pediatr. Infect. Dis. 4: 472-475.

Biggar, J. R. 1986. The AIDS problem in Africa. Lancet I:79-83.

Britton, C. B., and J. R. Miller. 1984. Neurologic complications in AIDS. Neurol. Clin. 2: 315-319.

Brun-Vezinet, F., C. Rouzioux, F. Barre-Sinoussi, D. Klatzmann, A. G. Saimot, W. Rozenbaum, D. Christal, J. C. Gluckmann, L. Montagnier, and J. C. Chermann. 1984. Detection of IgG antibodies to lymphadenopathy-associated virus in patients with AIDS or lymphadenopathy syndrome. Lancet I:1253-1256.

Burger, H., B. Weiser, W. S. Robinson, J. Lifson, E. Engleman, C. Rouzioux, F. Brun-Vezinet, F. Barre-Sinoussi, L. Montagnier, and J. C. Chermann. 1985. Transient antibody to lymphadenopathy-associated virus/human T-lymphotropic virus type III and T-lymphocyte abnormalities in the wife of a man who developed the acquired immunodeficiency syndrome. Ann. Intern. Med. 103:545-547.

Burke, D. S., W. Bernier, J. Voskovitch, R. Redfield, G. Jacobs, and J. Spiker. 1986. Prevalence of HTLV-III infections among prospective U.S. military recruits. P. 151 in Abstracts of the Second International Conference on AIDS, Paris, June 23-25, 1986.

Bygbjerg, J. C. 1983. AIDS in a Danish surgeon. Lancet I:925.

Castro, K. G., M. A. Fischl, S. H. Landesman, J. M. Johnson, J. C. Compas, and J. C. Desgrange. 1985. Risk factors for AIDS among Haitians in the United States. Paper presented at the International Conference on AIDS, Atlanta, Ga., April 14-17, 1985.

Centers for Disease Control. 1981a. Pneumocystis pneumonia—Los Angeles. Morbid. Mortal. Weekly Rep. 30:250-252.

Centers for Disease Control. 1981b. Kaposi's sarcoma and *Pneumocystis* pneumonia among homosexual men—New York City and California. Morbid. Mortal. Weekly Rep. 30:305-308.

Centers for Disease Control. 1982a. Persistent, generalized lymphadenopathy among homosexual males. Morbid. Mortal. Weekly Rep. 31:249-252.

Centers for Disease Control. 1982b. Update on acquired immune deficiency syndrome (AIDS)—United States. Morbid. Mortal. Weekly Rep. 31:507-514.

Centers for Disease Control. 1984. Hepatitis B vaccine: Evidence confirming lack of AIDS transmission. Morbid. Mortal. Weekly Rep. 33:685-687.

Centers for Disease Control. 1985. Revision of the case definition of acquired immunodeficiency syndrome for national reporting—United States. Morbid. Mortal. Weekly Rep. 34: 373-376.

Centers for Disease Control. 1986a. Apparent transmission of human T-lymphotropic virus type III/lymphadenopathy-associated virus from a child to a mother providing health care. Morbid. Mortal. Weekly Rep. 35:76-79.

Centers for Disease Control. 1986b. Recommendations for assisting in the prevention of perinatal transmission of human T-lymphotropic virus type III/lymphadenopathy associated virus and the acquired immunodeficiency syndrome. Morbid. Mortal. Weekly Rep. 34:721-726, 731-732.

Centers for Disease Control. 1986c. Acquired Immunodeficiency Syndrome Weekly Surveillance Report, September 9, 1986. Atlanta, Ga.: Centers for Disease Control.

Chamberland, M. E., J. R. Allen, and J. M. Monroe. 1985. Acquired immunodeficiency syndrome, New York City: Evaluation of an active surveillance system. JAMA 254:383-387.

Chido, F., E. Ricchi, P. Costigliola, L. Michelacci, L. Bovicelli, and P. Dallacesa. 1986. Vertical transmission of HTLV-III. Lancet I:739.

Clumeck, N., P. Van de Perre, M. Carael, D. Rouvroy, and D. Nzaramba. 1985. Heterosexual promiscuity among African patients with AIDS. Lancet II:182.

Cohn, D. C., and F. N. Judson. 1984. Absence of Kaposi's sarcoma in hemophiliacs with the acquired immunodeficiency syndrome. N. Engl. J. Med. 101:401.

Curran, J. W., W. M. Morgan, A. M. Hardy, H. W. Jaffe, W. W. Darrow, and W. R. Dowdle. 1985. The epidemiology of AIDS: Current status and future prospects. Science 229:1352-1357.

Dalgleish, A. G., P. C. L. Beverley, P. R. Clapham, D. H. Crawford, M. F. Greaves, and R. A. Weiss. 1984. The CD4 (T4) antigen is an essential component of the receptor for the AIDS retrovirus. Nature 312:763-767.

Daniel, M. D., N. L. Letvin, N. W. King, M. Kannagi, P. K. Sehgal, R. D. Hunt, P. J. Kanki, M. Essex, and R. C. Desrosiers. 1985. Isolation of T-cell tropic HTLV-III like retrovirus from macaques. Science 228:1201-1204.

Des Jarlais, D. C., M. Marmor, P. Thomas, M. Chamberland, S. Zolla-Pazner, and D. J. Sencer. 1984. Kaposi's sarcoma among four different AIDS risk groups. N. Engl. J. Med. 310:1119.

Drew, W. L., R. C. Miner, J. L. Ziegler, J. H. Gullett, D. I. Abrams, M. A. Conant, E.-S. Huang, J. R. Groundwater, P. Volberding, and L. Mintz. 1982. Cytomegalovirus and Kaposi's sarcoma in young homosexual men. Lancet II:125-127.

Evatt, B. L., R. B. Ramsey, D. N. Lawrence, L. D. Zyla, and J. W. Curran. 1984. The acquired immunodeficiency syndrome in patients with hemophilia. Ann. Intern. Med. 100: 499-504.

Feorino, P. M., H. W. Jaffe, E. Palmer, T. A. Peterman, D. P. Francis, V. S. Kalyanaraman, R. A. Weinstein, R. L. Stoneburner, W. J. Alexander, C. Raevsky, J. P. Getchell, D. Warfield, H. W. Haverkos, B. W. Kilbourne, J. K. A. Nicholson, and J. W.

Curran. 1985. Transfusion-associated acquired immunodeficiency syndrome. Evidence for persistent infection in blood donors. N. Engl. J. Med. 312:1293-1296.

FitzGerald, F. 1986. A reporter at large: The castro—1. New Yorker 62:34-70.

Francis, D. P., P. M. Feorino, J. R. Broderson, H. M. McClure, J. P. Getchell, C. R. McGrath, B. Swenson, J. S. McDougal, E. L. Palmer, A. K. Harrison, F. Barre-Sinoussi, J. C. Chermann, L. Montagnier, J. W. Curran, C. D. Cabradilla, and V. S. Kalyanaraman. 1984. Infection of chimpanzees with lymphadenopathy-associated virus. Lancet II:1276-1277.

Friedland, G. H., B. R. Saltzman, M. F. Rogers, P. A. Kahl, M. L. Lesser, M. M. Mayers, and R. S. Klein. 1986. Lack of transmission of HTLV-III/LAV infection to household contacts of patients with AIDS or AIDS-related complex with oral candidiasis. N. Engl. J. Med. 314:344-349.

Gagnon, J. H., and W. Simon. 1973. Sexual Conduct: The Social Sources of Human Sexuality. New York: Aldine.

Gallo, R. C., S. Z. Salahuddin, M. Popovic, G. M. Shearer, M. Kaplan, B. F. Haynes, T. J. Palker, R. Redfield, J. Oleske, B. Safai, G. White, P. Foster, and P. D. Markham. 1984. Frequent detection and isolation of cytopathic retroviruses (HTLV-III) from patients with AIDS and at risk for AIDS. Science 224:500-503.

Ginzburg, H. M., and S. H. Weiss. 1986. The human T-cell lymphotropic virus type III (HTLV-III) and drug abusers. Background paper. Washington, D.C.: Committee on a National Strategy for AIDS.

Gonda, M. A., F. Wong-Staal, and R. C. Gallo. 1985. Sequence homology and morphologic similarity of HTLV-III and visna virus, a pathogenic lentivirus. Science 227:173-177.

Groopman, J. E., P. I. Hortzband, L. Schulman, et al. 1985. Antibody seronegative, HTLV-III infected patients with acquired immunodeficiency syndrome or related disorders. Blood 66:742-744.

Groopman, J. E., J. L. Sullivan, C. Malder, D. Ginsberg, F. H. Orkin, C. J. O'Wara, K. Falchuck, F. Wong-Staal, and R. C. Gallo. 1986. Pathology of B-cell lymphoma in a patient with AIDS. Blood 67:612-615.

Henderson, D. K., A. J. Saah, B. J. Zak, R. A. Kaslow, H. C. Lane, T. Folks, W. C. Blackwelder, J. Schmitt, D. J. LeCamera, H. Masur, and A. S. Fauci. 1986. Risk of nosocomial infection with human T-cell lymphotropic virus type III/lymphadenopathy-associated virus in a large cohort of intensively exposed health care workers. Ann. Intern. Med. 104:644-647.

Hite, S. 1976. The Hite Report. A Nationwide Study on Female Sexuality. New York: MacMillan.

Hite, S. 1981. The Hite Report on Male Sexuality. New York: Knopf.

Ioachim, H. C., M. C. Cooper, and G. C. Hellman. 1985. Lymphomas in men at high risk for acquired immune deficiency syndrome (AIDS). A study of 21 cases. Cancer 56:2831-2842.

Jaffe, H. W., K. Choi, P. A. Thomas, H. W. Haverkos, D. M. Auerbach, M. E. Guinan, M. F. Rogers, T. J. Spira, W. W. Darrow, M. A. Kramer, S. M. Friedman, J. M. Monroe, A. E. Friedman-Kien, L. J. Laubenstein, M. Marmor, B. Safai, S. K. Dritz, S. J. Crispi, S. L. Fannin, J. P. Orkwis, A. Kelter, W. R. Rushing, S. B. Thacker, and J. W. Curran. 1983. National case-control study of Kaposi's sarcoma and *Pneumocystis carinii* pneumonia in homosexual men: Part I. Epidemiologic results. Ann. Intern. Med. 99:145-151.

Jaffe, H. W., W. W. Darrow, D. F. Echenberg, P. M. O'Malley, J. P. Getchell, V. S. Kalyanaraman, R. H. Byers, D. P. Drennan, E. H. Braff, J. W. Curran, and D. P. Francis. 1985a. The acquired immunodeficiency syndrome in a cohort of homosexual men. A six-year follow-up study. Ann. Intern. Med. 103:210-214.

Jaffe, H. W., M. G. Sarngadharan, A. L. DeVico, L. Bruch, J. P. Getchell, V. S. Kalyanaraman, H. W. Haverkos, R. L. Stoneburner, R. C. Gallo, and J. W. Curran. 1985b. Infection with HTLV-III/LAV and transfusion associated acquired immunodeficiency syndrome. Serologic evidence of an association. JAMA 254:770-773.

Johnson, R. E., D. N. Lawrence, B. L. Evatt, D. J. Bregman, L. D. Zyla, J. W. Curran, L. M. Aledort, M. E. Eyster, A. P. Brownstein, and C. J. Curran. 1985. Acquired immunodeficiency syndrome among patients attending hemophilia treatment centers and mortality experience of hemophiliacs in the United States. Am. J. Epidemiol. 121:797-810.

Kalter, S. P., S. A. Riggs, F. Cabanillas, J. J. Butler, F. B. Hagemeister, P. W. Mansell, G. R. Newell, W. S. Velasquez, P. Salvador, B. Barlogie, A. Rios, and E. M. Hersh. 1985. Aggressive non-Hodgkin's lymphomas in immunocompromised homosexual males. Blood 66:655-659.

Kalyanaraman, V. S., M. G. Sarngadharan, M. Robert-Guroff, I. Miyoshi, D. Blayney, D. Golde, and R. C. Gallo. 1982. A new subtype of human T-cell leukemia virus (HTLV-II) associated with a T-cell variant of hairy cell leukemia. Science 218:571-573.

Kanki, P. J., J. Alroy, and M. Essex. 1985a. Isolation of a T-lymphotropic retrovirus related to HTLV-III/LAV from wild-caught African green monkeys. Science 230:951-954.

Kanki, P. J., R. Kurth, W. Becker, G. Dreesman, G. McLane, and M. Essex. 1985b. Antibodies to simian T-lymphotropic retrovirus type III in African green monkeys and recognition of STLV-III viral proteins by AIDS and related sera. Lancet I:1330-1332.

Kinsey, A. C., W. B. Pomeroy, and C. E. Martin. 1948. Sexual Behavior in the Human Male. Philadelphia: W. B. Saunders.

Klatzmann, D., F. Barre-Sinoussi, M. T. Nugeyre, C. Danquet, E. Vilmer, C. Griscelli, F. Brun-Veziret, C. Rouzroux, J. C. Gluckmann, J. C. Chermann, et al. 1984a. Selective tropism of lymphadenopathy associated virus (LAV) for helper-inducer T lymphocytes. Science 225:59-63.

Klatzmann, D., E. Champagne, S. Chamaret, J. Gruest, D. Guetard, T. Hercend, J. C. Gluckman, and L. Montagnier. 1984b. T-lymphocyte T4 molecule behaves as the receptor for human retrovirus LAV. Nature 312:767-768.

Kreiss, J. K., D. Koech, F. A. Plummer, K. K. Holmes, M. Lightfoote, P. Piot, A. R. Ronald, J. O. Ndinga-Achola, L. J. D'Costa, P. Roberts, E. N. Ngugi, and T. C. Quinn. 1986. AIDS virus infection in Nairobi prostitutes: Spread of the epidemic to east Africa. N. Engl. J. Med. 314:414-418.

Krupp, L. B., R. B. Lipton, M. L. Swerdlow, N. E. Leeds, and J. L. Levy. 1985. Progressive multifocal leukoencephalopathy: Clinical and radiographic features. Ann. Neurol. 17:344-349.

Lancet. 1984. Needlestick transmission of HTLV-III from a patient infected in Africa. Lancet II:1376-1377.

Letvin, N. L., M. D. Daniel, P. K. Sehgal, R. C. Desrosiers, R. D. Hunt, L. M. Waldron, J. J. MacKey, D. K. Schmidt, L. V. Chalifoux, and N. W. King. 1985. Induction of AIDS-like disease in macaque monkeys with T-cell tropic retrovirus STLV-III. Science 230:71-73.

Levy, J. A., A. D. Hoffman, S. M. Kramer, J. A. Landis, and J. M. Shimabukuro. 1984. Isolation of lymphocytopathic retroviruses from San Francisco patients with AIDS. Science 225:840-842.

Lifson, A. R., and M. F. Rogers. 1986. Vertical transmission of human immunodeficiency virus. Lancet II:337.

Lifson, A. R., K. G. Castro, J. P. Narkunas, A. Lekatsas, T. E. Ksell, and R. S. Fox. 1986. "No identified risk" cases of acquired immunodeficiency syndrome. P. 99 in Abstracts of the Second International Conference on AIDS, Paris, June 23-25, 1986.

Mann, J. M., H. Francis, T. C. Quinn, P. K. Asila, N. Bosenge, N. Nzilambi, K. Bila, M.

Tamfum, K. Ruti, P. Piot, J. McCormick, and J. W. Curran. 1986a. Surveillance for AIDS in a central African city: Kinshasa, Zaire. JAMA 255:3255-3259.

Mann, J. M., T. C. Quinn, H. Francis, N. Nzilambi, N. Bosenge, K. Bila, J. B. McCormick, K. Ruti, P. K. Asila, and J. W. Curran. 1986b. Prevalence of HTLV-III/LAV in household contacts of patients with confirmed AIDS and controls in Kinshasa, Zaire. JAMA 256:721-724.

Mann, J. M., H. Francis, T. C. Quinn, R. L. Colebunders, P. Piot, J. W. Curran, N. Nzilambi, N. Bosenge, M. Malonga, D. Kalunga, M. M. Nzingg, and N. Bagala. In press. HIV seroprevalence among hospital workers in Kinshasa, Zaire. JAMA.

Marion, R. W., A. A. Wiznia, G. Hutcheon, and A. Rubenstein. 1986. Human T-cell lymphotropic virus type III (HTLV-III/LAV) embryopathy. A new dysmorphic syndrome associated with intrauterine HTLV-III infection. Am. J. Dis. Child. 140:638-640.

Marmor, M., L. Laubenstein, D. C. William, A. E. Friedman-Kien, R. David Byrum, S. D'Onofrio, and N. Dubin. 1982. Risk factors for Kaposi's sarcoma in homosexual men. Lancet I:1083-1087.

Marmor, M., A. E. Friedman-Kien, S. Zolla-Pazner, R. E. Stahl, P. Rubinstein, L. Laubenstein, D. C. William, R. J. Klein, and I. Spigland. 1984. Kaposi's sarcoma in homosexual men: A seroepidemiologic case-control study. Ann. Intern. Med. 100:809-815.

McCray, E. 1986. Occupational risk of the acquired immunodeficiency syndrome among health care workers. N. Engl. J. Med. 314:1127-1132.

Melbye, M. 1986. The natural history of human T lymphotropic virus-III infection: The cause of AIDS. Br. Med. J. 292:5-12.

Melbye, M., R. Biggar, P. Ebbesen, C. Neuland, J. J. Goedert, V. Faber, I. Lorenzen, P. Skinhoj, R. C. Gallo, and W. A. Blattner. 1986. Long-term seropositivity for human T-lymphotropic virus type III in homosexual men without the acquired immunodeficiency syndrome: Development of immunological and clinical abnormalities. Ann. Intern. Med. 104:496-500.

Metroka, C. E., S. Cunningham-Rundles, M. S. Pollack, J. A. Sonnabend, J. M. Davis, B. Gordon, R. D. Fernandez, and J. Mouradian. 1983. Generalized lymphadenopathy in homosexual men. Ann. Intern. Med. 99:585-591.

Pape, J. W., B. Liautaud, F. Thomas, J. R. Mathurin, M. M. St. Amand, M. Boncy, V. Pean, M. Pamphile, A. C. Laroche, and W. D. Johnson, Jr. 1986. Risk factors associated with AIDS in Haiti. Am. J. Med. Sci. 29:4-7.

Parks, W. P., and G. B. Scott. 1986. An overview of pediatric AIDS: Approaches to diagnosis and outcome assessment. Background paper. Washington, D.C.: Committee on a National Strategy for AIDS.

Peterman, T. A., G. R. Lang, N. J. Mikos, S. L. Soloman, C. A. Schable, P. M. Feorino, J. A. Britz, and J. R. Allen. 1986. HTLV-III/LAV infection in hemodialysis units. JAMA 255:2324-2326.

Petito, C. K., B. A. Navia, E. S. Cho, B. D. Jordan, D. C. George, and R. W. Price. 1985. Vacuolar myelopathy pathologically resembling subacute combined degeneration in patients with the acquired immunodeficiency syndrome. N. Engl. J. Med. 312:874-879.

Piot, P., T. C. Quinn, H. Taelman, F. M. Feinsod, K. B. Minlangu, O. Wobin, N. Mbendi, P. Mazebo, K. Ndangi, W. Stevens, K. Kalambayi, S. Mitchell, C. Bridts, and J. B. McCormick. 1984. Acquired immunodeficiency syndrome in a heterosexual population in Zaire. Lancet II:65-69.

Poiesz, B. J., F. W. Ruscetti, A. F. Gazdar, P. A. Bunn, J. D. Minna, and R. C. Gallo. 1980. Detection and isolation of type C retrovirus particles from fresh and cultured lymphocytes of a patient with cutaneous T-cell lymphoma. Proc. Natl. Acad. Sci. USA 77:7415-7419.

Polk, B. F., R. Fox, R. Brookmeyer, and S. Kanchanaraksa. 1986. Case-control study of incident AIDS in a cohort of seropositive gay men. P. 103 in Abstracts of the Second International Conference on AIDS, Paris, June 23-25, 1986.

Popovic, M., M. G. Sarngadharan, E. Read, and R. C. Gallo. 1984. Detection, isolation, and continuous production of cytopathic retroviruses (HTLV-III) from patients with AIDS and pre-AIDS. Science 224:497-500.

Redfield, R. R., P. D. Markham, S. Z. Salahuddin, D. G. Wright, M. G. Sarngadharan, and R. C. Gallo. 1985. Heterosexually-acquired HTLV-III/LAV disease (AIDS-related complex and AIDS). Epidemiologic evidence for female to male transmission. JAMA 254: 2094-2096.

Redfield, R. R., D. C. Wright, P. D. Markham, S. Z. Salahuddin, R. C. Gallo, and D. S. Burke. 1986a. Frequent bidirectional heterosexual transmission of HTLV-III/LAV between spouses. P. 125 in Abstracts of the Second International Conference on AIDS, Paris, June 23-25, 1986.

Redfield, R. R., D. C. Wright, and E. C. Tramont. 1986b. The Walter Reed staging classification for HTLV-LAV infection. N. Engl. J. Med. 314:131-132.

Rutherford, G. W., D. F. Echenberg, P. M. O'Malley, W. W. Darrow, T. E. Wilson, and H. W. Jaffe. 1986. The natural history of LAV/HTLV-III infection and viraemia in homosexual and bisexual men: A 6-year follow-up study. P. 99 in Abstracts of the Second International Conference on AIDS, Paris, June 23-25, 1986.

Safai, B., M. G. Sarngadharan, J. E. Groopman, K. Arnett, M. Popovic, A. Sliski, J. Schupbach, and R. C. Gallo. 1984. Seroepidemiological studies of human T-lymphotropic retrovirus type III in acquired immunodeficiency syndrome. Lancet I:1438-1440.

Salahuddin, S. Z., P. D. Markham, R. R. Redfield, M. Essex, J. E. Groopman, M. G. Sarngadharan, M. F. McLane, A. Sliski, and R. C. Gallo. 1984. HTLV-III in symptom-free seronegative persons. Lancet II:1418-1420.

Salahuddin, S. Z., P. D. Markham, M. Popovic, M. C. Sarngadharan, S. Orndorff, A. Fladagar, A. Patel, J. Gold, and R. C. Gallo. 1985. Isolation of infectious human T-cell leukemia/lymphotropic virus type III (HTLV-III) from patients with acquired immunodeficiency syndrome (AIDS) or AIDS-related complex (ARC) and from healthy carriers: A study of risk groups and tissue sources. Proc. Natl. Acad. Sci. USA 82:5530-5534.

Saltzman, B. R., C. A. Harris, R. S. Klein, G. H. Fredland, P. A. Kahl, N. H. Steigbigel, et al. 1986. HTLV-III/LAV infection and immunodeficiency in heterosexual partners of AIDS patients. P. 125 in Abstracts of the Second International Conference on AIDS, Paris, June 23-25, 1986.

Sarngadharan, M. G., M. Popovic, L. Bruch, J. Schupback, and R. C. Gallo. 1984. Antibodies reactive with human T-lymphotropic retroviruses (HTLV-III) in the serum of patients with AIDS. Science 224:506-508.

Schoeppel, S. C., R. T. Hoppe, R. F. Dorfman, S. J. Horning, A. C. Collier, T. G. Chew, and L. M. Weiss. 1985. Hodgkin's disease in homosexual men with generalized lymphadenopathy. Ann. Intern. Med. 102:68-70.

Schorr, J. B., A. Berkowitz, P. D. Cummings, A. S. Katz, and S. G. Sandler. 1985. Prevalence of HTLV-III antibody in American blood donors. N. Engl. J. Med. 313:384-385.

Scott, G. B., M. A. Fischl, N. Klimas, M. A. Fletcher, G. M. Dickinson, R. S. Levine, and W. P. Parks. 1985. Mothers of infants with acquired immunodeficiency syndrome. Evidence for both symptomatic and asymptomatic carriers. JAMA 253:363-366.

Sodroski, J., W. C. Goh, C. Rosen, K. Campbell, and W. A. Haseltine. 1986. Role of HTLV-III/LAV envelope in syncytium formation and cytopathicity. Nature 322:470-474.

Sonigo, P., M. Alizon, K. Staskus, D. Klatzman, S. Cole, D. Danos, E. Retzel, P. Tiollais, A. Haase, and S. Wain-Hobson. 1985. Nucleotide sequence of the visna lentivirus: Relationship to the AIDS virus. Cell 42:369-382.

Sprecher, S., G. Soumenkoff, F. Puissant, and M. Degueldre. 1986. Vertical transmission of HIV in 15-week fetus. Lancet II:288-289.

Stewart, G. J., J. P. P. Tyler, A. L. Cunningham, J. A. Barr, G. L. Driscoll, J. Gold, and B. J. Lamont. 1985. Transmission of HTLV-III virus by artificial insemination by donor. Lancet II:581-583.

Stricof, R. L., and D. L. Morse. 1986. HTLV-III/LAV seroconversion following a deep intramuscular needlestick injury. N. Engl. J. Med. 314:1115.

Teich, N. 1984. Taxonomy of retroviruses. Pp. 25-207 in RNA Tumor Viruses: Molecular Biology of Tumor Viruses, 2nd ed., R. Weiss, N. Teich, H. Varmus, and J. Coffin, eds. Cold Spring Harbor, N.Y.: Cold Spring Harbor Laboratory.

Temin, H. M. 1986. Mechanisms of cell killing cytopathic effects by retroviruses. Background paper. Washington, D.C.: Committee on a National Strategy for AIDS.

U.S. Department of Justice. 1983. Prisoners and Drugs: BJS Bulletin. No. NCJ-875-75. Washington, D.C.: U.S. Government Printing Office.

Van de Perre, P., D. Rouvroy, P. Lepage, J. Bogaerts, P. Kestelyn, J. Kayihigi, A. C. Hekker, J. Butzler, and N. Clumeck. 1984. Acquired immunodeficiency syndrome in Rwanda. Lancet II:62-65.

Vandepitte, J., R. Verwilghen, and P. Zachee. 1983. AIDS and cryptococcosis (Zaire, 1977). Lancet I:925-926.

Varmus, H., and R. Swanstrom. 1984. Replication of retroviruses. Pp. 369-512 in RNA Tumor Viruses: Molecular Biology of Tumor Viruses, 2nd ed., R. Weiss, N. Teich, H. Varmus, and J. Coffin, eds. Cold Spring Harbor, N.Y.: Cold Spring Harbor Laboratory.

Weissman, I. 1986. Approaches to understanding the pathogenic mechanisms in AIDS. Background paper. Washington, D.C.: Committee on a National Strategy for AIDS.

Winkelstein, W., J. A. Wiley, N. Padian, and J. Levy. 1986. Potential for transmission of AIDS-associated retrovirus from bisexual men in San Francisco to their female sexual contacts. JAMA 255:901.

Ziegler, J. B., D. A. Cooper, R. O. Johnson, and J. Gold. 1985. Postnatal transmission of AIDS-associated retrovirus from mother to infant. Lancet I:896-897.

3

The Future Course of the Epidemic and Available National Resources

Short- and long-term estimates of the magnitude, pattern, and trends of AIDS and other HIV-related conditions are crucial to health care planning efforts and to the design of prevention and treatment strategies. One of the major problems in planning these efforts has been that, because AIDS is a relatively new disease and HIV is an unusual virus, there is little previous experience on which to base predictions about the epidemic's behavior. This chapter describes what can be projected on the basis of present knowledge and the resources that can be brought to bear on current and anticipated problems. (Chapter 5 discusses the implications of current projections for the provision and financing of health care and psychosocial support for those with HIV-related conditions. Chapter 6 identifies epidemiologic and other areas of research that must be pursued so that better predictions can be made.)

PROJECTIONS BY THE PUBLIC HEALTH SERVICE

Following a June 1986 planning conference at Coolfont, Berkeley Springs, West Virginia, the Public Health Service (PHS) issued updated projections of the incidence and prevalence of AIDS by 1991 (see Appendix G). Following is a summary of the major projections made by the PHS:

• There are 1 million to 1.5 million Americans currently infected with HIV. Of these, 20 to 30 percent are expected to develop AIDS by 1991.

85

• By the end of 1991 there will have been a cumulative total of more than 270,000 cases of AIDS in the United States, with more than 74,000 of those occurring in 1991 alone.

• By the end of 1991 there will have been a cumulative total of more than 179,000 deaths from AIDS in the United States, with 54,000 of those occurring in 1991 alone.

• Because the typical time between infection with HIV and the development of clinical AIDS is four or more years, most of the persons who will develop AIDS between now and 1991 already are infected.

• The vast majority of AIDS cases will continue to come from the currently recognized high-risk groups.

• New AIDS cases in men and women acquired through heterosexual contact will increase from 1,100 in 1986 to almost 7,000 in 1991. This figure includes those heterosexuals reporting contact with people known to be infected or with people in known high-risk groups and heterosexuals who are presumed to have acquired the disease from contact with individuals not known to be in such groups.

• Pediatric AIDS cases will increase almost 10-fold in the next five years, to more than 3,000 cumulative cases by the end of 1991.

PROBLEMS IN MAKING PROJECTIONS

There are substantial uncertainties about such factors as the prevalence of HIV infection, the rate of transmission of the virus among various population groups, and the risks of disease among those infected. Accordingly, any projection of the future incidence and prevalence of AIDS (whether by the PHS or by others) will be subject to considerable uncertainty.

Nevertheless, empirical projections of the incidence, prevalence, and cost of AIDS, however crude or uncertain, are essential for planning a response to the epidemic. The critical issue is to identify the value and limitations of such projections and their policy implications so that improved projections of the burden of disease can be developed. Also, by assessing the limits of such models, the data that need to be collected can be identified.

The PHS estimates of the incidence of AIDS were derived from an empirical model based on a statistical trend analysis of AIDS cases reported to the CDC through May 1986 (Morgan and Curran, 1986). A very similar statistical model was used in earlier projections based on reported cases through mid-1985 (Curran et al., 1985; W. M. Morgan, Centers for Disease Control, personal communication, 1986). Such models depend on the assumption that observed trends in a disease, such as the distribution of cases by age, sex, geographic location, and risk group, will not change with time. They are adequate for reasonable short-term projections but are of far more limited use for long-term projections (e.g., more than five years).

Obviously, more complex models that incorporate known information on the sizes of populations at risk, viral transmission and infectivity, and the natural history of HIV infection and its associated diseases would be expected to yield more accurate, and thus more valuable, predictions. However, the data in those areas necessary to construct such models were considered by the committee's Epidemiology Working Group to be limited in the following ways:

1. There are no survey data that can be considered to accurately represent the general population. Surveys to date include those of blood donors seen at blood banks after voluntary deferral of donation by high-risk individuals was requested; applicants for military service, who are a disproportionately young, minority, and economically disadvantaged population; and members of high-risk groups. These groups are almost certainly not representative of the general population, and how to analyze data obtained from them to deduce what is happening in the general population is not known.

2. In high-risk groups (for example, homosexual men) there is wide variation among communities in the prevalence of disease and sero-positivity, based on location, age, and possibly frequency of high-risk behaviors (such as anal intercourse). This makes difficult the estimation of national prevalence in high-risk groups, or even estimates of the likely spread within these groups.

3. There are major differences as to the time when the virus was introduced into communities in various parts of the country, even among the same high-risk groups. Given the long and uncertain time lag between HIV infection and symptoms of that infection, this variation makes extrapolation from the number of AIDS cases meeting the CDC definition to the likely number of infected persons at a given time nationwide very tenuous.

4. The natural history of the disease is not yet fully defined. The proportion of infected persons who will develop AIDS or ARC is not yet known, nor is the time frame for the occurrence of these conditions. Thus, estimates useful in health care planning, such as hospital days required for treatment or days of work lost, are very difficult to derive.

Empirical models do not have to take into account these poorly understood factors to enable projections of the epidemic's future. However, they suffer from their own set of uncertainties. Though case reports to the CDC constitute the most reliable source of analysis of AIDS trends, such data have important limitations. First, the CDC criteria (Appendix

E) are undoubtedly too restrictive to include all serious manifestations of HIV infection. If the mix of manifestations of HIV infection changes over time, the predictions from empirical models will be inaccurate.

Second, cases of AIDS that meet the CDC criteria may be underreported, although the extent of underreporting is not known reliably. As long as underreporting rates have not varied over time, empirical analysis of time trends in reported AIDS cases would remain unbiased. However, increasing awareness of the main modes of acquiring AIDS and its decreasing novelty make it plausible that underreporting has increased as the disease has become more common, a phenomenon that has occurred with other diseases. If so, purely empirical models of AIDS trends will show a spurious deceleration of the epidemic.

Third, there are delays in reporting cases to the CDC. Accordingly, the time series of cumulatively reported cases understates the actual number diagnosed, especially for more recent months. In an empirical analysis of trends in the incidence of AIDS, the observed data on diagnosed cases need to be corrected for reporting lags. Because such corrections will mostly affect recent data, apparently minor changes in the correction method can significantly affect distant projections from time trend models. The method that CDC uses to correct for such delays assumes that the distribution of delays between the diagnosis and the report of the case to the CDC remains constant over time (Curran et al., 1985). Such an assumption needs careful and regular scrutiny.

Fourth, statistical confidence intervals (see Appendix G) surrounding future projections from empirical models are mathematically and biologically problematic because there is little basis for estimating the distribution of errors.

Fifth, projections of the prevalence of AIDS are based not only on projections of the incidence of AIDS but on estimates of the life expectancy of future AIDS victims. If changes in the natural history of the epidemic or improvements in medical care result in prolongation of life for AIDS patients, the prevalence of the disease would rise even faster than the incidence. The prevalence of disease is an indicator of the number of AIDS patients that will be alive and in need of health care.

Cases of AIDS that are diagnosed in the near future will reflect the consequences of past infection. Therefore, despite the uncertainties discussed above, the PHS projections (and those of other purely empirical models) are likely to be highly accurate in the short term. Consequently, despite the fact that current projection methods are crude, it is reasonable to assume that the rising incidence of AIDS will not soon reverse itself. Disease and death resulting from HIV infection are likely to be increasing 5 to 10 years from now and probably into the next century.

The committee believes that the PHS estimates are reasonable at this time and supports their use for planning purposes. However, its acceptance of these projections does not imply that they are precise, nor does it obviate the need to continue to acquire data that will permit the construction of more sophisticated models.

THE EPIDEMIC WITHIN AND BEYOND HIGH-RISK GROUPS

The populations at highest risk for HIV infection in the near future will continue to be homosexual men and IV drug users, but no accurate data exist on the size of these groups. It is also not known with what frequency homosexual men practice the behaviors (primarily receptive anal intercourse) that put them at high risk of HIV infection. Thus, the distribution of risk within the total group of men at risk because of homosexual activity is not known, nor can the likely rate of spread be calculated.

Estimates of the overall percentage of the male homosexual population infected with HIV must take into account the definition of the population under consideration. Lower estimates of the prevalence of seropositivity are usually associated with larger estimates of the total homosexual population (encompassing individuals who presumably have had fewer homosexual encounters). Given this consideration, the committee's Epidemiology Working Group estimated that seropositivity among male homosexuals ranges from over 50 percent in some areas for men who have had a large number of partners to under 20 percent for a population including any individual who has participated in homosexual activity.

By far the largest number of persons now seropositive in the United States presumably acquired their infection through homosexual activity. However, as discussed in Chapter 4, there is evidence that the spread of HIV through homosexual activity has slowed. The trend is attributed to behavioral change in response to the AIDS epidemic, but it may also be that many persons in the highest-risk subgroup (those with the most partners) have already been infected. HIV infection will probably continue to spread in homosexual males, although possibly at a slower rate because of the use by some of "safer sex" practices (e.g., avoidance of intercourse with infected persons, increased use of condoms, and avoidance of anal intercourse).

The numbers infected and at risk among IV drug users are even more difficult to estimate. The total number of IV drug users in the United States is not known, and persons move in and out of the group rather frequently. Although evidence indicates that there has been some modification of behavior in response to the AIDS epidemic, behavioral modification is much less pervasive in this high-risk group than among male homosexuals (see Chapter 4). In locales such as New York City where needles and syringes are extensively shared, many IV drug users may have already been exposed, but this may not be true for other urban centers. Continuing spread of HIV in IV drug users throughout the United States is expected in the future.

There is a broad spectrum of opinion about the extent of the likely spread in the United States of HIV infection in the heterosexual population, but there is strong agreement that the present surveillance systems have only limited capacity to detect such spread. Because of the much larger size of this population as compared with the recognized high-risk groups, there is potential for wide-ranging estimates. Opinions provided to the committee by members of the Epidemiology Working Group ranged from the estimate of HIV infection as a minor problem among heterosexuals to an estimate that perhaps millions of heterosexuals who have multiple sex partners or who patronize prostitutes will ultimately be affected.

In central Africa, bidirectional heterosexual transmission is believed to be the dominant mode of transmission (Mann, 1986). Interpretations of the data from Africa are complicated, however, by large numbers of sexual partners and by frequent prostitute contact among heterosexual African AIDS patients and by reports of repeated use of unsterile needles and syringes in many medical care settings.

Whatever the efficiency of heterosexual transmission, it is clear that the infection will continue to be amplified among populations in countries or regions with a high prevalence of infection by frequent transfusion of blood (unless screening of the blood supply begins), by the vertical transmission of infection to mother and child, and by the continued medical use of unsterile needles. Thus, the disease will continue to increase dramatically in those areas.

In the United States, where such amplification will generally not be present, it is presumed that heterosexual spread will be slower. However, IV drug use in some communities or groups may amplify sexual transmission. Much of the male-to-female spread of HIV infection in the United States has been associated with IV drug use and has been confounded by the possibility that the women are also IV drug users. The relatively high seropositivity in some prostitute groups has also been attributed to IV drug use. A small amount of data is beginning to appear on the proportion of male homosexuals who also have heterosexual contact. The figure may be as high as 10 to 20 percent, and these individuals represent a large reservoir for potential infection of women and their offspring and for further heterosexual spread of infection. In this regard, it should be noted that the PHS projections of the future number of heterosexually acquired cases are based on the observations of the heterosexual spread that has occurred thus far in the epidemic—predominantly heterosexual transmission from individuals who became infected through IV drug use or homosexual activity (as in the case of bisexuals).

It is not known how the infection will behave when spread in that segment of the heterosexual population which has no other risk factors (Winkelstein et al., 1986).

Overall, the committee concludes that over the next 5 to 10 years there will be substantially more HIV infections in the heterosexual population and that these cases will occur predominantly in those subgroups of the population at risk for other sexually transmitted diseases. These cases are expected initially to occur mainly in the geographic areas and among the demographic groups that already have a high frequency of AIDS or IV drug abuse. In addition, increased HIV infection in infants is expected as more women in their childbearing years become infected, but this may be moderated by screening, as discussed in Chapter 4. (See Chapter 6 for recommendations of studies that would track the course of the epidemic through heterosexual contact and permit interventions to be appropriately targeted.)

THE PROPORTION OF SEROPOSITIVE INDIVIDUALS WHO WILL DEVELOP AIDS

Opinions in the Epidemiology Working Group varied widely regarding the proportion of seropositive persons who will eventually die of HIV-related causes. At this time, there are only five years of observations on which to base such predictions. The data now available show that the proportion of a cohort of seropositive individuals that have progressed to AIDS is still rising five years after infection. Furthermore, once infected, a person may well remain at risk of clinical disease for life. With some of the less common clinical manifestations, particularly those that are neurologic, there may be a very long delay after infection.

The estimate provided to the committee by the Epidemiology Working Group was that 25 to 50 percent of seropositive persons will develop AIDS as defined by the CDC within 5 to 10 years of seroconversion, and that a higher percentage cannot be ruled out on the basis of present studies. This estimate is consistent with but goes beyond that of the PHS, which projected that 20 to 30 percent of currently seropositive individuals will be diagnosed with AIDS within 5 years (Appendix G). In addition, there is an increasing number of reports of manifestations of HIV infection that fall outside the CDC definition of AIDS, which therefore modify projections upward.

LONG-TERM PROSPECTS

HIV infection is likely to continue to spread among those individuals who engage in behavior known to transmit the virus. HIV infection behaves somewhat like hepatitis B, but a number of factors make it difficult to predict whether it will reach or exceed the prevalence of that disease. These factors include the asymptomatic period after HIV infection, which facilitates "silent" spread of the virus, the presumed lifelong infectivity of all infected individuals, the lack of data on the efficiency of transmission, and the difficulty of predicting changes in behavior and transmission that education may generate. There is also insufficient knowledge at this time to predict how the virus will evolve in its apparently new (human) host. Therefore, it is impossible, whether by model or by analogy, to predict the long-term course of the epidemic with any degree of certainty.

It is clear, however, that reducing transmission is a difficult proposition. Because no vaccine is likely to become available in the near future (see Chapter 6) and because of the seriousness of the disease, the only prudent course of action is an immediate, major effort to stop the further spread of infection through public health measures, particularly education. Any delay will bequeath to future policymakers a problem of potentially catastrophic proportions and will condemn many thousands of individuals to infection and disease.

NATIONAL RESOURCES FOR DEALING WITH AIDS AND HIV

There are many organizations, groups, and individuals that could be drawn upon to address aspects of the public health measures (Chapter 4), health care (Chapter 5), or research (Chapter 6) related to AIDS and HIV infection. Additionally, the epidemic has prompted the development of new groups to address certain problems and the extension of existing groups into new areas. This is particularly true of male homosexuals, who have developed community support groups. Former drug users have also conducted educational efforts. There are many resources spread across both the public and private sectors; thus, many of the needed actions can and perhaps should be undertaken by groups at both levels.

A complete inventory of the national resources available for dealing with AIDS and HIV infection would include information on existing and potential activities or areas of concern (e.g., research, health care, education), on the nature of each resource (e.g., pharmaceutical company, community group), and on the level of activities (e.g., national, state, local, risk group). Appendix D lists various groups and organizations that are already active or that could be enlisted to work against AIDS and HIV infection.

Impediments to Involvement

Many of the groups and organizations listed in Appendix D have already been engaged in problems related to AIDS and HIV infection that are appropriate to their capabilities, often with considerable success. But, in the judgment of the committee, other important resources in both the public and private sector have not yet become appropriately engaged or have addressed relevant problems inadequately.

The reasons for noninvolvement vary, but they include the following:

- lack of awareness about the magnitude of the problem and the needs
- slowness in responding to obvious needs
- apparent reluctance or inability to pursue particular programs because of political, ideological, moral, or religious considerations, including the social stigma associated with some of the risk groups
- lack of appropriate recruitment efforts
- lack of funds or other resources (e.g., facilities) for pursuing promising opportunities
- lack of appropriate inducements to enter the field (e.g., stability of funding)
- perceptions regarding the availability of reagents or other resources necessary for productive research
- specific commercial disincentives (e.g., liability for vaccine-related injuries, uncertainty over market size and public health policy)
- insufficient development of the basic research data base upon which further commercial development might proceed
- uncertainty with regard to federal agency responsibilities

Some of these impediments may be removed by relatively simple actions recommended in other parts of this report. Others are more complex and may require new mechanisms or more time to be reduced.

Mechanisms for Coordinating Activities

Mechanisms exist for coordinating certain facets of the overall approach to AIDS and other HIV-related problems. Within the executive branch, the Public Health Service has developed a plan to guide its constituent agencies (Appendix G). The committee concurs in general terms with the overall goals and approaches outlined in this plan. However, the plan focuses on only part of the federal government's activities and potential. Though the Public Health Service is a significant resource, it represents only a portion of the national capacity to address the problems caused by HIV infection. Other groups, such as the military and the Department of Education, are also well situated to conduct certain types of epidemiologic or clinical research.

No individual in the Public Health Service currently has primary responsibility for identifying priorities in implementing the PHS plan, but a Public Health Service AIDS Task Force has been established and a coordinator appointed. Certain activities will require contributions from various federal agencies outside the PHS, such as the Department of Defense and the Department of Education. Furthermore, many activities outlined in the plan might be better conducted with broad participation of nonfederal groups. No formal mechanisms exist for ensuring efficient collaboration in these areas.

Certain task forces under the AIDS coordinator of the Public Health Service have responsibility for monitoring efforts conducted by the PHS agencies with their purview. The committee believes that while these task forces may promote communication within and between federal agencies, they sometimes have not sufficiently engaged or informed other relevant national resources and have not identified priorities and devised or articulated the strategic plans necessary to attain the desired goals in the shortest possible time.

In many areas, there are no mechanisms for ensuring concerted action against AIDS and HIV infection, especially where activities involve diverse public and private sector bodies. Five important areas where this is the case are (1) vaccine and drug development, (2) epidemiologic and natural history studies in the United States and abroad, (3) evaluation of models for the appropriate care of HIV-associated conditions, (4) the financing of that care, and (5) the U.S. contribution to international efforts. Each of these subjects is considered in detail in the chapters that follow.

There is a need to mobilize all existing resources through more effective interaction between the public and private sectors. To meet this need, and also to inform the American public, Congress, and the executive branch, the committee proposes the establishment of a National Commission on AIDS. Such a body should be advisory to existing administrative entities. (For fuller discussion of this recommendation, see Chapter 1.)

REFERENCES

Curran, J. W., W. M. Morgan, A. M. Hardy, H. W. Jaffe, W. W. Darrow, and W. R. Dowdle. 1985. The epidemiology of AIDS: Current status and future prospects. Science 229:1352-1357.

Mann, J. M. 1986. The epidemiology of LAV/HTLV-III in Africa. P. 101 in Abstracts of the Second International Conference on AIDS, Paris, June 23-25, 1986.

Morgan, W. M., and J. W. Curran. 1986. Acquired immunodeficiency syndrome: Current and future trends. Pub. Health Rep. 101:459-465.

Winkelstein, W., J. A. Wiley, N. Padian, and J. Levy. 1986. Potential for transmission of AIDS-associated retrovirus from bisexual men in San Francisco to their female sexual contacts. JAMA 255:901.

4

Opportunities for Altering the Course of the Epidemic

Because of the lag time—up to four years or longer—in the development of AIDS after HIV infection, approximately 50 percent of the AIDS cases diagnosed in 1991 will be in persons who are infected now but do not yet have AIDS (Morgan, 1986). Thus, about half of the AIDS cases diagnosed in 1991—and a growing proportion after that—can potentially be prevented. It is in this course of action that the greatest opportunities for altering the course of the epidemic lie.

As discussed in Chapter 6, the committee believes that a vaccine against HIV infection is not likely to be available for at least five years and probably longer. Drugs are now being tested in the hope that one can be found to safely arrest the progress of HIV infection. Whether that search will be totally successful is highly uncertain. Thus, neither potential vaccines nor drug therapies offer much hope in the near future for altering the course of the epidemic.

It is necessary in this situation to maximize the use of available means of controlling the epidemic. In a few short years a remarkable amount has been learned about HIV and how it is transmitted. This solid evidence provides the basis for reasonable decisions about actions that must be taken to mitigate the devastating impact of HIV infection.

The challenge to those entrusted with fashioning policies to protect the public health in this regard is massive (Jonsen et al., 1986; Levine and Bermel, 1985). There is no agent currently available to treat the underlying disease process, no one has been known to recover from AIDS, and those exposed to the virus must be presumed to be chronically infectious.

Furthermore, the main groups at risk are subject to social stigma and private discrimination, which complicates the picture for health officials seeking to identify those who are or may become infected and thus capable of transmitting the virus.

Traditional public health responses to infectious diseases have included identifying those who harbor the infection. Among the methods used to accomplish this are testing or screening, reporting cases and compiling registries of those who are infectious, and isolating, when necessary, the persons capable of transmitting infection. Such programs may rely either on the voluntary compliance of those at risk or on compulsory measures. Because compulsory measures compromise liberty, autonomy, and privacy (especially when such fundamental behavior as sexual activity is at issue), they must be carefully considered in light of the potential public health benefit. Many such programs have historically been shown to be invidious, ineffective, or discriminatory (Brandt, 1985). This chapter describes the opportunities available for protecting individuals from HIV infection in a society that values privacy and civil liberties.

PUBLIC EDUCATION

For at least the next several years, the most effective measures for significantly reducing the spread of HIV infection are education of the public and voluntary changes in behavior. There are many social ills for which public education is prescribed as a cure, especially where there are few specific responses available. Education can sometimes be a soft substitute for hard action. In contrast, public education about HIV infection is, and will continue to be, a critical public health measure, even if a vaccine or drug becomes available. Education in this instance is not only the transfer of knowledge but has the added dimension of inducing, persuading, and otherwise motivating people to avoid the transmission of HIV. While it would be unrealistic to believe or claim that the spread of HIV infection is likely to be stopped by educational efforts to induce behavioral change, the efforts can be entered into with a strong degree of conviction and hope. Carefully monitored preventive interventions for other health problems (e.g., to reduce smoking or heart disease or to improve diet) show that these can be effective when pursued intensively (Farquhar et al., 1984). The incentive to avoid risk of infection with HIV should also be strong given the higher probability of adverse outcome (if infected) and the closer temporal connection between the behavior and the threat to health. Hence, education to prevent HIV infection can be strongly expected to bear results. In addition, by accompanying it with behavioral research directed at improving the knowledge of how to induce more effectively the desired behavioral changes, its effect can be heightened.

The present level of AIDS-related education is woefully inadequate. It must be vastly expanded and diversified, targeted not only at the general public but at specific subgroups, such as those in which significant transmission can be anticipated, those in a position to influence public opinion, and those who interact with infected individuals.

What Should Be the Content of Public Education?

The epidemiology of AIDS clearly demonstrates that unprotected sexual intercourse (receptive anal or vaginal intercourse), the use of shared needles and syringes, and the transfusion of blood products contaminated by HIV represent the greatest danger of transmission of the virus. Discussion of alternative sexual and other behaviors that provide a measure of protection against transmission must be conveyed to those targeted for AIDS education (Darrow and Pauli, 1984).

If behavior modification is the goal of education about AIDS, the content of the material presented must address the behavior in question in as direct a manner as possible. Educators must be prepared to specify that certain sexual practices are activities in which there is a very high risk of HIV transmission. Admonitions that one must avoid "intimate bodily contact" and the "exchange of bodily fluids" while simultaneously averring the safety of "casual contact" convey at best only a vague message. For instance, they may be understood as implying that one must avoid all sexual activities, a program that few will be willing to follow. People also need reassurance that certain sexual practices involve little or no risk of infection.

There has been considerable debate among health professionals, public health officials, and homosexuals about what exactly constitutes "safe sex" and how best to convey information about the relative risk of various behaviors (Handsfield, 1985). Many have argued that it is more accurate to speak in terms of "safer sex," because the unknowns are still such that it would be irresponsible to certify any particular activity as absolutely safe. Much of this argument will be moot as a more sophisticated understanding of modes of transmission is gained from research and studies under way in this country and abroad.

Condoms have been shown under laboratory conditions to inhibit the transmission of HIV, as has been demonstrated with at least two other viruses of approximately similar size: cytomegalovirus and herpes simplex virus type 2 (Conant et al., 1986). More needs to be known, however, about the practical efficacy of condoms in blocking sexually transmitted diseases spread by anal intercourse. Is anal intercourse more likely to break or tear condoms? Does the type of lubricant affect the integrity of the membrane? Are certain materials more effective than others?

Prudishness about the use and promotion of condoms has inhibited their use. They need to be widely available in establishments that have the potential to foster sexual liaisons, such as bathhouses and singles bars. They should also be readily accessible in less sexually oriented establishments, both to maximize their availability and to minimize the stigma associated with their use. Sexually active youth (both homosexual and heterosexual, male and female), being less likely to have been infected with HIV, have the most protection to gain from the use of condoms.

Increased condom use has been demonstrated following explicit, focused educational campaigns in the past (Darrow, 1974). More needs to be done (Goldstein, 1986). Programs designed to encourage the use of condoms must take account of different motivational forces underlying their use as contraception versus their use in preventing sexually transmitted diseases. Campaigns to encourage use of condoms must also overcome people's belief that they diminish sexual pleasure—or at least make them aware of the benefits in such a trade-off. The increased availability of condoms probably will raise concerns about encouraging sexual activity by young people who are not sufficiently mature. Such concerns, while understandable, are overshadowed by the dire consequences of HIV infection.

An integral aspect of an education campaign must also be the wide dissemination of clear information about behaviors that do not transmit the virus. The public must be assured that ordinary standards of personal hygiene that currently prevail are more than adequate for preventing transmission of AIDS even between persons living within a single household; transmission will not occur as long as one avoids the relatively short list of dangerous sexual and drug-use practices that have been identified. Unreasonable alarm about so-called casual contact with individuals perceived as possibly infected with HIV has produced many needless instances of discrimination and distress in the workplace and elsewhere (Bayer and Oppenheimer, 1986). There remain persons so misinformed about the relationship between blood transfusion and AIDS that they are afraid to be blood donors, much less blood recipients. Polls have shown that as much as one-third of the general population believes that AIDS can be acquired through blood donation (Engel, 1986).

The currently available evidence indicates that there is considerable ignorance of the ways in which AIDS is transmitted. Surveys document substantial fractions of American adults who believe incorrectly that AIDS can be transmitted by such means as a sneeze or by sharing a drinking glass (Eckholm, 1985b). Public education programs must aim at reducing this ignorance both in the general population and in the groups that will be particular targets of public education—those at highest risk of contracting or transmitting the infection. In this regard, the committee is concerned about the Centers for Disease Control directive that empanels local review boards to determine whether materials developed for AIDS education are too explicit and in violation of local community standards—this is the so-called "dirty words" issue (*Medical World News,* 1985). The result of such a process could be to cut off frank, explicit information from areas where it is needed the most—in regions outside those urban centers that have large concentrations of homosexual men and IV drug users where awareness of the specifics of HIV transmission is already high.

The information media's coverage of AIDS has been extensive, and it has been not always easy to distinguish between urgency and alarm. Public officials have taken steps to allay unreasonable fears—for example, Margaret M. Heckler, then Secretary of the U.S. Department of Health and Human Services, was publicized shaking hands with an AIDS sufferer and donating blood. Yet such constructive efforts are undermined by media exaggeration.

Writers and editors torn between the dictates of accurate reporting and standards of good taste in family newspapers, magazines, and on television have described modes of transmission euphemistically. Although occasional stories in major newspapers discussed the relative risks of receptive anal intercourse in so many words early in 1983 (when information about transmission began to emerge from epidemiologic research), most accounts spoke in terms of "sexual" or "intimate" contact more generally.

The picture is changing, even in family newspapers. A review of media coverage of AIDS noted this evolution, as reflected in the following quotations from unsigned editorials in the *New York Times* (Diamond and Bellitto, 1986).

- "[The AIDS virus is transmitted] through the exchange of body fluids, as in sexual contact" (August 21, 1985).
- "AIDS is transmitted . . . by drug abusers sharing unclean needles or by homosexual relations" (September 3, 1985).
- "AIDS is spread in two main ways, anal intercourse and the sharing of unclean needles by drug addicts" (September 15, 1985). [Vaginal intercourse now needs to be added to these routes of transmission.]

AIDS sufferers can obtain much information about the prospects for new treatments from the lay press alone. Yet the media have sometimes provided a distorted view of hopes for success. This tendency unfortunately is abetted by the inclination of some scientists to herald results of clinical trials prematurely, sometimes in forums outside the mechanism of peer-reviewed journals (Check, 1985).

For those already diagnosed with an HIV-related condition, information should be available regarding the kinds of treatment and volunteer services available. AIDS sufferers have been desperate for information about the testing of new drugs. Equitable access to drugs being tested in clinical trials will depend in part upon HIV-infected individuals being aware of such endeavors.

What Are the Aims of Public Education?

Because HIV infection is transmitted by means of only a few specific types of behavior, a prime goal of education about AIDS is to modify or eliminate such behavior. Means must be found to overcome the major obstacles to achieving this goal. In matters of sexual behavior, such obstacles include poorly understood individual attitudes and preferences that may have arisen early in life and become relatively firmly fixed.

In dealing with IV drug users, the obstacles to educational success include both the attitudes of users and the laws that affect their conduct. It must be made clear that, short of abandoning the behavior entirely, the use of personal and sterile injection equipment is the only way to avoid participating in the chain of transmission of the virus. The sharing of injection equipment appears to be a ritual among many drug users, perhaps begun because of a lack of ready access to sterile equipment or because of laws proscribing sale and possession of equipment. Research is needed to identify the educational techniques that will be most effective in convincing users of the danger of needle sharing. Also needed are ways to impress women users that infection can be transmitted by them to their fetuses with disastrous results.

Another goal of educational activities should be to replace the atmosphere of hysteria and irrational fear that is found in some quarters with rational information that will engender a level-headed attitude about the disease and one's own risk of becoming infected with the virus. Since many diverse groups must be educated, an early activity in this campaign must be the training of trainers. A network of individuals who are firmly grounded in the facts of the disease and who are adept at transmitting those facts in diverse settings should be established.

Who Needs Education?

The most obvious targets for a campaign of education about AIDS are the presently identified high-risk groups: homosexual men, IV drug users, prostitutes, and sexual partners of those in high-risk groups. Some efforts have already been made in this direction, but in general the only efforts with any claim to success have been those conducted by homosexuals through voluntary activist organizations. Many of these efforts have been funded by local homosexual groups themselves. Homosexual men in high-incidence areas such as San Francisco and New York report a decrease both in the numbers of sexual partners and in risky sexual practices. These self-reported behavioral changes are consistent with the lower incidence of rectal gonorrhea reported in these areas (McKusick et al., 1985).

Although homosexuals, especially in urban areas, are frequently portrayed as highly organized and easily reached, it would be a mistake to assume that all men who engage in homosexual activities that may put them at risk perceive themselves as belonging to the homosexual community, read the homosexual press, or listen to homosexual leaders. It is important to communicate broadly the message that specific sexual practices involving infected persons are dangerous, not that homosexual men are at risk.

Beyond the segments of the population that are at high risk of infection, many other groups must receive education about AIDS. Heterosexuals, particularly those who have multiple partners, must be made aware of the risk to them. Health care professionals must acquire and constantly update their store of information to be helpful to their clients (not only those suffering from clinical consequences of the infection but also the "worried well," both infected and uninfected) and to others with whom they are in a position to communicate. Public officials, opinion makers, and the press represent other groups to which extensive education about AIDS must be targeted. Their influence on matters of public policy is of prime importance, and misinformation among these groups can counteract the beneficial effects of many other educational efforts.

The youth of the nation, emerging into the sphere of sexual activity and becoming potential customers in the illicit drug trade, must be alerted to the existence of the disease and to its mode of transmission. Surveys of high school students reveal an alarming degree of misinformation about AIDS. Even many students living in San Francisco, an AIDS epicenter, were seriously misinformed as late as 1986. In a survey of 1,300 high school students, 40 percent did not know that AIDS is caused by a virus. One-third believed that a person could contract the disease by merely "touching someone who has AIDS" or by "using a person's comb." Four in 10 students did not know that the use of a condom during sexual intercourse decreases the risk of transmitting HIV infection.

The need for educating the nation's youth about sexually transmitted diseases is well known. For example, in 1980, prior to recognition of AIDS, the U.S. Public Health Service (1980) published a document entitled *Promoting Health/Preventing Disease: Objectives for the Nation*, which included a set of goals for the decade ahead. Among them was one with relevance for the AIDS educational effort: "By 1990, every junior and senior high school student in the U.S. should receive accurate, timely education about sexually transmitted disease."

Sex education in the schools still must overcome considerable political opposition and bureaucratic intransigence. Nevertheless, at least nine states have passed statutes that permit or even mandate education on sexually transmitted diseases in the public schools. There are some exceptions to the general unwillingness to broach issues of sex, even homosexuality. The Oregon legislature established a special Venereal Disease Education Teachers' Scholarship Fund. Ohio's Department of Health has piloted an information package on AIDS for use in schools (Intergovernmental Health Policy Project, 1985). Public schools in New York City have integrated AIDS education into "family life" curricula and mandated that a two-lesson course be available to all students. Letters about the course were sent home to the parents of 2,800 students in one high school; the parents could request that their child be excused from the class—only three did so (Rimer, 1986).

Even if the dangers of HIV infection are not discussed in the context of sex, certainly these dangers can be discussed in school curricula dealing with the dangers of drug abuse. Moreover, groups such as the American Red Cross are more likely than groups identified with homosexuals to be permitted to discuss the risks of HIV transmission in the schools. Recently, the Red Cross has increased its AIDS education efforts considerably to embrace concerns beyond blood banking in educating the public at large.

Blacks and Hispanics comprise a disproportionately high percentage of AIDS cases, in spite of the media's frequent portrayal of the disease as a problem almost exclusively of white, middle-class, homosexual men. These groups require specially focused programs developed by health departments in areas having large black and Hispanic populations.

There is much confusion about the possibility of heterosexual transmission of HIV (in both directions) and about the degree of risk associated with heterosexual contact. Hotlines report increased numbers of calls from women. The public at large deserves to receive considerable attention.

The large proportion of IV drug users among AIDS sufferers represents a serious threat to themselves and to their sexual partners. Many IV drug users are already caught up in patterns of asocial and antisocial behavior that may make appeals meaningless to them. Self-preservation will need to be emphasized strongly for this group of people.

The lack of available treatment programs and facilities for IV drug users represents a serious problem. Drug treatment programs are greatly overtaxed at present, and a program that inspired widespread efforts at rehabilitation among IV drug users (to avoid AIDS) could swamp already strained facilities. Thus, efforts to achieve access to IV drug users must be coupled with realistic planning of ways to cope with success.

Who Should Do the Educating?

The range and diversity of education needed against AIDS make it obvious that the effort must take many forms and find support from many sources. Health professionals—doctors, nurses, health educators, public health officials—are all important links in the educational process. They must be taught through professional associations, academic curricula, and continuing education so that they, in turn, can teach their patients and associates.

Among members of high-risk groups, counseling by peers is likely to be the most effective source of information, and such counseling should be available for those at risk. Government at all levels, not only local officials in certain high-incidence areas, must be willing to support and fund efforts to educate members of high-risk communities.

Many governmental efforts will necessarily address the general public rather than special target groups and will probably be limited to activities such as the distribution of pamphlets, placement of advertisements, and organization of telephone "hotlines." These activities will be useful in maintaining public consciousness of the disease and in reinforcing more-specifically-targeted educational efforts performed by others. However, if nothing else is done, these general educational efforts will be grossly inadequate.

Government must prepare to fund targeted education through grants and contracts to private organizations that can communicate with special groups, in language appropriate to those groups, about relevant aspects of the disease. These include homosexual organizations (among which appropriate educational work has already begun in some areas), schools and colleges, women's groups, youth groups, prisons, prostitutes' groups, and any type of organization with access to the IV drug user population.

A massive, coordinated educational program intended both to interrupt transmission of the virus and to allay public fears will not be cheap. Although funding by the federal government for AIDS-related activities has recently increased, the amounts budgeted total less than $25 million; many times that amount could usefully be spent (Fineberg, 1986; Jenness, 1986).

Although there is need for much greater involvement of foundations and private sector organizations with expertise in health promotion, such participation would not relieve the government of a fundamental responsibility in funding and implementing educational programs.

The most fundamental obligation for AIDS education rests with the federal government, which alone is situated to develop and coordinate a massive campaign to implement the educational goals outlined above.

Assessing Educational Interventions

The effects of educational programs will not be immediately reflected in declines in the incidence of AIDS cases. As noted earlier, AIDS incidence rates reflect infections contracted several years prior to the onset of the disease. If there were reliable data on seropositivity in representative samples of the target populations, these data could provide an indicator of the effectiveness of such programs. But even such up-to-date indicators of the spread of the infection would be of limited value, because seropositivity incidence rates can change for reasons unrelated to the effects of education programs. Such aggregate data would not identify who has been exposed to particular educational programs. Moreover, the likelihood of infection for an individual can change with the prevalence of infection in the population. For example, an individual may practice "safer sex" and greatly reduce his number of sexual partners as the result of exposure to an education program, but his likelihood of infection may nonetheless rise if the prevalence of the infection increases among his partners. This has been the case in San Francisco, where dramatic changes in sexual practices among homosexual men have been undermined by skyrocketing seropositivity rates (Centers for Disease Control, 1985b).

In addition to measures of disease and incidence and knowledge about disease transmission as reflected in polling data, it will be crucially important to obtain reliable indicators of changes in the incidence of behaviors that involve risk of infection. Such measurements will pose a considerable methodological challenge. Survey questions that ask whether respondents have changed their behavior because of the AIDS epidemic are open to serious doubts as to their validity. In particular, these questions—especially when asked in the context of an education program that reinforces notions about the dangerousness of the disease—have a potential for biasing estimates of the proportion of people who have changed their behavior. This source of bias will require careful study (using probing questions, alternate forms of questionnaires, and so on), and it may be especially crucial in studies of high-risk groups.

Evaluating the effects of different educational programs will require that relevant longitudinal data be gathered from participants in the programs and from control groups. Longitudinal data are necessary because only long-term changes in behavior patterns will be effective in controlling the spread of the epidemic. For example, with the relatively recent advent of HIV antibody testing, little is known about how individuals who test positive will react to this knowledge (see section on "Voluntary Testing," below).

The launching of a massive and decentralized education program will have many unique elements, and it may involve a slow learning process with considerable trial and error. Rigorous evaluations of these education programs will be important if we are to learn from experience and thereby improve the programs.

The technology and basic conceptual framework for conducting reasonable evaluation studies already exist. The evaluation of AIDS education programs should be conducted by a group independent of those responsible for developing and implementing the programs, and the evaluators should provide for strong centralized oversight and quality control of their work. Past experience with large-scale, decentralized social research and evaluation programs indicates that research may be of poor quality without such oversight.

A Special Case—Changing Behavior Among IV Drug Users

Although IV drug users have been recognized as a unique "at risk" group, they have not attracted as much media attention as other groups. Understanding of this group is critical, however, not only because they are the second largest group to have developed AIDS in the United States, but because they are the primary source for heterosexual transmission to their sexual partners and fetuses. Moreover, the large differences in seropositivity prevalence rates among IV drug users in different parts of the country mean that there is a tremendous opportunity to halt the further spread of infection by changing behavior among IV drug users.

Drug abusers in general and IV drug users in particular do not belong to organized support, self-help, or advocacy groups. On the contrary, these groups have been identified as reservoirs of medical problems (such as hepatitis) and social ills; IV drug use is traditionally regarded as being associated with self-destructive activities.

Generally, IV drug users are identified in one of two circumstances: when they seek treatment or when they are arrested. Yet many IV drug users are not regular users, nor are they readily identified by either the health care or the criminal justice system. Treatment for drug-related problems may be provided by the general medical care delivery system without the patient's ever being labeled an IV drug user. Frequently, IV drug users present with clinical signs of depression or other psychiatric illnesses, and these, rather than substance abuse, may be the reported clinical diagnosis. Most important, many persons abuse or misuse drugs and never receive any therapeutic intervention. As a rule, the general medical community has preferred not to treat either the social or the medical ills of IV drug users. Instead, society has relied upon the substance abuse treatment system, separate from the mainstream health care delivery system, to provide services for IV drug users.

In terms of the natural history of HIV infection, IV drug users engage in a wide variety of behaviors that affect the immune system. They are thus performing natural experiments that may teach much about cofactors in AIDS. From a behavioral science perspective, IV drug use has traditionally been considered one of the most difficult behavior patterns to alter permanently, so that the amount and types of changes in response to the threat of AIDS may provide important information about drug addiction at both the individual and societal levels.

The importance of studying AIDS among IV drug users is countered by the great practical difficulties in conducting research in this group. The institutionalized distrust between IV drug users and conventional authorities makes establishing rapport very problematic. Moreover, the unstable life-styles of many IV drug users make longitudinal research very difficult.

Because the majority (93 percent) of AIDS patients are men, the importance of this disease among women has often been overlooked. Yet women represent 20 percent of all heterosexual intravenous drug users with AIDS. Heterosexual acquisition of HIV infection and the development of AIDS have also been reported among female sexual partners of men at risk. Many men who use intravenous drugs are sexual partners with women who do not—one study revealed that 80 percent of male IV drug users had such a primary sexual relationship. Furthermore, among women who themselves have injected heroin, those seeking treatment for their dependency problems are likely to become fertile, as heroin produces anovulation whereas methadone does not.

Preventing AIDS among the sexual partners of IV drug users will clearly be a necessary part of overall public health control of the epidemic. But the behavior changes needed to prevent heterosexual and *in utero* transmission will be difficult to make and to maintain. Disruption of ongoing sexual relationships and the decision to forgo having children involve considerable psychological costs. These behavior changes would require more intensive prevention resources than those needed for simple dissemination of information. Sexual partners of IV drug users who do not themselves use drugs may also be harder to reach, because they will not necessarily come in contact with treatment centers or with the criminal justice system.

Although rapid and widespread dissemination of HIV through a drug-using community has occurred in several areas, it may not be inevitable. For instance, seropositivity rates vary dramatically by geographic proximity to New York City. The farther the distance from New York City, the lower the prevalence of seropositivity among IV drug users. A city within five miles of downtown New York had a seropositivity rate of 56 percent among its clients in a methadone maintenance treatment program. A similar program in a city approximately 100 miles from downtown New York had a seropositivity rate of 2 percent. Two cities at intermediate distances had intermediate rates. Sharing of paraphernalia was common among the IV drug users in all four cities. Overall, more than 95 percent of these drug users reported some needle-sharing behavior in their lifetime. It is assumed that those farther from New York City are at serious risk of soon being infected with HIV, underscoring the urgency of instituting massive educational and prevention programs immediately.

There appear to be two primary factors associated with rapid dissemination of HIV among drug users in New York City. Prior to concerns about AIDS, the sharing of equipment for injecting drugs was almost universal among IV drug users. Sharing was associated with initiation into IV drug use, it served as a social bonding mechanism among IV drug users, and it also occurred for practical reasons—because the drug user did not have enough money to purchase an unused needle and syringe, because fear of arrest kept users from carrying their own apparatus, or because unused equipment was simply not available. As a result of this sharing, the frequency of drug injection has been found to be a strong predictor of seropositivity in the New York City area.

Another factor, which may be a critical determinant of the speed of viral spread, is sharing of injection equipment across friendship groups. Clearly, if IV drug users confined their sharing of equipment to limited friendship groups, there would be limited transmission of the virus from one group to another. In New York City the sharing of equipment across friendship groups occurs most frequently in places where IV drug users can rent previously used equipment. In other cities the sharing across friendship groups may occur more frequently with a spare set of equipment kept by a drug dealer for customers to use immediately after purchasing the drug.

There is a stereotypical notion that IV drug users are so driven by their habits that they have no regard for the health consequences of injecting drugs. (This stereotype is accompanied by a view of IV drug users as a homogeneous group, although in fact people from all walks of life use IV drugs, some on an occasional basis.) Research on IV drug users in New York City, however, clearly shows that concern about dying from AIDS is great enough to change the behavior of many drug users. One study of patients in methadone treatment found that more than 90 percent knew that AIDS was transmitted through sharing injection equipment. Of these patients, 59 percent reported behavior change to reduce their risk of contracting AIDS. Other studies have confirmed this finding, with the most common behavior changes including increased use of sterile needles, reductions in sharing equipment, and reductions in drug injection.

Confirmation of these self-reported behavior changes comes from studies of the illicit market in sterile needles in New York City. This market has increased greatly since the AIDS epidemic began, and there has been some distribution of "free" sterile needles and syringes as a sales strategy by drug dealers.

Drug Abuse Treatment Programs

The ideal method of prevention of HIV infection among IV drug users would be to stop people from using IV drugs in the first place. While a drug-free society is a laudable goal, programs must be designed with the understanding that this is not a short-term possibility. Architects of social programs designed to combat drug abuse are faced with some difficult ethical and policy questions: Should programs focus only on drug injection (the AIDS danger), or should they be broader and include any use of such drugs as cocaine and heroin, or broader still and focus on any illicit drug use? Preventing noninjected drug abuse is a valid public health goal in itself, but it may dilute efforts to reduce the AIDS-specific problem of drug injection.

Educational programs about the dangers of AIDS and IV drug use are already being developed in some junior and senior high schools. These programs are clearly needed, but there are also limitations on their likely effectiveness. Drug prevention programs based on arousing fear have not been successful in the past, particularly if the fear is associated with a low-probability event. Moreover, many persons who eventually become IV drug users drop out of school well before they make decisions about injecting drugs. Prevention programs targeted at reducing initiation into IV drug use may have to operate outside of school settings and focus on resisting social pressures to begin injecting drugs (similar to the cigarette-smoking prevention programs that focus on teaching skills to resist initiation into cigarette smoking). Such programs are undoubtedly more expensive than are the in-school programs, but they are no less critical.

Fear of AIDS, among other reasons, will undoubtedly lead significant numbers of IV drug users to seek treatment for their drug use. For the United States as a whole, however, the availability of treatment was significantly less than the demand for treatment even before the AIDS epidemic. The committee heard dramatic testimony about users willing to sign up for treatment such as methadone maintenance, only to be told of waiting periods of months (R. Newman, Beth-Israel Hospital, Boston, Mass., personal communication, 1986).

Expanding the treatment system could significantly reduce IV drug use and the transmission of HIV. Users who had not been infected before entering such programs would greatly reduce their chances of being infected, and users who had already been infected would greatly reduce their chances of exposing others. The possibility exists for saving money as well as lives. At a purely economic level, treating AIDS costs anywhere from $50,000 to $150,000 per case (Chapter 5), whereas providing drug abuse treatment costs as little as $3,000 per patient per year in certain nonresidential programs.

Unfortunately, there are factors in addition to finances that currently limit the availability of drug abuse treatment. The notion of drug abuse treatment may have general approval until it involves treatment facilities in one's own neighborhood. Any public association of IV drug use with AIDS is likely to exacerbate the difficulties in finding acceptable locations for new drug abuse treatment programs. In addition, methadone maintenance treatment, which tends to be the most acceptable treatment modality for large numbers of IV drug users, also tends to have the lowest degree of public acceptance, and is controversial even among health care professionals.

Finally, using drug abuse treatment to reduce HIV transmission poses complex ethical and epidemiologic questions. If there is not, as is currently the case, sufficient treatment capacity for all persons who might want to enter treatment because of the AIDS epidemic, questions of triage arise: Who should be given priority among IV drug users? Should those with AIDS be treated first? Or those who have been infected but exhibit no symptoms yet? Or those who are seronegative?

The ethos of medical practice would seem to require that all IV drug users with AIDS be provided with whatever substance abuse treatment they need. Also, providing treatment to seropositive persons during the early part of an HIV epidemic in a local geographic area might dramatically slow the spread of the virus in that area. But should special outreach efforts be made to recruit such persons at the expense of providing treatment for seronegative persons? What is the appropriate mix of treatment modalities during (or preferably before) an AIDS epidemic among IV drug users in a community? Although questions of priority are important, limitations on resources are not an acceptable excuse for not using drug abuse treatment to halt further spread of infection.

Distribution of Sterile Needles and Syringes

Clearly it will not be possible to persuade all IV drug users to abandon drugs or to switch to safer, noninjectable drugs. Many may wish to reduce their chances of exposure to HIV but will neither enter treatment nor refrain from all drug injection.

Whether legal restrictions on the sale and possession of sterile hypo- dermic needles and syringes should be removed in order to reduce transmission of HIV among IV drug users has been the subject of much public discussion in New York, New Jersey, and other states (Sullivan, 1986; Waldholz, 1985). Increasing the legal availability of hypodermic needles has received some support among public health officials, but generally has been opposed by law enforcement officials, who predict that it would lead to more IV drug use.

The actual effects of increasing the legal availability of sterile needles are unknown. Almost no data have been collected on the relationship between the legal availability of sterile needles and levels of IV drug use prior to the AIDS epidemic, and it is doubtful that data collected prior to the awareness of AIDS would be applicable today.

AIDS has had sufficient impact on the sale of illicit drugs to encourage the use of sterile, disposable needles and syringes as a marketing device by drug sellers. Unfortunately, in some cases such supposedly sterile equipment has been counterfeited by resealing already used equipment (Black et al., 1986; Des Jarlais et al., 1985). Innovative model programs involving the distribution of sterile injection equipment by public health officials have taken place in other areas such as Amsterdam, The Netherlands. The actual effects of increased legal availability of sterile needles and syringes on reducing HIV transmission and levels of IV drug use may depend on the specific methods of changing the legal availability and the simultaneous presence of other AIDS prevention efforts. It is time to begin experimenting with public policies to encourage the use of sterile needles and syringes by removing legal and administrative barriers to their possession and use.

Recommendations

• For at least the next several years, the most effective measure for significantly reducing the spread of HIV infection is education of the public with respect to modes of transmission of the virus. The present effort is woefully inadequate. It must be vastly expanded and diversified, aimed particularly at population subgroups such as those in which significant transmission has already occurred or can be anticipated, those in a position to influence public opinion, and those who interact with infected individuals.

• The major aim of AIDS education is modification of certain behavior with respect to sexual and drug use practices, such as unprotected anal and vaginal intercourse with those who are infected or at risk of being infected and sharing of injection equipment. In order to achieve this aim, educators and educational materials must be free to use clear and direct, possibly colloquial, language that will be understood by those being addressed. The committee recognizes that the reluctance of governmental authorities to address issues of sexual behavior reflects a societal reticence regarding open discussion of these matters. However, it believes that governmental officials charged with protection of the public health have a clear responsibility to provide leadership and guidance when the consequences of certain types of behavior have serious health consequences.

• Discussion of alternative sexual behavior that provides at least a large measure of protection against transmission of the virus must be conveyed to those targeted for AIDS education. The proper use of condoms, in particular, should be stressed, and condoms must be widely and readily available to the public. It can no longer be assumed that unprotected heterosexual intercourse is safe. It probably is safe only in such situations as a long-term exclusive relationship in which both partners have not engaged in risk-taking behavior or where both partners test negative for HIV infection after six months of refraining from risk-taking behavior.

• Special efforts must be made to educate the population of intravenous drug users and their sexual partners about HIV transmission both by sharing of injection equipment and by sexual intercourse. This population is one of the least cohesive subgroups in the nation, and innovative methods for reaching it educationally must be developed.

• The total educational effort is the combined responsibility of all levels of government, and the private and philanthropic sectors must also participate significantly in this activity. Government agencies that are reluctant to use direct and colloquial language in the detailed content of education programs must be able to accomplish their educational goals by contractual arrangements with private organizations not subject to the same inhibitions.

• Special attention must be paid to AIDS education for young people in schools and colleges, many of whom are entering periods of experimentation with sex and drugs. Frank discussion of behaviors that do and do not transmit HIV has become an urgent necessity for this target population.

• Consideration should be given to establishing an office or appointment under the Assistant Secretary for Health in the U.S. Department of Health and Human Services with the responsibility for developing a massive campaign to implement the educational goals listed above. The office should encourage and coordinate governmental and private sector efforts at AIDS education.

• The legal provisions that prevent the Centers for Disease Control from paying for advertising should be altered by the Congress to permit greater access to the media for the purpose of AIDS education; the threat of HIV infection requires more than public service announcements at odd hours.

• One of the most difficult high-risk groups to deal with in the current AIDS epidemic is IV drug users. More research, methadone and other treatment programs, detoxification programs, and testing and counseling services related to drug treatment programs are needed. If there are legal barriers to the implementation of such programs, these barriers should be dismantled.

• Efforts to reduce sharing of injection equipment should include experimenting with removing legal barriers to the sale and possession of sterile, disposable needles and syringes.

• AIDS education should be pursued with a sense of urgency and a level of funding that is appropriate for a life-or-death situation. Greatly expanded educational programs to effect behavioral change are necessary for high-risk groups and the public at large. These efforts should be supported not only by the government, but also by experts in advertising and the media. The total budget for AIDS education and public health measures from governmental and private sources combined should approximate $1 billion annually by 1990 (see section on "Funding for Education and Other Public Health Measures," below).

PUBLIC HEALTH MEASURES

Traditional methods that public health officials use to check the spread of disease include surveillance for epidemiologic purposes, screening of high-risk persons possibly exposed to infection, and isolation or quarantine of infectious individuals. Perhaps no aspect of the issues surrounding HIV infection has caused more controversy than the use of these methods for reporting and attempting to control the infection. Of the available methods, only surveillance has been employed on a large scale. Mandatory screening programs in the strict sense have not yet been employed with free-living populations, nor have isolation or quarantine.

The debate about the use of traditional public health measures with HIV infection must take note of certain factors that distinguish it from other diseases in degree, if not in kind. The stigma associated with AIDS, ARC, and seropositivity far exceeds that of other venereal diseases in most cases. The fear and threat of discriminatory action based on misunderstanding of such conditions are real. Moreover, several types of behavior associated with the spread of infection are illegal in some if not most states. Such behaviors include consensual sexual relations between males, IV drug use for nontherapeutic purposes, and prostitution. Further complicating the public health picture with regard to HIV infection are the facts that infection seems to be lifelong and that no vaccine (for prevention of infection) or satisfactory therapy currently exists.

Tests for Infection with HIV

The availability of screening tests for antibodies to HIV (see Appendix B) has generated new and vexing questions about their use within blood banks and beyond that realm. The utility and use of the tests remain controversial for reasons pertaining to the public perceptions and concern about AIDS, the technical limitation of presently available testing methodologies, and the sheer magnitude and diversity of the tests' present and projected applications. While blood-screening tests have provided an invaluable tool in the epidemiologic understanding of the course and transmission of AIDS, they present, at once, an essential tool in the successful limitation of the spread of HIV infection and a focus for divisive social forces that may inhibit the most expeditious realization of that goal.

Only two years have passed since the discoveries that provided the basis for HIV screening tests, but the newly developed blood tests are employed more than 20 million times a year, or about 80,000 times per working day. While the tests are not perfect, they have made the nation's blood supply much safer (National Institutes of Health, 1986).

The standard tests used to identify individuals who have been infected with HIV detect antibodies to the virus in the serum. Antibodies to HIV can be detected by several techniques, including enzyme-linked immunosorbent assays (ELISA), immunofluorescent assays, and Western blot analysis. Each of these techniques, when performed by expert technicians, is very accurate at detecting antibody either to the whole virus or to viral subcomponents.

Of the available techniques for antibody testing, ELISA-based tests are by far the most widely used. The popularity of this technique has as much to do with its cost and ease as with its accuracy. ELISA tests to HIV antigens have recently been developed by several private companies under license to the federal government.

ELISA tests react by turning color in the presence of antibodies—the more intense the color, the more antibodies present. A test is deemed positive when a predetermined level of intensity is observed. When the cutoff set by the laboratory is low so that faint specimens are labeled positive, the chance of detecting HIV infection despite a weak antibody response is increased. However, setting the cutoff point low involves a certain trade-off, because at the same time it increases the chance of "false positives"—i.e., positive samples that do not contain antibodies but that nevertheless produce a reaction to the test.

The importance of protecting the blood supply has meant that the threshold for the ELISA test has been set low enough that the blood of infected individuals is very likely to yield a positive result (a testing measure known as sensitivity). Yet the blood of those who are not actually infected will occasionally test falsely positive. In blood banks, where those at risk of HIV infection have already been asked to refrain from donating blood for transfusion, the uninfected greatly outnumber the infected. This group of uninfected persons produces the largest number of positive test reactions, because even a small fraction of false-positive results outnumbers the positive reactions of the few individuals who actually are infected with HIV. Thus, in the blood donation context, the likelihood is that a test result judged "positive" on a single initial test is from a person not actually infected.

Because of the severe stigma attached to positive test results, more specific confirmatory testing is recommended in most cases. This is usually done by performing other tests, such as immunofluorescent assays or Western blot analyses. These tests usually provide a sufficient level of resolution to permit an accurate determination of the presence or absence of specific reactivity with HIV. The combination of ELISA and other tests increases the positive predictive value of the serologic determination.

It is possible to isolate the virus from a large proportion of individuals who have antibodies to HIV (Gallo et al., 1984; Jaffe et al., 1985). Hence, any individual with antibodies confirmed by Western blot or other testing should be considered to represent risk to unprotected sexual partners or to others through blood, sperm, or organ donations.

As indicated above, tests for the detection of HIV antibodies (like all other serologic tests), while quite accurate, are not perfect. As discussed in Chapter 2, the majority of infected individuals develop antibodies relatively quickly; HIV antibodies appear by six months in most of these cases. Nevertheless, some recently infected individuals have been reported to be antibody negative but actively infected.

Currently available initial and confirmatory tests actually rank quite high in accuracy in relation to other tests used in medical screening and diagnosis. It should be emphasized that the task of deciding upon sensitivity and specificity cutoff points is never solely technical and always will involve value judgments. For example, blood banks must balance the medical and social costs of falsely identifying noninfectious units (wasting the blood and stigmatizing the donor) versus missing infectious units and imperiling the blood supply.

Blood Banking

Soon after the first descriptions of AIDS among homosexual men appeared, the first cases of AIDS in recipients of blood transfusions were reported. The likely, and exceptionally worrisome, conclusion that AIDS could be transmitted by a bloodborne infectious agent of unknown character heralded a challenge of unprecedented nature and scope to blood-banking services. Since that time, the practice of transfusion medicine and the use of the HIV blood-screening tests have become one of the most complex and emotional aspects in the AIDS epidemic (Goldsmith, 1985). Yet remarkable progress has been made in ensuring the safety of the nation's blood supply (National Institutes of Health, 1986).

It is almost universally agreed that screening tests are of paramount importance in the context of blood, plasma, and tissue banking. The blood-banking enterprise has a formidable challenge in educating the public. People must be taught that the notion that blood donation itself places a donor at risk for AIDS is patently false, and they must be reassured that the capacity to test for HIV antibodies, coupled with voluntary self-deferral, has increased the safety of the blood supply.

Yet all infected donors will not be detected by currently available diagnostic tests. The small fraction of false-negative test results and the length of time between infection with the virus and the appearance of antibodies underscore the need for those who have engaged in high-risk behaviors to refrain from donation; even with available screening techniques, this is still of paramount importance. Blood and plasma collection centers are urged to establish administrative systems to encourage such self-deferral while maintaining donors' privacy. Pioneered by groups such as the New York Blood Center, such mechanisms involve the use of "privacy booths" where donors who think they are at risk but who went to the donation center at the urging of colleagues or friends can limit the use of their blood to research rather than transfusion. The need for this provision and for increased educational efforts is highlighted by the fact that most recent seropositive donors, when followed up, have been found to be members of known risk groups, although some did not recognize this (National Institutes of Health, 1986).

The antibody test was introduced at blood centers despite concerns that results were not entirely accurate. Furthermore, it was feared that the availability of an accessible testing option provided at blood donation sites might ironically imperil the safety of the blood supply by encouraging members of high-risk groups to donate in order to learn their test results. To allay these concerns, the implementation of the test in blood banks was delayed briefly, and in some cases a moratorium of up to six months was declared on notification of donors of their test results.

The federal government also made approximately $10 million available to states as start-up funds to establish alternative testing sites, physically separated from blood banks, where persons could be tested for HIV antibodies. These were established in public health departments, hospitals, sexually transmitted disease clinics, and health service organizations for homosexuals. Typically, people who desire to be tested at an alternative site are counseled privately, and if they wish to be tested they are given an identifying number (such as date of birth) so that they can receive results anonymously.

In most blood banks an ELISA test must be reactive on two or more determinations with a serum specimen for the test to be considered positive. All sera positive by ELISA are then evaluated by Western blot analysis. The test subject is not notified unless the serum is positive by both techniques. In the initial phases of testing, donors whose blood tests positive by only a single test are added to local (but not national) deferral registries to alert blood bank administrators to not accept subsequent donations, and subsequent donations are discarded.

The ELISA screening methodologies most widely used at present in the screening of blood donors inevitably yield a small percentage of both false-positive and false-negative results. As discussed above, the cutoff point for definition of a positive test is a matter of judgment and is set within the specific context of test usage. The level of activity in the blood-banking community is such that in this sector alone there are more than 20 million tests for HIV antibodies annually. This means that with tests of the accuracy currently available, there may be about 17,000 blood donors annually who have a repeatedly reactive test, but only 4,000 of these may test positive by the Western blot test. Thus, the existence of even a small fraction of false-positive results has implications for many individuals. Being falsely labeled positive can have devastating personal implications in terms of sexual relations, childbearing decisions, and various forms of discrimination. These false positives ought to be taken into account in the public policy debates about the use of the tests.

A recent consensus conference sponsored by the National Institutes of Health has recommended that increased efforts be made to confirm the status of those whose test results are questionable and to bring them back into the donor pool if they are truly seronegative (National Institutes of Health, 1986). The consensus conference deemed inappropriate the practice of failing to notify persons who are ELISA-positive initially but negative by confirmatory tests and are nevertheless added to deferral registries. It also encouraged blood banks to assist in efforts to find and notify past recipients of blood from individuals who are currently seropositive and have a history of blood donation. The Red Cross has begun a "Look Back" program to do so.

The consensus conference also underscored the universal agreement that autologous transfusions (i.e., banking one's own blood for future use) are the safest forms of transfusion. The use of this process should be limited to elective surgery where patients can plan ahead to store their own blood, and it needs to be offered to all eligible patients. The consensus conference also discussed the practice of "directed donations," whereby specific individuals among a patient's family or friends are designated as donors. It found that no data have been adduced to demonstrate that the practice is any more or less safe than relying on blood from a general inventory that has been properly screened, and that there are "persuasive arguments against directed donations based on social and ethical considerations." The consensus conference also reiterated the need for protecting donor privacy while at the same time properly informing the individual of (even equivocal) test results and arranging for appropriate counseling.

Surveillance

Surveillance, which involves both passive reporting and the active seeking of information, provides data on the prevalence, incidence, and distribution of diseases or infection in the population. Such data can be used to monitor the spread of a disease, to shed light on the mechanisms of transmission, to help in designing public health measures to prevent the spread of a disease, to evaluate the effectiveness of interventions, and to guide planning for the provision of facilities. Data on HIV infection and related diseases are critical to all aspects of coping with the epidemic.

In all states, AIDS cases must be reported promptly to local and state health authorities. This action has been taken across the country in response to guidelines from the Centers for Disease Control under the CDC definition of AIDS. Nearly all of the states have taken this action by regulation or directive (such as letters from the state health department to local health authorities, hospitals, clinics, medical practitioners, and so on) rather than by formal legislative enactments. The Centers for Disease Control, which relies predominantly on a reporting system in tracking AIDS, has also done spot checks through retrospective reviews of death certificates and requests for experimental drugs used in treating AIDS to see whether such cases had been reported through normal channels.

The reporting of AIDS cases to local public health authorities and the Centers for Disease Control is a critical aspect of monitoring the course of the epidemic. The definition of AIDS adopted by the CDC for epidemiologic surveillance purposes has been refined, although it is widely recognized that this definition may not be appropriate for decisions about reimbursement or locus of care.

There is considerable stigma associated with AIDS. In some cases, this stigma has followed sufferers even beyond death, with morticians' refusing to bury victims. The result has been an increasing number of anecdotal accounts of underreporting of new AIDS cases and fatalities. Statistical and research techniques well known to epidemiologists are such that it is possible to gauge trends in the spread of diseases that have well-understood epidemiologic patterns without the reporting of each and every case. With HIV infection, however, it is desirable to have reporting that is complete or nearly so in order that more can be learned about the epidemiology of the disease—e.g., its spread in the heterosexual population.

Reporting Schemes

The reporting of seropositive individuals is currently required in only about six states, although such action is being considered in many others. The desirability of setting up schemes to list names and identifiers of those who test positive to HIV antibodies in the context of voluntary programs is another contentious area in the debate over public health aspects of AIDS.

In this regard, it is instructive to look at the rationale behind a program in the State of Colorado instituted by health department regulation in 1985 (Colorado Board of Health, 1985). This program, established in a relatively low-incidence state, has received considerable attention because of its novelty and because of the vigor with which those who instituted it have propounded it as a model for other states. Colorado established testing centers to which members of high-risk groups are encouraged to present themselves voluntarily. Test results are kept track of by a computer, programmed to provide a system of notification for follow-up tests and protected by an elaborate security system.

The arguments presented for the Colorado system are fourfold. First, it alerts health authorities to the presence of infected individuals. Second, it is linked to counseling, which outlines the test's implications for a person's health, sexual practices, and sexual contacts. Third, it may help monitor the incidence and spread of infection. Finally, by having a list of individuals, the state claims to be in a position to establish an order of priority of those to be contacted if and when a promising therapy becomes available (in the case of those who are positive) or if and when vaccines become available (in the case of those who are negative).

Despite the arguments proffered by the proponents of administrative schemes like Colorado's, the reporting of seropositive persons has not been requested by the Centers for Disease Control, and there are strong public policy arguments against it. Such data are not necessarily accurate in estimating the extent of infection across the country. The programs of diagnostic testing are currently still quite sparse throughout the country, so data collection would not provide an accurate baseline, especially since reporting requirements would encourage people to find a jurisdiction offering the test on an anonymous basis, thereby skewing the results. Most important, most public health authorities, civil rights groups, and groups representing certain high-risk populations insist that a legal requirement of reporting seropositive status would greatly discourage voluntary testing and would inhibit high-risk persons from seeking counseling and medical treatment out of fear of loss of privacy.

Contact Tracing and Notification

Closely related to reporting requirements are efforts by public health authorities to trace the contacts of infected persons. Such programs of contact notification or tracing are a traditional part of controlling sexually transmitted diseases.

There is very little public health contact tracing in the AIDS field at present. In areas with large concentrations of homosexual men who are already seropositive, it would be both difficult to undertake and very demanding on resources. However, San Francisco has established a small program involving bisexuals, in the hopes of reaching women who do not know they have been put at risk (especially those who may be of childbearing age and who thus could transmit infection perinatally).

Those in favor of anonymous (not merely confidential) testing systems have argued that only when such schemes are in place will those in high-risk groups come forward to receive the test. They claim that even where confidential systems have been set up to protect names and identifiers, it is the low level of "confidence in confidentiality" that is the critical factor. Moreover, even strong assurances of confidentiality can be undermined by future threats. Legislation can override original protections, and court subpoenas may seek data originally held to be confidential. Indeed, merely being seen at a testing center can stigmatize an individual, and even a negative test result might imply membership in a high-risk group. Test subjects may be encouraged to waive confidentiality protections "voluntarily" as part of seeking employment or insurance. Other possible threats include informal disclosure by any number of individuals who may have access to data (AIDS Action Council, 1986).

The existence of testing programs with lists of identifiers, or making receipt of health care contingent upon even highly confidential testing, might lead some people to seek care elsewhere and discourage others from seeking care at all. Some have argued that the existence of contact-tracing programs might actually foster anonymous sexual encounters by those fearful that names will be turned over to public health authorities. This would undermine the possibility of informal contact notification by infected individuals.

Groups with a public health orientation have argued that anonymous testing ought to be considered as a last resort, to be used only if it does not conflict with other efforts to ameliorate the epidemic. For many public health officials, anonymous testing and the failure to maintain registries and to keep track of patient identifiers represent lost opportunities of the greatest public moment. With anonymous testing the opportunity to follow up individuals for counseling, contact tracing, or epidemiologic research may be lost.

Mandatory Screening

Mandatory screening of the entire U.S. population for HIV infection at the present time would be impossible to justify on either ethical or practical grounds. The number of seropositive persons in the United States in mid-1986 is estimated to be between 1 million and 1.5 million. To identify these and newly infected persons, screening of the entire population would have to be instituted and repeated periodically—perhaps every year or six months—to track changes in antibody status.

Another policy option would be mandatory screening of selected subgroups of the population—for example, homosexual males, IV drug users, prostitutes, prisoners, or pregnant women. However, such screening may not be feasible for some of these groups. Persons whose private behavior is illegal are not likely to comply with a mandatory screening program, even one backed by strong sanctions. Furthermore, mandatory screening programs based on sexual orientation would at least appear to discriminate against entire groups. For example, some homosexual males have only one sexual partner or are not sexually active, whereas some heterosexuals have numerous sexual partners. Members of the latter heterosexual group are more likely to transmit HIV infection than members of the former homosexual group. In addition, with the exception of perinatal transmission and transmission by rape, the acquisition of HIV infection requires consensual behavior by the recipient.

For the aforementioned reasons, the committee is opposed to the mandatory screening of population subgroups. Furthermore, should an effective therapy for HIV infection be developed, mandatory screening of at-risk subgroups might prove unnecessary, because at-risk individuals would have much stronger incentives to step forward voluntarily for testing.

Screening of certain populations has been suggested in a number of specific situations. It has been proposed for a variety of professional, occupational, or client groups, such as health care workers, food handlers, or residents of prisons or jails. The Public Health Service has published extensive guidelines for health care workers, for workers generally, and for school and foster care children. None of the PHS guidelines recommends mandatory testing. They do, however, recommend voluntary testing where transmissibility has been shown to be a serious problem—e.g., the screening of donated blood and tissues and the screening of women at risk who might consider having children.

The justification for selective screening programs requires a clear demonstration that the benefit to health outweighs the considerable potential loss of privacy and damage to occupational, professional, or personal status that could result from disclosure of test results. Mandatory premarital screening for HIV infection is one program that has been debated and rejected by groups such as the American Medical Association. The committee believes that including HIV antibody testing as part of a mandatory premarital examination is inadvisable. It would counter a trend away from such testing generally, would yield few positive test results while labeling many thousands of individuals falsely positive, and would not extend to persons having sexual relations who do not intend to marry. Persons at high risk could be reached much more effectively by being encouraged to take part in voluntary testing programs.

HIV screening and testing programs should be examined in the context of the increasing use of medical tests in other arenas—e.g., genetic screening (Kolata, 1986). There are special considerations when a test yields ambiguous results or information about which there is little that can be done (Garreau, 1986). Tests for infection with HIV share certain characteristics with genetic screening tests that yield equivocal information or tell of increased risk of developing disease some decades hence. Obviously, testing for infection with HIV differs in that it involves an infectious disease with ramifications considerably different from those of inherited diseases and conditions.

One example of a mandatory testing program can be found in the military (U.S. Department of Defense, 1985). All recruit applicants are screened for HIV infection; those who test positive are ineligible for admission to any service branch. Active-duty personnel are also screened; seropositive individuals are limited to service in the continental United States and become part of large-scale epidemiologic research programs (Norman, 1986).

The military's rationale for testing is unique; considerable caution should be exercised in arguments about extending any such program to the private sector. Part of the armed forces' argument stems from concerns about military preparedness—that the nation needs soldiers who are fit to serve, which may entail their being stationed in areas where diseases unknown in this country might put immunocompromised persons at even greater risk. The military also claims that soldiers have provided blood for each other in battlefield transfusion emergencies, without time for extensive testing (although, admittedly, such occurrences are rare with the use of blood-volume expanders to stabilize the wounded). Other concerns involve immunocompromised inductees' susceptibility to live-virus vaccines, which are required for military personnel. There are also the political ramifications of the potential further spread of the disease to distant lands where servicemen are stationed and may have sexual relations with citizens of host countries. Finally, an unstated rationale for excluding seropositive applicants from recruitment likely includes the considerable health care and opportunity costs the military would have to bear if newly recruited personnel were to develop AIDS or ARC.

Voluntary Testing

In a therapeutic context the HIV antibody test allows physicians to determine whether their patients have been infected with HIV. Individual and aggregate data concerning antibody test results also enable epidemiologists to assemble baseline data for longitudinal studies monitoring the natural history of the disease. Furthermore, while there is no currently agreed-upon therapeutic intervention for those who test positive, knowledge of antibody status for those in high-risk groups may encourage adherence to safer sex practices and a reduction in or abstinence from drug use.

This last point is the assumption underlying the Public Health Service's recommendation that all those at risk voluntarily seek out testing. Actually, little is known about the short- and long-term adjustments to seropositivity undertaken by either those found to be positive or their loved ones. The potential certainly exists for dramatic impacts in terms of psychological and physical health, sexual behavior, social functioning, and prevention of the spread of infection. The committee urges that such effects be the subject of additional research studies in the context of programs of voluntary, confidential testing.

Knowledge of antibody status no doubt has differing implications for various subgroups of the population, though the ability to cope with this information depends on the individual's own personality and social support network as well as on the social and political context. Attitudes regarding testing have changed considerably in the short time during which the test has been available (Eckholm, 1985a). The behavioral relevance and influence of the knowledge of one's serologic status have presumably also evolved.

Few would argue that persons who wish to know their antibody status do not have the right to such information. Such an argument would fly in the face of decades of increased support for truth-telling in medicine, exemplified by a virtually complete reversal in physicians' willingness to share a terminal diagnosis with competent, adult patients. The most important implication of the knowledge of infection and likely infectivity is the added motivation to forgo behavior that may put others at risk (or that may put oneself at possible further risk). Persons in high-risk groups who know that they have risked infection in the past have reason to be aware of the dangers their behavior might represent to themselves or others. Yet screening programs might well uncover many who have had no reason to suspect their having been infected—blood donors who had no awareness of their sexual partners' bisexuality or drug use, for example.

How should information about seropositivity be imparted? Perhaps the best forum for such disclosure would be in the setting of a well-established physician-patient relationship. Yet this ideal might fall far short of reality for many of those at risk, such as IV drug users who have not been integrated into the health care system.

The difficulties in informing patients of a condition that may be fatal or of imparting information couched in probabilities and statistics have been encountered in other contexts. As described earlier in this chapter, there are very great challenges involved in encouraging behavioral changes among those who are asymptomatic, especially changes concerning sexual and drug abuse behavior motivated by biological, psychological, and cultural factors. Measures taken to reduce the likelihood of further spread of the virus may have a devastating impact on an individual's social relationships and mental health.

Pilot studies of blood donors who were notified of their positive status revealed that some of these persons had been left by their spouses or lovers after being apprised of blood test results. In describing the experience of prospective recruits who were refused induction into military service because of their seropositive status, newspaper accounts have told of a number of young men sent home with little understanding of the implications of their test results (Spolar, 1985). Some found their spouses or families unwilling to take them back, unable to understand why they could not continue their family heritage of military service, and wondering if their test results meant that they "had AIDS."

Social scientists have described systematic differences in the way people perceive risks and adopt strategies to avoid risks and minimize their own vulnerability. With HIV infection, risk perception may depend on one's identification with the problem. Homosexual men have been exposed to considerable information about HIV testing and are, of course, more likely to know personally someone who has succumbed to AIDS or is currently sick with HIV infection. Those not in high-risk groups may be less likely to know someone with AIDS but may have felt the impact of the widespread media attention that AIDS has attracted.

One 1985 study of homosexual men's attitudes toward testing, whether or not absolutely representative, points out some of the problems inherent in processing information about the HIV antibody test (Coates et al., 1985). The longitudinal study of 728 men in San Francisco included questions about antibody testing. More than two-thirds (69.2 percent) indicated that they would like to receive the test, because knowing whether they were infected would reduce anxiety or help them make decisions about behavioral changes. This majority view contradicted the advice of most opinion leaders in the local community, who raised concerns about the potential emotional damage from testing, the possible breach of confidentiality, and the ambiguity of the test. The most disturbing finding from the survey was the number of subjects (a majority) who believed that a positive antibody test somehow conferred immunity, that they had successfully "fought off" the virus.

The committee believes that the largely undesirable social response to the identification of individuals as being antibody positive argues for voluntary, anonymous systems of testing, but this would entail potential loss of certain public health benefits. Where such systems exist, individuals who believe that their behavior has placed them at risk may decide whether or not to avail themselves of antibody testing. For some, the specific knowledge of a positive test might encourage prudence in sexual or IV drug use activities that might put others at risk; knowledge of a negative test might encourage individuals to safeguard this status. All individuals who believe that they may be infected have an obligation to refrain from activities that put others at risk by adopting safe sex behaviors and following the related recommendations of public health services.

The question of whether to undergo testing should be a personal health care decision to be made by an individual, ideally following counseling by health care professionals. However, even though the committee believes that testing should be voluntary, it encourages the use of testing and advocates that it be widely available. The benefits that could accrue to the individual from such a system include the following: (1) a heightened alertness to the possibility of clinical manifestations of HIV infection, leading to more rapid diagnosis and the early institution of treatment; (2) identification of potential candidates for receipt of investigational or, eventually, licensed drugs; and (3) reinforcement of the motivation to adopt precautions to protect others. Even though further research will be needed to show whether knowledge of antibody status has a salutary impact on health-promoting behaviors, such knowledge may be helpful to many individuals. If voluntary testing were linked with confidential identifiers, certain public health benefits would also accrue: the spread of the epidemic could be effectively monitored, appropriate follow-up such as counseling could be provided, and opportunities for epidemiologic research could be pursued.

In arguing for a system of voluntary, confidential testing (but with provision for anonymous testing if desired), the committee simultaneously recommends that steps be taken to minimize any adverse or discriminatory ramifications of antibody testing so that those who might benefit from knowing their status can avail themselves of it without apprehension. This requires consideration of administrative mechanisms to protect confidentiality with regard to information about HIV infection. Additional or bolstered sanctions against unwarranted disclosure through state or federal laws or regulations may be necessary.

In no case should a test be made without the subject's prior knowledge (or that of a duly appointed proxy when the test subject's competence is questioned). The test should never be offered without substantial pre-test and post-test counseling. This is particularly important when knowledge of antibody status might result from donating blood or seeking entry into the military.

The committee believes that one critical area of voluntary testing involves perinatal transmission. As discussed in Chapter 2, HIV can be transmitted from infected women to their offspring during pregnancy or during labor and delivery. Breast-feeding has also been suggested as a potential mode of transmission. And while it is far from clearly established, some have suggested that pregnancy itself is associated with an increased likelihood of developing disease for HIV-infected women.

Because of these concerns, the Centers for Disease Control advises women at risk of HIV infection to consider delaying pregnancy until more is known about perinatal transmission of the virus and health risks to their offspring (Centers for Disease Control, 1985c). The low infection rates in the female population of childbearing age in general would not warrant routine screening, but women in high-risk groups should consider seeking antibody testing. This would include IV drug users, prostitutes, women who have had many sexual contacts in areas where HIV infection is prevalent, women with a history of multiple sexually transmitted diseases, or women who have had sexual contacts with men in high-risk groups. These women should have the opportunity to seek testing and counseling. Much of this advice would naturally be given in IV drug abuse

centers, comprehensive hemophilia treatment programs, sexually transmitted disease clinics, family planning centers, and so on. The health care
professionals staffing such institutions need to be aware of the risk of
infection, transmission, and the interpretation of test results. The committee recommends that associations of health care professionals who
deal with women as clients in such situations—for example, obstetricians
and gynecologists—develop guidelines detailing the situations in which to
offer voluntary testing and how best to counsel women at risk. The CDC
guidelines are recommended for those wishing more details on this issue
(Centers for Disease Control, 1985c).

Compulsory Measures

There have been a number of proposals involving coercive measures
with regard to members of risk groups, HIV-infected individuals, and
patients with AIDS. These have appeared in legislative proposals and on
editorial pages. They range from such unusual proposals as a call for
tattooing seropositive individuals to isolating or quarantining those at risk
of transmitting the virus. Frequently such proposals invoke control
measures traditionally used to contain certain airborne contagious diseases (e.g., tuberculosis), and even in such cases they were used only for
recalcitrant patients. Such proposals must, however, be viewed in the
light of knowledge about the predominant modes of HIV transmission,
which generally involve voluntary behaviors (with the exception of
perinatal transmission, rape, and blood and blood product transmission).
Moreover, while there have been a handful of celebrated cases involving
AIDS sufferers who continue to engage in risky sexual activity, the fact is
that those dying from AIDS do not pose the greatest danger in this regard.
Rather, greater spread is likely from the million or more persons who are
already infected and who are asymptomatic.

The active, voluntary cooperation and participation of members of
high-risk groups will be needed to curtail the epidemic. Coercive programs may not only be ineffectual, they may actually undermine individuals' sense of responsibility for the community. The committee
believes that coercive measures would be ineffective, if not counterproductive, in altering the course of the epidemic.

Probably because the general public has not fully or widely understood
the predominant modes of HIV transmission, there has been considerable
public concern about the likelihood of infection by other than the sexual,
parenteral, or perinatal routes. Given the potentially fatal nature of the
infection, such concern is understandable. Increasing awareness of the
modes of transmission has resulted in the development of policies to
protect the health of the public in settings where contact with infected

individuals may occur. Precautions appropriate to the workplace, schools, and health care institutions have been elaborated by the CDC (Centers for Disease Control, 1985a). The committee concludes that these guidelines represent a reasonable approach to protecting the public health and that they are soundly based on the available scientific evidence.

Despite the lack of potential for altering the course of the epidemic by isolation or quarantine, some states may seek special compulsory powers to deal with the unusual situation of a recalcitrant individual who is seropositive and who repeatedly refuses to follow reasonable public health control directives. No state has enacted special compulsory isolation or quarantine programs for AIDS cases, although at least one state—Connecticut—has amended a quarantine statute specifically to include AIDS. A quarantine of AIDS patients or carriers has been favored by as much as 40 percent of the general public when queried by pollsters.

All states have laws on the statute books or regulations promulgated by their public health departments to prevent, treat, and control communicable diseases in general and venereal diseases in particular. Many states enumerate specific venereal diseases, while others require health department officials to specify such a list for subsequent regulation. Many such statutes allow for criminal sanctions in the case of individuals who knowingly transmit disease. These sanctions are seldom imposed.

Historically, in all but a few states, physicians and private laboratories have been required to report the names of individuals with certain communicable or venereal diseases to departments of health. (This is a rare departure from the general rule of physician-patient confidentiality, prompted by concern for the health of third parties.) With syphilis, for example, a public health model of response has been developed that includes prompt treatment of the "index case" and the identification and notification of sexual partners through contact tracing.

In many states the definitions and lists of venereal diseases are decades old and do not reflect current concerns about such diseases as herpes and chlamydia. Most of the states have not, at least as of yet, designated AIDS or HIV infection as a sexually transmitted disease. Many state health authorities are of the opinion that they already have effective laws and regulations that could be made applicable to AIDS if and when necessary, but public health statutes concerning infectious diseases are outmoded and may not afford the civil rights protections adopted by American courts. States should review their statutes to ensure compatibility with current concepts of confidentiality.

The usefulness of traditional public health infection control measures to be taken by public health authorities is uncertain. As discussed above, because of the severe consequences of HIV infection, a few states have required that ARC and even seropositivity be reported. Since there is no generally accepted means of preventing the spread of AIDS other than education, the usefulness of reporting identifying information to public health authorities would be unlikely to outweigh the adverse social consequences of such identification.

Compulsory Measures Among Institutionalized Populations

Most of the compulsory actions taken to deal with AIDS have affected closed-community settings such as prisons and jails, mental hospitals, and residences for the mentally retarded. As mentioned, the U.S. armed forces have also instituted compulsory testing of voluntary recruits, active-duty personnel, and reservists.

Several prison and jail systems across the country have instituted compulsory serologic testing for HIV infection. When prisoners are found to have AIDS or ARC, they are often placed in isolation areas or transferred to other facilities where they can be treated. Prisoners who are seropositive are often segregated and discharged as soon as practicable under the requirements of the correctional system. Some prison systems, notably those in jurisdictions with a large number or proportion of prisoners who may be in high-risk groups (especially IV drug users), are considering establishing systems that would transfer seropositive inmates to special facilities more able to deal with such populations.

The public authorities who administer prisons, jails, mental hospitals, and similar residential centers have a special legal obligation to care for patients and residents by taking precautions to prevent the spread of dangerous infectious diseases in closed facilities.

Compulsory Closing and Regulation of Facilities

In a few parts of the country, notably New York City and San Francisco, public health authorities have taken action to close a few bathhouses and bars or taverns where multiple, usually anonymous, sexual encounters take place among male homosexual clientele. These closings have been done under special regulations or under existing legal powers (Rabin, 1986). Only a few such closings have taken place, and they have perhaps been largely symbolic, to aid in general campaigns meant to discourage the use of such places for sexual activities known to spread HIV infection and other sexually transmitted diseases.

Attempts to close the bathhouses resulted in pitched battles over what is for some a symbol of homosexual liberation, and for others, commercial establishments allowed to foster casual, anonymous sexual activity putting participants at the greatest risk of transmitting HIV infection. Critics in New York City have said that regulations closing the bathhouses are tantamount to the recriminalization of sodomy and that too broad regulations would allow closure of other bars, clubs, bookstores, and even hotels. In contrast, some public health officials have said that to allow such institutions to continue to operate in the face of the epidemic would be irresponsible.

Although high-risk sexual relations with many anonymous partners admittedly puts one at the greatest risk of HIV infection, opponents of bathhouse closure have argued that it is the type of behavior, not its locus, that presents the greatest danger. Closing such establishments might discourage such behavior. On the other hand, it could merely remove it to public parks or private houses. Moreover, a forum and an opportunity for public education to a targeted high-risk group could be lost.

Nevertheless, when applied conservatively and reasonably, these compulsory closings can be an effective public health measure. Furthermore, they would most likely be upheld in the courts as constitutional. If public health authorities should decide that compulsory closing or the regulation of facilities is appropriate as an extraordinary measure to stem the tide of AIDS, care must be taken not to transform such actions into the harassment of any facilities catering to a largely homosexual clientele for meals, entertainment, and social discourse; the constitutional protections afforded the freedom of association must be respected.

Compulsory closing of such facilities should be a last resort, following regulatory inspection programs of a more general nature to discourage sexual contact that may spread disease and to maintain environmental and sanitation standards (for example, through improved lighting and removal of private rooms). Such regulations should, of course, apply to any public facilities where sexual practices may be dangerous to health and may spread disease, whether the clientele is homosexual, heterosexual, or both.

Recommendations

• The decision of whether to be tested for antibody to HIV should remain a matter for individual discretion, given the array of potential risks and benefits that the test poses for those tested. Testing should be encouraged in light of its potential public health benefits. Mandatory screening of at-risk individuals is not an ethically acceptable means for attempting to reduce the transmission of infection. In addition, such a mandatory program would not be feasible in an open society.

• Testing programs should be coupled with strong guarantees of confidentiality. Such assurances should perhaps be backed by punitive sanctions for unauthorized disclosure of antibody test results. The committee does not recommend compulsory reporting of seropositive test results.

• The committee does not favor the establishment or the use of compulsory measures for isolation or quarantine of AIDS patients or seropositive persons in the general population. There may be need, however, to use compulsory measures, with full due process protection, in the occasional case of a recalcitrant individual who refuses repeatedly to desist from dangerous conduct in the spread of the infection.

• Special precautions against the spread of AIDS and the AIDS virus may be necessary in closed populations, such as in prisons, jails, mental institutions, and residences for the retarded. Such measures should be applied with caution and only as clearly necessary and should not be used or cited as models for compulsory programs among the general population.

• As a general policy, children with AIDS should be admitted to regular primary and secondary classes. The CDC guidelines are recommended for further reference in this area.

FUNDING FOR EDUCATION AND OTHER PUBLIC HEALTH MEASURES

Although the committee did not attempt to budget in detail the cost of the education and other public health measures needed to stem the spread of HIV infection, it recognizes that some estimate of the likely magnitude of resources is needed. These include funds for risk-reduction education, serologic screening, surveillance, and experiments with the greater availability of needles and syringes and drug use treatment aimed at preventing the spread of HIV. In some cases, as in the treatment of drug abuse or counseling associated with serologic testing, the line between expenditures on prevention and treatment is somewhat blurred.

Funds directed toward preventing HIV transmission presently come predominantly from federal and state sources. Federal funds for AIDS education and other public health measures are appropriated to the CDC and also flow via that agency to states through a variety of arrangements, including cooperative agreements, contracts, and grants for activities such as establishing alternative serologic testing sites and demonstration projects for risk-reduction education. The total funds allocated to the CDC for all AIDS-related public health measures are estimated to have been $64.9 million in FY 1986. (AIDS education may also be undertaken by the Office of the Assistant Secretary for Health.) For FY 1988, $107.1 million has been requested. The Public Health Service budget request to the Department of Health and Human Services for FY 1988 includes $68.8

million for all AIDS-related health education activities within a total request of $471.1 million.

The Intergovernmental Health Policy Project (1986) has recently reviewed the expenditures of states for AIDS prevention. According to the project, state expenditures have grown markedly in the last few years. In FY 1984-1985 total expenditures by the states and the District of Columbia were $9.6 million, and in FY 1985-1986 they were $33 million. For FY 1986-1987 a total of $65 million is projected. The latter total is for 21 legislatures and the District of Columbia. But five states (California, New York, Florida, New Jersey, and Massachusetts) account for 85 percent of the total expenditures since July 1, 1983 ($117.3 million), with California and New York jointly accounting for 66 percent. Of this $117.3 million, $5.2 million has come from redirection or reallocation of existing resources within state health departments—usually from communicable or sexually transmitted disease programs.

The states of California and New York together account for approximately 55 percent of all reported AIDS cases, with the New York and San Francisco SMSAs alone accounting for 40 percent of cases (as of August 1, 1986). Thus, there is a positive correlation between the state expenditures and the number of reported AIDS cases. However, funding future infection control efforts through a "formula" based on the number of AIDS cases in an area would be a grave mistake in light of the long lag time between infection and disease. Indeed, the Public Health Service has projected that 80 percent of all new AIDS cases in 1991 will occur outside of New York City and San Francisco. Approximately 50 percent of these cases are potentially preventable, and the others will occur in individuals already infected (Morgan, 1986). In subsequent years the proportion of cases potentially preventable is larger.

If efforts to stop the spread of infection are to be effective, they must start (or be expanded) immediately, not only in areas where there are now AIDS cases but also in areas where there are as yet few or no cases. Delaying such efforts until cases occur would make it likely that the problem of AIDS in those areas will subsequently be far greater. The opportunity to forestall the further spread of infection must not be lost.

Some examples illustrate the magnitude of funds needed for all the public health prevention efforts listed above:

• Testing at alternative test sites, including counseling, is estimated to cost approximately $40 per individual (J. Chin, California State Department of Health Services, personal communication, 1986), and although the numbers in the various AIDS risk groups are not precisely known, they may encompass as many as 10 million homosexual males, 1.5 million IV drug users, and probably millions of heterosexuals at some risk. Also, more than 5 million pregnancies occur every year, in some proportion of which women will be tested and counseled.

• The most successful education programs to date (exemplified by the experience in San Francisco) have occurred within small geographic areas where there are educated homosexuals. Programs for other groups, such as IV drug users, will face more difficult problems of access and motivation; they will therefore probably require more resources per capita. In addition, large groups such as sexually active heterosexuals who have had a number of partners will need to be reached and motivated to adopt risk-reducing behaviors.

• Newspaper, radio, and particularly television advertisements are influential means of communicating information to a mass audience, but the use of these media is expensive. One page of advertising in a major newspaper can cost around $25,000 per day, and a minute of national television time can cost between $60,000 and $400,000. Consequently, to influence the behaviors affecting HIV transmission, policymakers must begin to contemplate expenditures similar to those made by private sector companies to influence behavior—for instance, $30 million to introduce a new camera, or $50 million to $60 million to advertise a new detergent. Furthermore, advertising campaigns at these levels are judged successful even when they produce relatively modest shifts in behavior. The efforts needed to influence the behaviors that spread HIV will have to be greater and more sustained (Fineberg, 1986).

California has moved earlier than most states to provide funds for AIDS prevention, undoubtedly because the need for such actions has been reinforced by the occurrence of cases. (It is hoped that other states will not delay launching prevention efforts until they have the same stimulus.) Current annual state expenditures for AIDS prevention efforts in California average 65 cents per capita, and in San Francisco such expenditures approximate $5 per capita (D. P. Francis, California State Department of Health Services, personal communication, 1986). Extrapolated on a population basis for the entire United States, these figures would amount to state expenditures nationwide of approximately $150 million and $1 billion, respectively. The committee believes that the desirable level of state expenditures probably falls between these two figures. It bases this conclusion on the fact that although San Francisco has a sizable concentration of homosexual men, this group does not unduly bias the California population as a whole. In addition, the need for active prevention of spread among heterosexuals is only now becoming recognized, and efforts need to be directed to this group. The risk to heterosexuals is greater in areas of high prevalence, but prevention efforts will need to be relatively uniform nationwide.

The committee also believes that expenditures just from the states of the size mentioned above will be inadequate for a number of reasons. For one, the effectiveness of the educational message will be reinforced if it is delivered from a variety of agencies in a variety of settings. Thus, federal efforts should complement those of the states, which in turn should complement the local efforts of employers and private groups. Funds should be provided for these efforts at each level.

Recommendation

For the reasons listed above, the committee believes that a total national expenditure based on a per capita prevention expenditure roughly similar to that made in San Francisco by the State of California is a necessary goal. This suggests the need for approximately $1 billion annually for education and other public health expenditures within a few years. A major portion of this total should come from federal sources, because only national agencies are in position to launch coordinated efforts commensurate with the potential size of the problem.

The process of designing and implementing educational interventions to reduce the risk of HIV transmission, followed by evaluations of their effectiveness, will enable policymakers to evaluate over the next year or two the magnitude of effort needed to bring about a drastic reduction in the spread of HIV infection. It is possible that the amounts envisaged by the committee will not be sufficient to stem increases in the prevalence of infections, especially since some of the groups at risk are difficult to reach with conventional approaches and since, despite the expenditures noted above, the infection continues to spread in areas such as San Francisco, though at a reduced rate. More funding for prevention measures will be necessary if those envisaged here for 1990 do not prove sufficiently great to slow the epidemic.

DISCRIMINATION AND AIDS

The stigma associated with AIDS has led to unfortunate instances of discrimination in employment, housing, and access to social services. Sometimes this discrimination involves persons with AIDS or ARC— sufferers are discriminated against by those who misunderstand the modes of transmission and harbor unfounded fear of the risk of infection from mere casual contact. In other cases disputes arise because of underlying prejudices about those at risk for AIDS (for example, over services for IV drug users or in using AIDS to rationalize antihomosexual bias). Although the precise extent of such occurrences is difficult to document, a recent report by the New York Commission on Human

Rights found AIDS as the basis of a number of allegations of anti-homosexual bias and violence (City of New York Commission on Human Rights, 1985).

Legal disputes involving AIDS are arising constantly (Curran et al., 1986; Lambda Legal Defense and Education Fund, Inc., 1984; Tarr, 1985). One report on the mediation of AIDS disputes used the number of requests to legal aid services in high-incidence areas as a barometer of the social disquiet occasioned by AIDS (Stein, 1986). In 1985 the San Francisco Bay Area Lawyers for Individual Freedom (BALIF) received 1,400 requests for legal assistance. Gay Men's Health Crisis (GMHC) has more than 3,000 pending requests for legal consultation and expects 1,000 new queries throughout 1986. GMHC's title belies its present ecumenical nature: 30 percent of its requests were from the heterosexual community.

Questions may arise in the workplace about testing prospective employees for infection with HIV; about hiring or firing someone who has AIDS, ARC, or is seropositive; or about the refusal of employees to work alongside or to provide services to someone who has AIDS (Leonard, 1985).

A number of major employers, led by a group in the San Francisco area, have begun to establish programs to educate employees about the risk of AIDS, along with policies clarifying the status of persons with AIDS or ARC in the workplace.

Several states have enacted laws of various types to prevent discrimination against persons with AIDS. Several of the laws also cover seropositive persons on the same basis. These laws, statutes, and city ordinances generally deal with discrimination in employment and housing. Some of the laws prevent employers from requiring HIV testing of employees and job applicants. In several jurisdictions, the state antidiscrimination commission or agency has designated AIDS and HIV infection as protected under their programs.

On the federal level, one federal circuit court has found infectious diseases, and by implication AIDS and possibly HIV infection, covered under federal law preventing discrimination against the handicapped (*Arline* v. *School Board of Nassau County*, 1985). The U.S. Supreme Court has accepted this decision for review, and a ruling on this issue can be expected soon. The statute in question, the Rehabilitation Act of 1973 (U.S. Congress, 1973), provides that no otherwise-qualified individual shall, solely by virtue of his or her handicapping condition, be excluded from participation in or from receiving benefit under any program receiving federal financial assistance. (The statute does not cover private businesses or schools.) A recent federal memorandum from the Office of Legal Counsel of the U.S. Department of Justice takes the position that discrimination against persons suffering from the disabling effects of

. AIDS would violate the federal law, but that firing or refusing to hire someone because of fear of the spread of AIDS would not be prohibited, even if unfounded.

Recommendations

• The committee believes that discrimination against persons who have AIDS or who are infected by HIV is not justified, and it encourages and supports laws prohibiting discrimination in employment and housing as formal expressions of public policy. The committee also supports a federal policy to include AIDS as a handicapping condition under the federal law prohibiting improper discrimination against the handicapped.

• Any form, direct or indirect, of discrimination against vulnerable high-risk groups for AIDS should be discouraged and prohibited by state legislation and, where appropriate, by federal regulation and statute. In a positive manner, participation by representatives of high-risk groups in policymaking bodies should be encouraged where appropriate and practicable, and the help of organizations representing high-risk groups should be enlisted for public service programs such as health education, personal counseling, and hospital and home treatment services.

REFERENCES

AIDS Action Council. 1986. Consensus Statement on HTLV-III Antibody Testing and Related Issues. Washington, D.C., May 30, 1986.

Arline v. *School Board of Nassau County*, 772 F. 2d 759 (11th Cir. 1985).

Bayer, R., and G. Oppenheimer. 1986. AIDS in the work place: The ethical ramifications. Business and Health Jan./Feb.:30-34.

Black, J. L., M. P. Dolan, H. A. DeFord, J. A. Rubenstein, W. E. Penk, R. Rabinowitz, and J. R. Skinner. 1986. Sharing of needles among users of intravenous drugs. N. Engl. J. Med. 314:446-447.

Brandt, A. M. 1985. No Magic Bullet: A Social History of Venereal Disease in the United States Since 1880. New York: Oxford University Press.

Centers for Disease Control. 1985a. Education and foster care of children infected with HTLV-III/LAV. Morbid. Mortal. Weekly Rep. 34:517-521.

Centers for Disease Control. 1985b. Self-reported behavioral change among gay and bisexual men. San Francisco. Morbid. Mortal. Weekly Rep. 34:613-615.

Centers for Disease Control. 1985c. Recommendations for assisting in the prevention of perinatal transmission of human T-lymphotropic virus type III/lymphadenopathy-associated virus and acquired immunodeficiency syndrome. Morbid. Mortal. Weekly Rep. 34:721-726, 731-732.

Check, W. 1985. Public education on AIDS: Not only the media's responsibility. Hastings Center Reports 15:27-31.

City of New York Commission on Human Rights. 1985. The Gay and Lesbian Discrimination Documentation Project. Second Report Covering Nov. 1983-Oct. 1985. New York: City of New York Commission on Human Rights.

Coates, T. J., L. McKusick, S. F. Morin, K. A. Charles, J. A. Wiley, R. D. Stall, and M. A. Conant. 1985. Differences among gay men in desire for HTLV-III antibody testing and beliefs about exposure to the probable AIDS virus. Paper presented at the annual meeting of the American Psychological Association.

Colorado Board of Health. 1985. Rules and Regulations Pertaining to Communicable Disease Control. Denver: Colorado Board of Health.

Conant, M., D. Hardy, J. Sernatinger, D. Spicer, and J. A. Levy. 1986. Condoms prevent transmission of AIDS-associated retrovirus. JAMA 255:1706.

Curran, W. J., L. O. Gostin, and M. E. Clark. 1986. Acquired Immunodeficiency Syndrome: Legal and Regulatory Analysis. Contract No. 282-86-0032. Washington, D.C.: Department of Health and Human Services.

Darrow, W. W. 1974. Attitudes towards condom use and the acceptance of venereal disease prophylactics. Pp. 1-292 in The Condom: Increasing Utilization in the U.S., M. H. Redford, G. W. Duncan, and D. S. Prager, eds. San Francisco: San Francisco Press.

Darrow, W. W., and M. L. Pauli. 1984. Health behavior and sexually transmitted diseases. Pp. 65-73 in Sexually Transmitted Diseases, K. K. Holmes, P. A. Mardh, P. F. Sparling, and P. J. Weisner, eds. New York: McGraw-Hill.

Des Jarlais, D. C., S. R. Friedman, and W. Hopkins. 1985. Risk reduction for the acquired immunodeficiency syndrome among intravenous drug users. Ann. Intern. Med. 103:755-759.

Diamond, E., and C. M. Bellitto. 1986. The great verbal cover up: Prudish editing blurs the facts on AIDS. Washington Journalism Rev. 8:38-42.

Eckholm, E. 1985a. City, in shift, to make blood test for AIDS virus more widely available. New York Times, December 23, B-8.

Eckholm, E. 1985b. Poll finds many AIDS fears that the experts say are groundless. New York Times, September 12, B-11.

Engel, M. 1986. Fears of AIDS limit blood donations. (Report of American Association of Blood Banks survey.) Washington Post Health Supplement, January 15, 15.

Farquhar, J. W., N. Macoby, and D. S. Solomon. 1984. Community applications of behavioral medicine. Pp. 437-480 in Handbook of Behavioral Medicine, W. D. Gentry, ed. New York: Guildford Press.

Fineberg, H. V. 1986. Statement to the Senate Committee on Labor and Human Resources, Washington, D.C., April 16, 1986.

Gallo, R. C., S. Z. Salahuddin, M. Popovic, G. M. Shearer, M. Kaplan, B. F. Haynes, T. J. Palker, R. Redfield, J. Oleske, B. Safai, G. White, P. Foster, and P. D. Markham. 1984. Frequent detection and isolation of cytopathic retroviruses (HTLV-III) from patients with AIDS and at risk for AIDS. Science 224:500-503.

Garreau, J. 1986. Is medical testing worth the cost in our freedoms? Washington Post, June 29, C-1.

Goldsmith, M. F. 1985. HTLV-III: Testing of donor blood imminent; complex issues remain. JAMA 253:173-181.

Goldstein, R. 1986. Rubber soul: The condom makes a comeback. Village Voice, March 4, 17-19.

Handsfield, H. H. 1985. AIDS and sexual behavior in gay men. Am. J. Publ. Health 75:1449.

Intergovernmental Health Policy Project. 1985. A Review of State and Local Initiatives Affecting AIDS. Washington, D.C.: The George Washington University.

Intergovernmental Health Policy Project. 1986. An Overview of State Funding for AIDS Program and Activities. Washington, D.C.: The George Washington University.

Jaffe, H. W., P. M. Feorino, W. W. Darrow, P. M. O'Malley, J. P. Getchell, D. T. Warfield,

B. M. Jones, D. F. Echenberg, D. P. Francis, and J. W. Curran. 1985. Persistent infection with human T-lymphotropic virus type III/lymphadenopathy-associated virus in apparently healthy heterosexual men. Ann. Intern. Med. 102:627-628.

Jenness, D. 1986. Testimony on FY 1987 Appropriation for AIDS before the Subcommittee on Labor, Department of Health and Human Services, Education and Related Agencies of the House Appropriations Committee. U.S. Congress, May 5, 1986.

Jonsen, A. R., M. Cooke, and B. A. Koenig. 1986. AIDS and ethics. Issues Sci. Technol. II:56-65.

Kolata, G. 1986. Genetic screening raises questions for employers and insurers. Science 232:317-319.

Lambda Legal Defense and Education Fund, Inc. 1984. AIDS Legal Guide. New York: Lambda Legal Defense and Education Fund, Inc.

Leonard, A. S. 1985. Employment discrimination against persons with AIDS. U. Dayton Law Rev. 10:681-703.

Levine, C., and J. Bermel, eds. 1985. AIDS: The Emerging Ethical Dilemmas. Hastings Center Reports Symposium. New York: The Hastings Center.

McKusick, L., W. Horstman, and T. J. Coates. 1985. AIDS and sexual behavior reported by gay men in San Francisco. Am. J. Publ. Health 75:493-496.

Medical World News. 1985. $1.2 million goes to AIDS education but explicit programs shunned. November 25, 36.

Morgan, W. M. 1986. HIV (HTLV-III/LAV) and AIDS: Current and future trends. Presented at the PHS Conference on Prevention and Control of AIDS, Coolfont, Berkeley Springs, W. Va., June 4-6, 1986.

National Institutes of Health. 1986. The Impact of Routine HTLV-III Antibody Testing of Blood and Plasma on Public Health. Draft report of a consensus conference. Bethesda, Md., July 7-9, 1986.

Norman, C. 1986. Military testing offers research bonus. Science 2:818-820.

Rabin, J. A. 1986. The AIDS epidemic and gay bathhouses: A constitutional analysis. J. Health Politics, Policy Law 10:729-747.

Rimer, S. 1986. High school course is shattering myths about AIDS. New York Times, March 5, B-1.

Spolar, C. 1985. Recruits fault Navy's AIDS policy; sailors with virus antibodies resent facing dismissal. Washington Post, November 23, A-1.

Stein, R. E. 1986. The Settlement of AIDS Disputes: A Draft Report for the National Center for Health Services Research. Grant No. HS-005597-01. Washington, D.C.: National Center for Health Services Research.

Sullivan, J. F. 1986. Jersey "willing" to give addicts clean needles. New York Times, July 24, A-12.

Tarr, A. 1985. AIDS: The legal issues widen. Natl. Law J., November 25, 1.

U.S. Congress. 1973. Rehabilitation Act of 1973, Sec. 2 et seq., 504, as amended, 29 U.S.C.A., Sec. 701 et seq., 794.

U.S. Department of Defense. 1985. Policy on Identification, Surveillance, and Disposition of Military Personnel Infected with Human T-Lymphotropic Virus Type III (HTLV-III). Washington, D.C.: U.S. Department of Defense.

U.S. Public Health Service. 1980. Promoting Health/Preventing Disease: Objectives for the Nation. Washington, D.C.: U.S. Public Health Service.

Waldholz, M. 1985. New York City's health unit urges easier syringe rule. Wall Street Journal, September 3, A-14.

5

Care of Persons Infected with HIV

The medical care of patients infected with HIV is a problem involving a complex, multisystem disease process, multiple hospitalizations, invasive diagnostic testing, and an extremely high mortality rate. Hospital-based medical services are particularly strained by these clinical features, and community-based services are strained additionally by the inadequate financial and social reserves of many patients and by the lingering fear of contagion associated with the epidemic. The background paper prepared for the committee by Green et al. (1986) provides more detail on the strains likely to be imposed on hospital services.

This chapter, particularly the sections devoted to health care and psychosocial support, lays out what the committee feels is desirable for persons infected with HIV, particularly those with AIDS. Their needs for care in some instances are similar to those of other patients with catastrophic or terminal illnesses, such as cancer. While focusing on needs related to HIV, the committee believes that the health care system should strive to provide a desirable level of care for all patients.

ROLES OF HEALTH CARE PROVIDERS

The newness of AIDS and the concentration of cases in a few geographic areas have hindered evolution of the most appropriate overall medical management of patients with HIV-associated conditions. HIV infection is a new condition, but the associated opportunistic infections and cancers occur in other situations.

No satisfactory treatment for HIV infection is yet available, although a number of experimental drugs are undergoing testing in clinical trials (see section on "Antiviral Agents" in Chapter 6). While methods for the management of opportunistic infections and cancers in AIDS patients are evolving, thus far they have not significantly lengthened the survival time of these patients.

Most physicians have not yet treated persons infected with HIV. However, physicians in all areas need to be aware of signs and symptoms of HIV infection so that early diagnosis can be made, enabling all infected individuals to receive prompt care and counseling to reduce transmission.

As the AIDS epidemic grows, a variety of practitioners are becoming identified as "AIDS specialists"; not surprisingly, most to date have been infectious-disease specialists and oncologists. In addition, growing numbers of clinical immunologists, pediatricians, and psychiatrists are undertaking the management of HIV-infected patients. Other practitioners who will probably develop expertise as AIDS specialists are neurologists and obstetricians.

Because of the widening spectrum of disease manifestations associated with HIV infection and the variety of therapeutic skills that are needed to treat such patients optimally, it appears likely that a diverse group of practitioners will continue to provide care for AIDS patients. Most specialists currently involved in treating AIDS patients are hospital-based physicians. As the epidemic grows, practitioners in health maintenance organizations and in private practice will increasingly need to provide primary care to patients.

Recommendations

• Medical specialty and professional organizations should undertake educational activities—for example, the distribution of materials designed to alert physicians, dentists, and other health professionals to the signs and symptoms of HIV infection, and the preparation of informative material for patients.

• The National Center for Health Services Research and Health Care Technology Assessment should commission representatives from the relevant medical and health care specialties to assess periodically the treatment of HIV infection and associated conditions, to suggest optimal treatment, and to disseminate this information to health care providers.

• Medical and dental education programs from the undergraduate through graduate and postgraduate levels should begin to incorporate both academic and practical training concerning HIV infection into their courses of study.

• Because HIV infection is now geographically concentrated in a relatively few areas of the country, it may be desirable for selected health care providers from other areas to have short-term training in high-incidence areas before the epidemic spreads to their purview.

HEALTH CARE SETTINGS FOR AIDS PATIENTS

Hospital Care

The clinical course of AIDS is characterized by a progressive decline in immune competence and by repeated episodes of severe opportunistic infections, which lead to hospitalization for diagnosis and therapy. No single system of inpatient care will work equally well in all hospitals. Factors that influence the optimal system of hospital care include the type of hospital, the patient mix (as between homosexuals and IV drug users), and the number of AIDS patients cared for by the hospital.

Some hospitals dealing with large numbers of inpatients with AIDS have established centralized, dedicated units for the purpose of delivering AIDS care (Volberding, 1985). Modeled largely on the first AIDS unit, located at San Francisco General Hospital, these units are similar in many respects to oncology wards. Typically, patients with AIDS are cared for in a discrete area of the hospital with nurses and psychosocial support staff trained for the task. However, as the epidemic grows, those hospitals with such units will not be able to house all of the AIDS and ARC patients who need care unless capital investment is undertaken to expand their facilities. Therefore, in the future such units may increasingly be used for only the sickest patients. Alternatively, other forms of care, such as that provided by AIDS teams, may be deemed more appropriate. However configured, a system where the care of AIDS patients is distributed among attending physicians and house staff is probably desirable because of the diverse medical needs of these patients. Such distribution of care can also help ensure adequate education of all medical personnel in what will become an increasingly common disease and prevent "burnout" of health care providers.

The hospital epidemiology service (which has responsibility for infection control) is often the organizational unit in the hospital responsible both for formal AIDS training of physicians, nurses, and ancillary staff and for handling day-to-day crises involving AIDS patient care and other employee concerns, such as contagion. These units are becoming increasingly overburdened by such demands. It is important that they be able to increase their personnel so that other functions crucial to overall hospital infection control are not compromised. The designation of a single infection-control practitioner as the AIDS contact person has been a successful approach in several hospitals.

An important function of inpatient AIDS care is the efficient planning of patients' discharges from the hospital. Because the greatest costs for the overall care of patients with AIDS occur during hospitalization, reducing the hospital stay should reduce overall costs (Scitovsky et al., 1986). To do this, the AIDS staff can coordinate plans for eventual patient discharge and integrate these plans with the outpatient clinic and available community agencies.

Outpatient Care

The care of patients with a progressive and complex disease such as AIDS, if it is to be both comprehensive and cost-effective, must be directed as much as possible to the community. Yet this care must also include access to appropriate inpatient facilities when hospitalization is required, as it is in essentially all cases. These functions can best be served by a carefully coordinated approach to the outpatient medical management of patients with ARC or AIDS.

Outpatient medical care of AIDS patients must take into account the multidisciplinary medical nature of the disease, the many psychosocial difficulties experienced by patients, and the social setting in which the disease occurs. For hospitals dealing with appreciable numbers of patients with HIV-related disease, outpatient care is best delivered through a dedicated AIDS clinic. Such a clinic can, in its most developed form, bring together complementary medical subspecialists, such as infectious-disease, oncology, dermatology, and pulmonary medicine specialists. This organization both takes advantage of the specialists' expertise and facilitates exchange between them to improve the evaluation and treatment of the broad spectrum of HIV-related problems. A dedicated AIDS clinic with multidisciplinary representation can also decrease compliance problems and the duplicate ordering of typically expensive laboratory and invasive diagnostic procedures.

A dedicated AIDS clinic can effectively use physicians trained in general internal medicine and family practice, who can provide an important broad base of patient care. These physicians can serve as models for the care of AIDS patients in private medical practice and in areas of the country with relatively small numbers of patients, where dedicated AIDS facilities are not yet required.

An important element in the medical care of AIDS outpatients is the use of nursing staff and nurse practitioners (LaCamera et al., 1985). Nurse practitioners, for example, can provide extensive routine patient care, under appropriate guidance and supervision from physicians expert in the clinical aspects of AIDS. Furthermore, nursing staff provide an important role in patient education, often providing essential counseling services.

The overall needs of patients cannot be met unless the various outpatient services function in a well-coordinated manner. For this coordination to occur, the specific needs of the clinic's population must be considered, and key representatives of the professional staff must meet on a regular basis to review these needs. Another direct effect of this integration of medical care is the efficient use of both inpatient and community-based care. Maintaining confidentiality in outpatient settings will need due attention.

Community-Based AIDS Care

The real power of coordinated AIDS care plans is found in the integration of hospital and outpatient care with those facets of patient care based in the community (Abrams et al., 1986). Community-based care can be broadly defined as care occurring at a patient's residence to supplement or replace hospital-based care. At best, this care includes the administration of medications with nursing supervision, the use of home-based infusion of fluids and antibiotics, and home hospice programs delivering social support and palliative care in the terminal stages of the disease.

In San Francisco, a third function in addition to nursing and hospice support has been added to the services available to patients with AIDS. Shanti, a volunteer community agency concerned with death counseling, organized a program known as the Shanti Project that, together with the City of San Francisco, provides small-group housing for patients with AIDS who otherwise would be unable to stay in independent residences. In this program, several patients share an apartment that is regularly monitored by volunteer Shanti staff members. These staff members assess the adequacy of support services for residents and of contact agencies, including visiting nurse services and a home hospice program, to alter services as the conditions of residents change. Also, residents can help care for each other, decreasing the need for attendant and homemaking services, which can be difficult to reimburse. (The situation in San Francisco is somewhat different from that in most other areas in that homosexual men constitute a higher proportion of AIDS cases, and there are few problems relating to addicted patients. It is also different in the degree of acceptance and cohesiveness of the homosexual community, which results in a large pool of volunteers to complement medical care.)

Care of AIDS patients at their place of residence is possible even in very complex cases. However, it requires a substantial commitment from service agencies involved in delivering this care and careful integration of this care with more traditional systems of hospital-based care.

As might be anticipated from the complex nature of the medical conditions caused by HIV, the potential demands on home nursing agencies are very large. At their most basic level, they include such essential home functions as shopping, cleaning, preparing meals, and maintaining personal hygiene. In most cases some of these services can be provided by the patient or by family, friends, and neighbors. Where such personal resources are nonexistent, services must be supplied.

In some communities, volunteer agencies have provided many of these services. The Gay Men's Health Crisis in New York City, the Shanti Project and the San Francisco AIDS Foundation in San Francisco, and AIDS Project/LA in Los Angeles are prime examples of such agencies. In cities or in patient groups where sufficient volunteer support is lacking, these services must be provided and funded by private or public means. A serious limitation in many cases where basic services are needed is the amount of such care provided by insurance coverage (insurance issues are discussed later in this chapter). In many instances, insurance coverage is limited to services provided by registered or licensed nursing personnel, even though the true need may be for less specialized and less expensive attendant and homemaking care.

In addition to relatively straightforward assistance in performing daily activities, AIDS patients at home often require more sophisticated and specialized nursing intervention. For instance, patients may require IV hydration because of persistent fevers, sweats, and/or diarrhea; they may need IV antibiotics for the treatment of AIDS-associated opportunistic infections; or they may require parenteral narcotics for the control of pain. For these and similar services, nurses are required, even if the need is sporadic. While many insurance policies cover such services, other sources of reimbursement, such as Medicaid, either do not cover them or do not provide enough reimbursement to allow efficient use of such services.

As patients with AIDS become progressively more ill, the nature of their care often changes from aggressive management of AIDS-related illnesses to palliative support in anticipation of death. As this change occurs, management should ideally move from a conventional medical model to a hospice-oriented approach, which has been demonstrated to be very effective in the care of patients with malignant diseases (Martin, 1986). In the hospice system, treatment is designed to palliate symptoms rather than to reverse underlying disease processes.

As with other community-based systems, some hospice support can be provided by volunteer agencies. In most cases, however, these are inadequate, and paid programs play a more central role. Here, as in all aspects of community-based care, reimbursement is an issue and can be problematic. Because reimbursement for hospice care is not provided by most insurance policies or by the government (excepting Medicare, with certain limitations), specific sources of support must be sought, often from city or state agencies.

The several components of community-based care—residential-facility support, home attendant and homemaking care, home nursing care, and home hospice care—obviously overlap so extensively that coordination of service planning is critical. To some degree this coordination should occur during the careful planning of responsibilities of involved agencies to minimize overlap. Still, communications between agencies are critical and can best be facilitated by regular meetings of key members of these groups. To further optimize this planning, hospital personnel representing both inpatient and outpatient care should also be included. In this way, as outpatient or inpatient nursing personnel recognize new needs of patients, these needs can be brought to the attention of community-based agencies for efficient planning.

The care of patients with AIDS and other HIV-related conditions needs to take account of the fact that a significant proportion of patients (homosexuals or IV drug users) may not have access to the support traditionally provided by family members. Further, it may pose problems in small communities where the range of health care services for any condition may be limited.

In some areas of high incidence, models of care entailing extensive community and peer support have been successful in shortening the length of hospitalization required by AIDS patients. Two major programs, funded by the Robert Wood Johnson Foundation and the Health Resources and Services Administration, are being established to investigate the transferability of models of care entailing extensive community support to other areas of the country and other population groups.

Recommendations

• Actions should be stepped up to cope with the projected burden of HIV-related illness on the medical care system.

• Although more research is needed to define the best approaches to care in different settings, experience thus far favors inpatient care by units or teams with a nursing and psychosocial support staff trained in AIDS care and integrated with outpatient and community-based staff.

• For areas with a high incidence of HIV infection, where the financial impact of AIDS on health care systems will be great, attention should be given to the development of AIDS-dedicated outpatient clinics. These units should have a staff of pertinent medical specialists, generalists, nurses and nurse practitioners, and specialists in psychosocial problems. Nurses and other professionals with responsibilities for AIDS care should receive special training and social support.

- Systems of community-based care should be provided, where needed, for AIDS patients. Such systems should be able to provide attendant or homemaking services up to 24 hours daily as needed and nursing staff able to provide IV hydration, IV antibiotics (including use of experimental agents in certain cases), parenteral narcotics, and basic physical assessments of additional HIV-related diseases requiring medical intervention. Social work professionals should also be available to provide guidance and patient advocacy on housing, financial, legal, and insurance problems.

- Home-based hospice support should be provided for the terminally ill. Such support should include assessment and palliative treatment of symptoms, including fevers, pain, and diarrhea; psychological support and bereavement counseling for patients, lovers, family, and friends; and assistance in the disposition of the deceased.

- Arrangements should be made to provide housing support, including small-group housing facilities and/or supervised hotel accommodations, and transportation of patients between medical facilities and place of residence.

- The use of volunteer agencies to assist in patient care and counseling should be encouraged (but services must be rendered by paid providers if volunteers are not forthcoming).

- Representatives of existing agencies and health care providers should organize AIDS care groups to coordinate presently fragmented efforts.

NEEDS OF SPECIFIC PATIENT POPULATIONS

All AIDS patients present great demands on the systems of medical care. However, these demands are amplified even further in some patients, including those with AIDS who use IV drugs, infants with AIDS, patients with severe dementia, and patients who are institutionalized.

In contrast to other AIDS risk groups, IV drugs users typically are socially and economically disadvantaged, with minimal, if any, social supports. Thus, the burden of their care falls almost totally on the medical system, with little expectation of assistance from family, friends, or volunteers. Durations of hospitalization for IV drug users with AIDS are said to be much longer than for homosexual men with AIDS. Also, their often-continuing use of narcotics makes the use of community-based group care settings much more difficult.

Infants with AIDS may be the most tragic of all AIDS cases. Often born to mothers who use IV drugs, they frequently have no family support for their medical care and social needs. This situation is now reaching crisis proportions in New York City and Newark, New Jersey. In certain hospitals in these areas, 15 percent of pediatric beds are already occupied by AIDS cases (M. Heagarty, Harlem Hospital, personal communication, 1986). There is a critical shortage of foster care families who are willing to accept these children, and many are therefore spending their entire lives in the hospital. Tragically, even children who are only seropositive, or who are seronegative but are known to have drug-addicted mothers, are difficult to place due to widespread fear of AIDS. During its deliberations, the committee was told that there are increasing numbers of children in New York City whose mothers and younger siblings have AIDS, who are themselves seronegative, and who are facing the loss of their entire families (Stoller, 1986). There is an urgent need for community social agencies to respond to this situation.

Another set of patients who pose special problems are those suffering from neurologic complications. Patients infected with HIV have an extremely high incidence of central nervous system disease (Navia et al., 1986; Perry and Jacobsen, 1986; Snider et al., 1983). In the majority of cases, the resulting encephalopathy remains mild until death occurs from some other complication. But in some, and perhaps with increasing incidence, this encephalopathy progresses to severe and often fatal dementia over a period of several months.

During this time continuous custodial care may be required. Irrespective of the level of family or social support, these patients can almost never receive adequate care in a community-based setting, because they require 24-hour-a-day surveillance. Because extended care facilities, in almost all cases, refuse admittance to patients with AIDS, dementia will lead to extended use of acute care hospital beds unless alternatives are found.

Most mental health professionals have the training and expertise to help patients with dementia. The problem therefore is not so much what should be done, but where and by whom. The chronic care inpatient and outpatient facilities available for such patients are already under pressure in terms of space and funding, and this pressure will only increase in the next few years as the number of AIDS cases increases.

In some settings, particularly where the number of cases is high, problems may arise in staffing because of the psychological stresses involved in caring for terminally ill patients. These may be reduced by rotation of staff through particularly stressful situations and/or selection of staff who handle such situations well.

Along with the usual problems associated with medical inpatients and outpatients, additional problems are posed when an individual with AIDS or an HIV-related disorder is institutionalized (for instance, in a psychiatric hospital, penal facility, or hospice). The authorities responsible for such institutions have a responsibility for the health of all internees. However, the institution may not have the capacity to treat the patient's medical and psychiatric problems, and other patients, inmates, or care-takers may have a fear of acquiring AIDS (Douglas et al., 1985; Polan et al., 1985). No single remedy is applicable to all situations, but in most settings such patients can participate with others in general activities without posing a danger to themselves or others. Whatever the solution in a particular situation, there is no doubt that the cost of providing care in these facilities will increase as more patients with AIDS and HIV-related disorders are institutionalized.

Overall, adequate inpatient and outpatient facilities are simply not yet available for many AIDS patients who lack insurance, financial resources, or a supportive network, especially in areas where the prevalence of AIDS is high (Nichols, 1985). This situation must be remedied. Moreover, chronic care facilities are often reluctant to accept patients with AIDS either because of the patients' medical requirements or because of fears of contagion (Cassens, 1985; Christ et al., 1986). As a result, some patients often stay for a prolonged period of time in a general hospital, increasing the cost both to the individual and to the public.

PSYCHIATRIC AND PSYCHOSOCIAL SUPPORT

Needs of Patients with AIDS

In terms of general psychiatric management, patients with AIDS who are most severely ill pose the least perplexing problems. The problems may be severe, but they are familiar to mental health professionals who regularly see patients in the general hospital. For instance, a prominent psychiatric problem is depression (Holland and Tross, 1985; Tross, 1985). This depression is not simply a normal grief response to having a fatal illness, but rather a pathological process characterized by alienation, irrational guilt, diminished self-esteem, and, at times, pronounced sui-cidal thoughts (Perry and Markowitz, in press). These symptoms are related to conscious and unconscious conflicts about the way in which the disease was acquired and what it means to the particular patient. Psychotherapy, antidepressant medication, and precautions to prevent suicide may all be necessary.

The psychiatric interventions for patients suffering from dementia are similar to those for the general management of mental disorders. A therapist can help these patients establish structure in their daily living, set limits appropriate to the patient's current capacities, decrease hypo-chondriacal preoccupations with reasonable reassurance, reduce self-destructive or impulsive acts, and help the patient with financial matters, including the preparation of a will. If available, family members should be counseled about providing the patient with custodial care and arranging for eventual institutionalization if necessary, although these facilities will be increasingly difficult to obtain. Psychopharmacologic agents may be of help in severe cases (Perry and Markowitz, in press).

Some AIDS patients may remain unreasonably hopeful about recovery despite the presence of their fatal illness. When the denial has become so extreme that it interferes with the patient's receiving palliative medical care or when it jeopardizes others because the patient refuses to practice risk-reducing behaviors, the denial must be confronted and treatment instituted.

Compounding the psychological problems posed by AIDS (coping with death in a young adult, disfigurement, physical weakness, and pain) are psychosocial stresses that are more particular to the AIDS epidemic. These include ostracism by family, friends, and some physicians; lack of a supportive social network; and the paucity of facilities, funding, and health care providers (Morin et al., 1984). In addition, most of these individuals realize that not only are they infected, but they are infectious. The realistic and irrational concerns about transmitting the virus to others places an enormous burden on an individual already profoundly concerned about his or her own health.

Most trained mental health professionals with a basic knowledge of AIDS can provide the support, psychotherapy, and, if necessary, psychopharmacotherapy to treat the anxiety, grief, depression, hypochondriacal preoccupations, alienation, and avoidance behavior experienced by these patients. More of a problem is finding clinicians available for this task as the epidemic becomes more pervasive. Existing voluntary agencies (such as the Gay Men's Health Crisis in New York City or the Shanti Project in San Francisco) have limited resources, and similar agencies are not available in most other locations. Although cost-efficient self-help groups are valuable for many, they are not applicable for all; some individuals have unique problems or are too concerned about issues of confidentiality to participate in a group process. In addition, public and private organizations have been sluggish in responding to the psychosocial needs of these individuals, in part because the epidemic has been largely confined to homosexual men and IV drug users.

Needs of Patients with ARC

ARC patients present particularly difficult problems because of ARC's complex spectrum. Some patients with severe ARC, who may suffer from problems such as dementia, cachexia, and intractable diarrhea, may be more incapacitated than some patients with AIDS.

Longitudinal studies have been conducted in which homosexual patients with AIDS or ARC have been psychologically assessed using standardized instruments over a one-year period and compared with healthy homosexual men (Tross, 1985). Not surprisingly, all three groups show a high level of distress. Interestingly, however, the ARC group showed the greatest psychological problems. For patients with ARC, physical symptoms that previously would have been ignored—a dry mouth, a mild cough, a slight rash—could respectively be an early sign of thrush, an opportunistic pneumonia, or Kaposi's sarcoma. Some ARC patients even express a sense of relief when a disease process diagnostic for AIDS is found.

ARC patients may be incapacitated by anxiety. Especially in patients with mild ARC, the health care provider must encourage appropriate, but not excessive, use of medical facilities.

Needs of Patients with Subclinical HIV Infections

Patients with HIV infection but no clinical symptoms are often referred to as being "asymptomatically" seropositive. However, they often experience extreme anxiety and depression when they learn of their positive antibody status (Pindyck et al., 1986). Overall, however, no conclusive data are yet available regarding the psychological effects of antibody testing. Nor are data available to document that the results of antibody testing reduce risk-related behaviors over an extended period of time. The available preliminary data from the American Red Cross, the military, the Greater New York Blood Center, and the California alternative testing sites indicate that although individuals who are informed that they are seropositive are understandably distressed, the immediate consequences of such information have not been dire. The proportion having immediate suicidal thoughts or intent is low. Furthermore, many individuals find the information helpful in that it relieves uncertainty about whether or not they are seropositive, helps them in family planning, and encourages seronegative individuals to maintain their seronegativity. Mentioning these potential benefits is in no way intended to minimize the acute and chronic stress imposed by antibody testing.

A positive antibody test may increase a person's use of medical services. As with ARC patients, these individuals understandably may be more concerned that a viral upper-respiratory-tract infection or bronchitis may be due to a potentially fatal infection. Thus, medical attention may be sought, and the health care provider, also anxious about the possibility of more serious disease, may perform more testing than otherwise would be warranted.

Appropriate medical care for otherwise well HIV-infected individuals is difficult to define. A balance must be struck between the rapid identification of serious disease processes and the tremendous burden on health care systems if the testing required to make these diagnoses is not used judiciously.

Needs of Seronegative Persons

Persons who do not have HIV antibodies but who are at risk for infection are often psychologically distressed despite their seronegativity. This distress, which is sometimes acute, may be related to the fear of impending seroconversion among individuals whose recent behaviors (e.g., IV drug use or "unsafe" sex) have placed them at risk of infection. Stress commonly also results from the fact that these persons must alter their future behavior to avoid infection (Holland and Tross, 1985; Morin et al., 1984).

Providing counseling and other psychiatric interventions for these individuals may reduce their psychological problems and also may help prevent the spread of the epidemic. Clinicians can counsel homosexual men about the need to practice safer sex, or they can use the psychological distress experienced by an IV drug user as a catalyst to promote rehabilitation for this disorder. However, resources for IV drug users such as methadone maintenance clinics have become increasingly limited, and referral for such care may be difficult until appropriate resources become available (see Chapter 4).

Seronegative individuals who are not in high-risk groups may also need assistance in coping with the epidemic. For example, the care of patients with HIV-related disorders places an inordinate stress on providers of care (Christ et al., 1986). Factors contributing to this stress include the relative youth of these patients, fears of contagion, prejudice against high-risk groups, unfamiliarity with AIDS-related issues, the intensive care required for patients with AIDS, and the high prevalence of this disorder in some geographical areas, which limits training in the treatment of other medical conditions (in some hospitals in New York, 25 percent of the medical beds are taken by patients with AIDS). Psychiatric interventions for these providers of care include workshops to educate them about the disease, rotations to services with fewer HIV-related disorders, and opportunities to express their rational and irrational fears and despair regarding the care of patients with HIV-related disorders. These interventions should not be restricted only to those involved in direct patient care but should be extended to those ancillary caretakers (e.g., attendants, nurses' aides, dieticians, janitors, morticians) who are also stressed by the presence of these patients and may have unwarranted concerns that lead to inappropriate behavior and rejection.

Family members, lovers, and friends are also stressed by their involvement with individuals who have an HIV-related disorder. For example, the parents of children with AIDS may be ostracized from the community, feel guilty about keeping their child's status a secret so that he or she may attend school, or have concerns about becoming infected themselves. Because the problems experienced by these associates vary enormously, no single approach is appropriate. The important point is that the psychosocial needs of these individuals should not be ignored.

Many persons with no known risk factors develop an inordinate concern about having AIDS or getting it and may present to clinicians, insisting upon laboratory tests to rule out HIV-related disorders. The management of these patients is similar to the well-described management of hypochondriasis and other somatoform disorders. The unwarranted fear of acquiring AIDS in many individuals is determined in part by ignorance, displacement, and the newness and uncertainty of the AIDS epidemic. This fear can lead to irrational concerns, to irrational recommendations such as quarantine, or to frequent visits to physicians for vague complaints. Those overwhelmingly preoccupied with the disease may require psychotherapy (Perry and Markowitz, in press). Efforts to increase public understanding of the disease should, however, ameliorate these problems to some extent.

Recommendations

The committee believes that the following measures would help in planning for the provision of effective psychosocial interventions for those affected by HIV infection:

- The efficacy and cost-effectiveness of various psychosocial interventions should be assessed for seropositive and seronegative populations, for those with psychopathological reactions to having AIDS or ARC, and for those who are not in high-risk groups (e.g., family, friends, caretakers, the general public).
- Educational material should be developed and tested for use with those psychosocially stressed by AIDS-related disorders.
- The impact of psychosocial interventions on different categories of high-risk individuals should be measured to determine which groups are preferable targets of effort to limit the spread of HIV.
- Psychiatry staff must be able to assess patients' mental status so that the courts can determine competence in cases of dementia.
- Additional funding will be necessary to provide sufficient chronic care facilities, partial hospitalization, outpatient units, drug rehabilitation centers, and home care to meet the psychosocial requirements of those with HIV-related disorders and to provide the additional staffing and

support in existing facilities because of the unique psychosocial requirements of patients with HIV-related disorders.

ETHICAL ASPECTS OF PROVIDING CARE

The AIDS epidemic presents many situations in which ethical considerations are pertinent (Jonsen et al., 1986). Patients with AIDS, ARC, and other manifestations of HIV infection have a right to an adequate level of health care just as all other members of society do. (The implications of society's obligations in regard to the financing of care are discussed briefly at the end of this chapter. A fuller discussion of these issues can be found in the report of the President's Commission for the Study of Ethical Problems in Medicine and Biomedical and Behavioral Research (1983b).)

Health professionals also have an ethical obligation not to avoid infected persons or to discriminate against them in providing care, as discussed by the American College of Physicians and Infectious Diseases Society of America (1986). In the early days of the AIDS epidemic, a minority of health professionals shunned AIDS patients or inappropriately publicized the character of patients' diagnoses. There continue to be isolated reports of health care providers who refuse to care for AIDS patients, seropositive individuals, or even patients who are merely members of high-risk groups.

Those at risk of transmitting HIV also have an ethical obligation to protect others from becoming infected. In the health care context, this means refraining from donating blood, semen, body tissue, or organs. Patients who are potentially infectious should also notify health care providers so that they can take proper precautions. In the context of personal relations, this obligation means taking precautions, such as adopting "safer sex" practices or not sharing IV injection equipment, to prevent passing the virus to others (see Chapter 4). This obligation pertains both to those known to be infected and to those at risk of being infected (unless there is certainty that they do not harbor the virus).

As epidemiologic evidence has accumulated on the extremely low risk of health care workers' being infected by AIDS or ARC patients or seropositive individuals, many of the initial fears of health professionals have been allayed. The best available evidence suggests that HIV is less infectious than hepatitis B, cytomegalovirus infection, or tuberculosis. Standard precautions against exposure to blood and body fluids are prudent and will protect health care workers (Public Health Service, 1985).

A second implication of society's obligation to provide care for persons infected with HIV has ramifications for both health care providers and the health care system. During the final months of their tragically shortened lives, AIDS sufferers should be provided with appropriate terminal care according to their wishes (a patient, of course, has a right to refuse care). A critical factor in fulfilling this obligation is respect for the wishes of patients about their treatment. There are a variety of legal and practical mechanisms for effectuating patients' wishes regarding terminal care. These range from discussions with friends, family members, or care givers to a more formal recording of a "living will," a document recognized in many states to allow a patient to make his wishes known while still competent to do so (Lo et al., 1986; Raffin et al., 1986).

In virtually all states, legislation exists making possible a durable power of attorney, but in some states this may not specifically mention terminal health care. It is desirable that, where necessary, legislation be amended or introduced to specifically allow a patient to designate others as proxies to make decisions about terminal care in the event that the patient becomes mentally incompetent. This is especially important with many homosexual patients with AIDS, who may wish to invest a friend or lover with such decision-making authority, where otherwise only family members would have legal standing.

Finally, there is the question of when in terminal care treatment should be stopped, particularly if there is not an expressed wish, a living will, or a durable power of attorney. The committee recognizes all these ethical issues as important and recommends the report of the President's Commission for the Study of Ethical Problems in Medicine and Biomedical and Behavioral Research (1983a) to those wishing to consider them further.

The neurologic complications and dementia frequently associated with HIV infection underscore the need to determine early in the course of the illness the patient's wishes in regard to respiratory assistance, cardiopulmonary resuscitation, admission to intensive care units, and other forms of aggressive therapy. At San Francisco General Hospital, for example, physicians are encouraged to discuss "Do not resuscitate" orders with patients within 72 hours of admission. A survey of 118 homosexual patients at that institution revealed that most had thought about life-sustaining treatment, wanted to discuss their views with care givers, and could cope emotionally with such discussions. Moreover, it was found in this small initial study that it would be difficult to predict patients' preferences without such discussions (Steinbrook et al., 1986). That these talks do not always take place may be a function of the reticence of either party or a feeling that broaching such issues might undermine confidence of patients in care they are to receive. Some, especially outpatients, may deny the gravity of their illness. Another barrier to discussion may be the diffusion of responsibility among various care givers.

The committee regards it as highly desirable that AIDS patients be given specific opportunity and encouragement to make their wishes regarding terminal care known to those providing their care. Hospitals, other settings for terminal care, and health care providers should offer this opportunity early in a patient's illness.

Another factor in fulfilling society's obligation to provide care is the provision of a variety of settings in which AIDS patients can spend their final days. These settings should include their own homes, specially created group homes, hospices, and long-term care facilities. The city and county of San Francisco have demonstrated how such systems of terminal care can be developed for middle-class AIDS patients. The challenge for the future will be to adapt appropriately the San Francisco model and to test other models in other settings where AIDS patients come from a diversity of ethnic and socioeconomic backgrounds.

COSTS OF HEALTH CARE FOR HIV-RELATED CONDITIONS

The direct health care costs resulting from HIV infection include those attributable to the following:

- pre-test and post-test counseling associated with serologic testing
- detection of infection by serologic testing and confirmation
- monitoring of asymptomatic infected individuals
- diagnosis of the range of conditions associated with ARC and AIDS and their treatment, including ambulatory care, inpatient acute care, chronic care in hospices and custodial facilities (e.g., for dementia), and the various forms of extensive outpatient support

The cost of treating manifestations of HIV infection in any particular case will vary with the marked differences in signs and symptoms and length and severity of illness among various patients. Costs also differ among approaches to case management in different settings.

Information is lacking for calculating costs for the spectrum of conditions associated with HIV infection. Some attempts have been made to determine these costs, but the efforts have mostly been directed to costs of inpatient treatment in acute care hospitals. Much less is known about costs in outpatient hospital clinics, physicians' offices, and long-term care facilities. Little is known about the costs of home-based services. Still less is known about the value of the services provided by family members, lovers, friends, and others in support of the terminally ill person's basic activities of daily living. Though such supportive care is generally not classified as personal health service, it requires diversion of economic resources that substitute for long-term institutional care or home-based care by health professionals. Except for some evidence on the costs of screening and first-time counseling, very little is known about the use of health care services among persons who are seropositive but do not necessarily have signs or symptoms of overt disease.

Direct Costs of Care for AIDS Patients

A range of estimates has been made of the costs of care for AIDS patients. Most studies have focused on direct health care costs, including patient care in and out of the hospital, physician services, drugs, laboratory services, nursing, and home health care.

Researchers have computed both incidence-based and prevalence-based measures of health care costs for AIDS victims. In the incidence-based approach, the average lifetime cost per case is estimated from date of diagnosis to date of death. By contrast, prevalence-based analyses estimate the average cost per unit time incurred by a patient alive at any time during that particular time period. Incidence-based computations are useful for assessing the financial burden of a diagnosis of AIDS on any given person. Prevalence-based estimates are useful for assessing the aggregate cost of AIDS care in a particular month or year. Estimates of the average lifetime cost per AIDS case, from diagnosis to death, range from about $50,000 to about $150,000 (in current dollars). Estimates of the average annual cost per prevalent case of AIDS range from about $20,000 to about $60,000 (in current dollars) (Hardy et al., 1986; Kizer et al., 1986; Meskin and Klemm, 1986; Scitovsky et al., 1986). The wide range of estimates reflects differences in data sources and methodology. The low estimates derive from California data and the higher estimates from New York sources (reflecting in part a large proportion of IV drug users, who typically have underlying illness).

There is considerable evidence that the inpatient treatment of AIDS varies by region of the country. The average length of inpatient stay, in particular, is markedly lower in San Francisco than in New York City, Boston, and even in other parts of California (Scitovsky et al., 1986). Whether the costs of treatment outside the acute care hospital show a similar geographic variability is unknown.

There is evidence that at certain acute care hospitals, the real costs of inpatient treatment for an average episode of opportunistic infection among AIDS patients may have declined over time. Among the explanations for such a decline are diminished use of private hospital rooms for isolation, increased training and experience of physicians and nurses, increased use of separate inpatient facilities dedicated to AIDS care, and earlier discharge to home or other health care facilities. It remains unknown whether other types of medical care expenditures have shown a similar trend.

Several factors have been identified as contributing to the high costs of treating AIDS patients. These include successive hospital admissions; long lengths of stay due to severe medical complications; more-intensive nursing care; greater use of intensive care units; greater use of pharmaceuticals, many of which are expensive and/or experimental; greater use of specialized diagnostic and therapeutic equipment; greater use of supplies to maintain infection control; and lack of alternative control systems (Boufford, 1985).

The treatment of AIDS patients in the hospital requires the use of certain procedures and precautions that generate additional expense for the hospital (Green et al., 1986). Special infection-control precautions necessary to prevent transmission of AIDS to health care workers and other patients require greater use of protective clothing similar to that recommended for hepatitis. Personnel must be trained in the prevention of transmission of bloodborne infections. Additional costs include the disposal of contaminated articles and infectious waste, which requires greater use of special equipment and bags than for non-AIDS patients. Although the Centers for Disease Control has stated that private rooms are not necessary for AIDS patients unless the patient's illness precludes the practice of good hygiene, many hospitals have elected to use private rooms. This additional expense is not usually covered by insurance and must be absorbed by the hospital (Green et al., 1986).

Several studies have examined the additional staff requirements for AIDS patients and have suggested that more nursing time is required for these patients than for others. A majority of this additional time is spent on hygiene, a task that could be performed by ancillary staff (Belmont, 1985; Greater New York Hospital Association, 1986).

The costs of treating hospitalized AIDS patients vary according to the patient. Generally, costs have been found to be considerably higher when associated with the treatment of *Pneumocystis carinii* pneumonia. Patients with Kaposi's sarcoma often require fewer hospital admissions, and their treatment can often be handled on an outpatient basis (Arno and Lee, 1986; Belmont, 1985; Scitovsky et al., 1986).

The type of patient—whether homosexual, IV drug user, or pediatric—also influences costs. IV drug users usually have underlying poor health when entering the hospital and tend to have a higher rate of opportunistic infections. Both IV drug users and pediatric cases tend to have longer hospital stays (cumulatively) due to lack of support systems and alternative care facilities (Belmont, 1985).

Studies of costs so far have pieced together data collected from individual investigations, resulting in a fragmentary picture. The estimate by Hardy et al. (1986) of lifetime hospital costs, which was estimated from New York City data on the number of days of hospitalization following initial admission, is now recognized as being high primarily because no comprehensive data were available on the total length of hospitalization. The computations of Scitovsky et al. (1986) represent unbiased estimates of health care costs for AIDS patients of different types at San Francisco General Hospital during a specific year. Whether they are applicable to other patient populations at other time periods is not clear. Even Scitovsky's estimates, as the author acknowledges, are subject to substantial measurement uncertainty.

Another limitation of the current data concerns the present manner in which information on the cost of treating HIV-associated conditions is recorded in most hospital or state data systems. This recording does not now lend itself to easy compilation for analysis. To take an obvious example, AIDS patients are not often identified as such. A study by the California Department of Health Services (1986) reports that a major impediment to data collection and cost analyses is the lack of any specific ICD (International Classification of Disease) code for AIDS or other HIV-related conditions.

In addition, with the exception of Scitovsky's study, all of the studies have been limited mostly to costs associated with inpatient treatment in acute care hospitals. Much less is known about the use of and the costs associated with outpatient clinics, physicians' offices, long-term care facilities, and home health services for AIDS patients.

Costs of Care for ARC Patients and Seropositive Individuals

Comprehensive calculation of the costs resulting from HIV infection would include not only those associated with AIDS but those associated with ARC patients and persons who are clinically asymptomatic but seropositive for HIV. Virtually nothing is yet known about these costs, but there are several reasons, including the following, to believe that they may be substantial:

• Even though the cost of care for a seropositive individual or ARC case may be lower than that for an AIDS case, the much larger numbers of the former (Curran et al., 1985) mean that the aggregate costs associated with them may be greater.

• The costs of care for these patients may be incurred for many years, whereas AIDS is usually fatal within one to two years.

• With increased use of the serologic test for HIV antibodies, a much larger proportion of the 1 million to 1.5 million people currently estimated to be infected with HIV in the United States will become aware of their serologic status, and many of these individuals will subsequently have regular contact with the health care system. The total number of infected persons will also increase.

• The neurologic and psychological manifestations of HIV infection can be severe, and the provision of care for such conditions is expensive.

Indirect Costs of HIV-Related Conditions

In addition to the direct costs of health care for individuals infected with HIV, there are undoubtedly large indirect costs associated with HIV-related conditions. These include the loss of wages for sick individuals and the loss of future earnings for persons who are permanently incapacitated or die prematurely because of illness. Estimating these losses, however, is subject to problems in choosing what to include in a comprehensive calculation. For instance, should levels of anticipated earnings be included? Should the savings in health care expenditures when a person dies prematurely be taken into account? How are social security and pensions to be taken into account?

The committee is unaware of any studies that attempt to estimate the future magnitude of indirect costs associated with AIDS or ARC patients or seropositive individuals. Because of the methodological problems inherent in such estimates and because of the limited time and resources available to it, the committee did not attempt to measure these costs, but it has no doubt that they will be substantial.

Cost Implications of Projected AIDS Cases

The Public Health Service has estimated that 71,000 individuals with AIDS will be alive at the beginning of 1991 and that 74,000 new cases will be diagnosed in that year (see Appendix G). It assumed that underreporting or underascertainment of cases will amount to 20 percent of the total reported AIDS cases, adding 29,000 more AIDS cases to the total for 1991. For these 174,000 AIDS patients alive at some point during 1991, the Public Health Service has estimated that the total costs of care in that year will be $8 billion to $16 billion. The $8-billion figure is based on unit costs from Scitovsky et al. (1986). The $16-billion figure represents adjustments to produce a worst-case scenario. It takes into account that the estimates by Scitovsky for San Francisco may be on the low side nationally, that the population projections are midrange, and that the earlier cost estimates (Hardy et al., 1986) have been higher.

In all likelihood, the $8-billion to $16-billion projection represents a low estimate for the total annual costs in 1991 associated with HIV infection. It does not include the costs associated with ARC patients and seropositive individuals and does not take into account the fact that many of the AIDS patients alive in 1991 may be receiving experimental therapies. In addition, should treatments become available that extend life but do not cure the underlying disorder, costs will be even greater.

Other questions have also emerged regarding the future financial burden posed by AIDS. As methods of treating opportunistic infections become more effective, thus prolonging life expectancy, what will be the increased burden in terms of costs? What will be the burden on those cities having large numbers of AIDS cases—specifically, on public or charity hospitals that will undoubtedly have a disproportionate share of AIDS patients who are IV drug users with little or no financial support? What additional drain on health care resources will be imposed by the apparent shift in presenting clinical manifestations (Volberding, 1986)? For instance, will there be less Kaposi's sarcoma and more neurologic damage and dementia?

Projected Hospitalization Facilities

In a background paper prepared for the committee, the impact of the AIDS epidemic on hospital resources was assessed in terms of bed need and hospital costs (Green et al., 1986). Based on the PHS projections of the number of AIDS cases by 1991, inpatient data on the average length of stay, lifetime hospitalization, and inpatient and outpatient treatment costs (as estimated by Scitovsky et al., 1986), Green and co-workers (1986) derived the following estimates.

Nationally, by 1991 AIDS cases alone will probably require more than 1 percent of all available hospital beds and amount to more than 3 percent of total hospital costs. This approaches what is being experienced in New York City in 1986. In absolute terms, the 145,000 AIDS cases expected to be alive in 1991 (unadjusted for underreporting; see Appendix G) will use 4.6 million hospital bed days, with the majority of this use occurring outside of San Francisco and New York City. This total (4.6 million) is in excess of the number of bed days devoted to lung cancer (3.36 million) or motor vehicle accidents (3.54 million) in 1980. In San Francisco, AIDS cases will use 9.5 percent of available hospital beds, with 19 cents of every dollar spent on inpatient and outpatient treatment going to the care of AIDS patients. In New York City, more than 4 percent of all hospital beds will be occupied by AIDS patients by 1991, with much of this use concentrated at municipal and charity hospitals, and care for AIDS patients will consume more than 8 percent of total hospital treatment costs for the area.

AIDS patients often require more emotional support from nursing staff than do non-AIDS patients, as well as more direct patient care. AIDS patients also require more nursing care in intensive care units than do non-AIDS patients because of the frequent development of multisystem failures. Additional costs of treating AIDS patients are incurred in other hospital service areas, including housekeeping and dietary services. An AIDS patient's room takes much longer to clean than that of a non-AIDS patient. Ancillary procedure rooms also take longer to clean after use for AIDS patients.

For reasons explained in Chapter 3, uncertainty surrounds the projections of future numbers of AIDS cases, but they are based on the best available data and are indicative of the magnitude of the problems to be expected. The implications of these future demands on available resources are especially striking when compared with present levels. For San Francisco the projected use of hospital beds and total hospital treatment costs for 1991 are nearly five times the present requirements; for New York City the consumption levels are more than double those for 1986. Those cities and other urban areas that will handle a large number of AIDS cases will have to provide a great deal of additional care. Hospital beds may be available in some areas of excess capacity, but the strain on general resources for care is likely to be considerable. For cities having large numbers of IV drug users, the strain will be particularly great on their municipal hospitals. In New York City, AIDS patients who are IV drug users may occupy more than 10 percent of municipal hospital beds by 1991.

By illustrating the magnitude of the problem to be faced, only a small part of which is presently avoidable, such projections reemphasize the need for immediate planning to cope with the AIDS epidemic.

Conclusions and Recommendations

The costs of care for AIDS and other HIV-related conditions will add a large and unavoidable burden to the U.S. health care budget into the next century. To design an efficient and reasonable scheme for financing these expenditures, a sound data base is needed to ascertain the relative costs and effectiveness of inpatient hospital treatment, outpatient and home care, hospice care, and other types of health services.

• Ways should be sought to facilitate the collection of information on all aspects of the costs of care for HIV-related conditions, especially AIDS and ARC, with complete confidence that patient confidentiality is ensured. Collection of information can probably best be helped by the design and use of specific diagnostic categories for AIDS and HIV-related conditions. Studies of the costs and effectiveness of alternative forms of care need to distinguish among various manifestations of HIV infection, including Kaposi's sarcoma, opportunistic respiratory and gastrointestinal infections, and neurologic disorders.

• All demonstration projects or other approaches to the provision of care for HIV-associated conditions should be designed so that it is possible to compare outcomes (longevity, quality of life) and thus the effectiveness of care. The National Center for Health Services Research and Health Care Technology Assessment (possibly in conjunction with other organizations—e.g., the Health Care Financing Administration) should commission an appropriate group to provide advice on the minimal data collection requirements to evaluate care modalities in demonstration projects or major centers providing care. Guidelines for data collection should, at a minimum, address (1) patient demographic data, (2) medical status at study entry, and (3) outcome measures (possible measures include longevity or the number of days spent out of the hospital as a surrogate for quality of life). Establishment of such guidelines is urgently required in light of the imminent funding of a number of major projects. Also, it is desirable to rapidly establish optimal modalities for cost-effective care before the anticipated large increases in the number of patients take place.

• Funding for the health services research described above should be provided by the federal government, by the states, and by other organizations such as foundations and providers of health insurance.

FINANCING OF HEALTH CARE FOR HIV-RELATED CONDITIONS

The financing of care for AIDS patients must be examined in the context of how other medical and health services are financed. In the United States, financing for health care is accomplished through a variety of arrangements, both public and private. Public programs include Medicaid, Medicare, the Veterans' Administration, the Indian Health Service, and other special programs. Private programs encompass a variety of insurance plans.

Sources of Financing

Medicaid

Most of the public funds that presently finance care for AIDS patients flow through the Medicaid program. The Health Care Financing Administration has estimated that 40 percent of AIDS patients are being served under state Medicaid programs at any given time (Smith, 1986). In some areas, up to 69 percent of AIDS patients are receiving Medicaid benefits (Boufford, 1985). AIDS patients primarily qualify for Medicaid by being classified as disabled and by meeting income and asset criteria established for Supplemental Security Income (SSI) (Smith, 1986).

A 1983 directive by the Social Security Administration's Office of Disability Programs enables a person who has met the CDC definition of AIDS to be presumed disabled for purposes of SSI eligibility. If a patient meets income standards, he or she can qualify for this program and in most states can receive Medicaid benefits through a shortened determination process. Two-thirds of the states have adopted this procedure. If persons with AIDS do not qualify for the SSI program, they may become eligible for Medicaid through the spend-down process in those states that have a medical indigence program (Smith, 1986).

Federal regulations prohibit a state Medicaid agency from creating special services or expanding benefits for those with a specific disease. However, for AIDS patients eligible for Medicaid, a cluster of services can be offered to resemble a similar service that is not reimbursable (e.g., a hospice-like package). The Consolidated Omnibus Budget Reconciliation Act of 1985 (U.S. Congress, 1986) allows state Medicaid offices to provide hospice care as an optional service.

Under Medicaid, states can implement alternative approaches to providing care, such as case management and home- and community-based and hospice-like care programs, through waivers that are subject to review and approval by certain federal agencies (e.g., the Health Care Financing Administration) (Smith, 1986). To obtain agency approval for these waivers, states must (1) document the cost-effectiveness of the project, (2) describe the effect of the project on recipients, and (3) describe what the project hopes to achieve and how it is consistent with the Medicaid program.

Funding of home-, community-, and hospice-based care, in conjunction with hospitalization as necessary, is generally a more appropriate (and probably more cost-effective) approach to providing care for individuals with AIDS and other HIV-related conditions than is prolonged hospitalization. However, as of June 1986 no state had applied to the Health Care Financing Administration for the waivers necessary for such care to be covered through the Medicaid Program (Smith, 1986).

The committee is concerned that pursuit of funding to support community-based care be a priority goal in the provision of health care for HIV-related conditions, including AIDS. States are urged to negotiate with all possible sources of support for such care (e.g., Medicaid, the Health Care Financing Administration, insurance companies) to develop mutually advantageous and cost-effective reimbursement strategies that adequately cover such care.

The present and future impact on the Medicaid system from financing AIDS care has not been thoroughly assessed. However, the Health Care

Financing Administration has established that the federal share of Medicaid coverage of AIDS patients in 1985 was $50 million. This amount is expected to double in 1986, but the figure still represents less than 0.5 percent of the total federal share of the Medicaid budget for 1986 (Meskin and Klemm, 1986).

A study by the California Department of Health Services (1986) of AIDS patients covered by Medi-Cal (the California Medicaid program) estimated that the amount paid for AIDS patients in FY 1984-1985 was $4.5 million. If the costs of care for HIV-infected patients not meeting the CDC definition of AIDS are included, this amount becomes $5.3 million. Based on projections of the number of AIDS cases in California through 1991, Medi-Cal reimbursements for AIDS patients are expected almost to double annually, reaching $96.3 million in FY 1990-1991. This estimate assumes that 12 percent of all AIDS patients in California will be covered under Medi-Cal.

Similar projections for Medicaid financing of AIDS patients in New York State are not available. However, in New York the burden on Medicaid could be much higher because of the larger number of AIDS cases in New York and the significantly larger proportion who presently receive Medicaid benefits (Scitovsky et al., 1986).

Notwithstanding changes that might occur in the eligibility status of AIDS patients, it is clear that public financing mechanisms frequently do not fully meet the costs incurred in treating these patients. Some hospitals report that the uncompensated costs of care for AIDS patients can be four times higher than for other patients (Belmont, 1985; McHolland and Weller, 1985). The reimbursement rate under Medicaid is estimated to be as much as 60 percent less than the actual costs incurred from the treatment regimen for an AIDS patient (Belmont, 1985; Boufford, 1985). For municipal hospitals in some areas, such as New York City, the difference must be met by city revenues. In other areas these unrecovered costs are compensated for by hospitals' increasing charges for private patients.

To date, 40 percent of the national total of approximately 24,500 AIDS cases have occurred in New York City and San Francisco. In these locations, provision of care has often been through particular centers. Where the level of reimbursement is less than actual costs, this may place a particular burden on these institutions and on the revenue systems that support them. However, the Public Health Service has estimated that by 1991, 80 percent of the cumulative total of 270,000 AIDS cases will be outside these two cities (see Appendix G). Thus, the increase in absolute numbers of cases outside the centers presently affected will be dramatic. Similar problems will therefore arise in many parts of the country.

Medicare

Medicare contributes to financing health care costs of the elderly (those over 65), the permanently disabled who meet disability insurance eligibility requirements, and those with end-stage renal disease. Because of the demographics of HIV-related disease (which currently affects individuals primarily between ages 20 and 45), AIDS or ARC patients would only qualify for Medicare under its disability program. To be eligible for Medicare under the Social Security Disability program, disabled workers must first meet the requirements for "insured status" by having made, as employees, certain contributions to the disability trust fund. They then must be considered disabled according to the social security definition: that is, they must be unable to engage in any substantial gainful activity by reason of an impairment that can be expected to result in death or to last for a continuous period of not less than 12 months.

After receiving social security cash benefits for two years, disabled beneficiaries may begin to receive benefits under Medicare. However, due to the often rapid progression from a diagnosis of AIDS to death, few AIDS patients survive the 24-month waiting period and are therefore ineligible for Medicare benefits. Presently, only 1 to 3 percent of AIDS patients are being served under Medicare (Smith, 1986). However, Medicare could become a significant source of payment if changes were made in the disability waiting period or if new drugs or other patient management improvements prolong survival past the two-year waiting period.

Private Insurance

An estimated 85 to 88 percent of all Americans have health insurance coverage. This coverage is provided through a wide variety of plans offered by insurance companies, Blue Cross and Blue Shield plans, and health maintenance organizations. In a background paper prepared for the committee by Lifson and Lierberman (1986), these forms of coverage are described in detail. Private insurance covers a significant proportion of the costs for AIDS care, ranging from 13 to 65 percent in various hospitals (Scitovsky et al., 1986).

Improving the Coverage of Health Care Costs

Although many individuals have health insurance, 50 million Americans have inadequate coverage and 30 million under the age of 65 have none (Congressional Research Service, 1986). Generally, the reasons for this inadequate coverage are lack of employment, jobs without fringe benefits, or the fact that these individuals are poor medical risks. In addition, one in five American families, 16 million families altogether, incur medical costs that exceed 5 percent of their gross income (Congressional Research Service, 1986). The burden of paying for health care that is not covered by insurance falls on the recipients directly, on health care providers, and on existing public finance systems.

Several legislative proposals have been introduced in Congress in recent years to address these issues. Of the proposals that have passed, the Consolidated Omnibus Budget Reconciliation Act of 1985 (U.S. Congress, 1986) is the most pertinent to AIDS. This act makes persons whose employment has been terminated, in most circumstances, eligible for 18 months of continued health insurance coverage, for themselves and their dependents, at 102 percent of the employer's cost if they worked for an employer with more than 20 employees. At the end of the continuation period, a conversion policy will generally be available. The provisions of this legislation could be used by ARC or AIDS patients whose employment was terminated. However, its usefulness is limited by the requirement of prior employment. In addition, a U.S. Department of Health and Human Services task force is currently examining various options for dealing with catastrophic health costs and incomplete coverage (Bowen, 1986). Among the options under consideration are the following:

• Expanding Medicare and Medicaid to serve a broader population or, specifically through Medicaid, offering otherwise ineligible persons the option of purchasing some form of catastrophic protection;
• Authorizing "medical individual retirement accounts";
• Implementing catastrophic provisions in employee health insurance plans;
• Providing federal subsidies for nonfederal catastrophic policies;
• Providing low-cost, subsidized coverage to uninsured low-income and unemployed persons through state insurance pools; and
• Imposing a small federal tax to allow state payment of catastrophic illness policies for persons incurring expenses exceeding 20 percent of family income.

Emerging Issues

The health insurance covering the majority of Americans, whether private companies or public programs, is seldom specific to a particular disease. A major exception is the end-stage renal disease (ESRD) program of Medicare (Eggers et al., 1984).

Consideration of financing AIDS care raises a number of questions. For example: Are the problems and costs associated with AIDS (or, more broadly, HIV-related conditions) sufficiently compelling for it to be singled out for some special form of financial treatment, as with end-stage renal disease? If so, what types of care should be covered? If not, how can the current arrangements be improved to better cope with the problems that AIDS and other diseases pose? What manifestations of HIV infection other than AIDS might need specific financial consideration? Would such coverage arise from local or national sources, from private or public sources? What criteria or principles should govern public policy decisions affecting such coverage? In the application of such principles, what epidemiologic, clinical, and economic data would be relevant?

Issues that are emerging in relation to the financing of care for HIV-related conditions include the following:

- Many affected individuals, particularly IV drug users, may have no health insurance.
- Some individuals seeking health insurance coverage may be aware that their behavior has put them at risk for HIV infection, but may not wish to reveal this if it affects their likelihood of obtaining insurance.
- Providers of insurance, when entering into insurance contracts, would like to be able to assess the financial risk the contract entails for them and to be permitted to use reasonable "tools" to ascertain this.
- Gaps may exist in the coverage provided by insurance or public programs. For example, many programs have exclusions, will not pay for care provided while a patient is receiving experimental therapy (as much of AIDS therapy presently is, since it is a new disease), or may not cover community-based services such as home care.
- Use of the CDC surveillance definition of AIDS as a criterion for eligibility for certain types of financing (e.g., Medicaid) is limiting because it excludes other severe HIV-associated conditions that may be equally disabling.
- The two-year waiting period to qualify for Medicare disability excludes most individuals with AIDS because most of them do not survive that long.
- Coverage of the costs of medical care for ARC patients and seropositive individuals has received little study and remains unclear.
- The unreimbursed costs of care for AIDS patients at some hospitals seem to be higher than average for patients generally, imposing a disproportionate burden on certain geographic areas and institutions.
- AIDS is a particularly costly illness, and those whom it affects may not have accumulated resources to offset these expenses.
- Pediatric AIDS is becoming a significant problem; society has

traditionally accepted a special responsibility for the health of children, especially if their parents are unable to provide for their needs.

• AIDS is a new problem that has rapidly added a considerable and unequally distributed burden to the health care financing system, a burden that will grow greatly in the next few years.

• Even those AIDS patients with extensive health care coverage may be impoverished by the loss of employment and the costs of routine daily care. Although the majority of these patients are ambulatory during all but the most acute phases of the disease, few of them can sustain gainful employment, even during periods when their disease is relatively quiescent. Though no quantitative data are available on the extent of workdays lost, Scitovsky et al. (1986) have suggested that AIDS sufferers can work no more than 40 percent per year. Hardy et al. (1986) have suggested that this figure is only 14 percent, based on a review of other studies. Therefore, a proper analysis of insurance for AIDS victims also needs to consider disability, wage replacement, and possibly death benefits as well as medical care coverage.

AIDS and other HIV-related conditions present multiple financial burdens to society, the cost of medical care constituting only one component of these, albeit a large one. Many of the issues that arise in connection with financing AIDS care are not unique to it, but reflect problems inherent in the present system for financing care. These problems are posed at a time when federal and state governments and others are grappling with their respective responsibilities and the best mechanisms for meeting the health care costs of the poor, the uninsured, and the underinsured. This is also a time when there is considerable pressure to contain health care costs (and the costs such as employee fringe benefits that depend on them). However, in the opinion of the committee, there is one aspect of the financing of care for AIDS that deserves special consideration. This relates to the way in which the concerns of employers or the providers of insurance might affect the motivation of individuals in groups at risk of infection to step forward and participate in efforts to stem the spread of infection.

So long as the claims of insured AIDS patients constitute a relatively small fraction of the total claims of all insured people in employment-based plans, there will not be major increases in the costs of such plans. However, increases in the proportion of AIDS cases among insurance claims will cause increases in costs. Insurers will charge higher premiums to employers, and employers will have an incentive to exclude infected or high-risk persons from employment in an attempt to contain their contributions to the costs of benefits packages.

When insurance companies are writing individual or small-group policies, they have an actuarial incentive to identify and possibly exclude persons who are at risk of HIV infection or who are already seropositive, because these people pose the threat of potentially very large expenditures. A few states or jurisdictions have enacted special antidiscrimination laws that bar insurance companies from denying insurance to persons who are at high risk or seropositive for HIV infection (Intergovernmental Health Policy Project, 1986). Some of these laws also bar required testing for HIV infection and questions asking whether an insurance applicant has been tested. At an earlier time, when the data on the disease suggested that very few seropositive persons would experience the severe form of the disease, these provisions seemed to many legislative bodies to be appropriate. In more recent months, data have indicated a considerably higher conversion to serious disease. Under these conditions the use of screening devices (such as the HIV antibody test) for the underwriting process may be more reasonable. Other tests are used routinely as tools in assessing an individual's risk of disease.

Incentives to identify and exclude high-risk persons are not eliminated by laws that prevent discrimination in employment or insurance coverage. Even if screening tests specific for HIV infection were barred, and even if discrimination on the basis of sexual orientation were illegal, employers and insurers would still have strong incentives to screen persons by any imperfect means at their disposal. Anecdotal evidence suggests that surrogate blood tests, histories of sexually transmitted disease, and other substitute measures have been considered or may already be in use. These surrogate measures invariably have lower predictive value than antibody testing and in some cases very little, if any, predictive value at all. If any test is used, it should be the most predictive. However, the committee recommends that final decisions on the permissibility of using screening devices in underwriting be postponed pending the outcome of deliberations regarding the establishment of a mechanism to ensure coverage of health care costs of HIV-infected individuals, as discussed below.

The general threat of discrimination in employment or insurance to provide for the costs of medical care may deter individuals in high-risk groups from being tested to ascertain their antibody status. Since knowledge of antibody status may prompt some individuals to adopt healthier behavior, social disincentives to testing should be minimized.

As noted earlier in this chapter, the committee believes that society has an obligation to ensure that all sick individuals receive adequate medical care. An implication of this belief is that all individuals should have access to some form of "insurance" (public or private) that will finance their care, if needed. Those who can afford it should pay premiums so that they are insured, but those who cannot have a right to expect public provision.

However, coverage for the cost of care for AIDS and other HIV-related conditions may be subject to misperceptions. If they become ill, IV drug users and homosexual men would in effect be entitled to benefits, and the facile interpretation that other insured persons or society at large would be paying for a "chosen" life-style needs to be directly confronted. "Insurance" coverage for AIDS means covering the costs of a disease and not support of a life-style, just as coverage for the treatment of lung cancer does not support the life-style of smokers. Increased awareness that AIDS is spreading in the sexually active heterosexual population will reduce this problem of misperception somewhat. However, the real question is whether differences of opinion over the morality or advisability of certain behavior should affect a sick person's access to health care. The committee believes that perceptions as to a person's culpability for an illness are irrelevant to the question of access to medical care and the opportunity to make provision for covering its costs. (This opinion is consistent with the position of the President's Commission for the Study of Ethical Problems in Medicine and Biomedical and Behavioral Research (1983b) as discussed in the report *Securing Access to Health Care*.)

If some "insurance" mechanism were available as a last resort whereby any individuals (even if at risk of infection, seropositive, or already ill) could make provision or otherwise be assured that their future health care costs would be covered, then much of the tension between the interests of insurers and individuals at risk of infection would be eliminated.

The range of problems associated with AIDS and HIV-related care financing illustrate shortcomings in the general health care financing system. Thus, it is desirable that provisions for ensuring coverage of AIDS care costs be encompassed in a scheme that resolves general problems in financing rather than be AIDS-specific.

There are a number of mechanisms available to deal with the problems faced by potential patients and insurers whereby last-resort coverage might be provided. These include federal catastrophic health insurance or state pools for medically high-risk individuals. The committee did not have the time or resources to deliberate on the relative benefits of these or other approaches (or on the question of whether a categorical scheme, analogous to Medicare ESRD coverage, just for HIV-related conditions was justified in case the establishment of other general mechanisms proved to be too slow or not entirely satisfactory). Planning for financing of care for AIDS and other HIV-related conditions must begin immediately, because creative new approaches may be needed and putting such schemes into place takes considerable time, as illustrated by the length of time taken to resolve questions with respect to financing of care for end-stage renal disease—a decade (Rettig, 1980).

Policy Issues

A variety of eligibility questions would need to be answered in the process of developing any scheme of the type discussed above. These include questions involving the criteria for allowing individuals to participate in the scheme, the HIV-related (or other) conditions that would be covered, and the grounds for revision of eligibility criteria. Some experience with the categorical ESRD coverage indicates that the rapid expansion of total ESRD costs during the 1970s and 1980s resulted not from changes in the incidence of renal disease but from changes in the standards of eligibility for dialysis (Eggers et al., 1984).

An issue in the design of health insurance schemes—both private and public—is the question of what methods of providing benefits impart the most appropriate incentives to both providers and patients. If treatment of AIDS in settings outside of acute care hospitals generally proves to be more cost-effective than longer hospitalizations, then coverage of treatment in these settings is desirable and lack of coverage provides an inappropriate incentive to use hospitals, which would raise total costs. If reimbursements for care for AIDS and other HIV-related conditions fall substantially below the actual cost of care, then hospitals and other facilities may have incentives to turn away AIDS patients. Another aspect of this issue is the way the scheme affects incentives to seek care. If medical treatment or knowledge of cofactors were to improve substantially, early incentives to seek care could be critical.

Incentives to seek care are relevant not only to treatment of HIV infection but also to its prevention. In this regard, it is critical to examine ways in which the current system or any new system of health care financing might be modified to help persons at risk avoid infection. Of special concern is funding for the treatment of IV drug use, which is likely to be effective in prevention of HIV transmission. Incentives to be tested for HIV antibodies might help slow the spread of infection when coupled with counseling. Also, outpatient clinics for the care of sexually transmitted diseases, for example, may be effective sites for education about HIV transmission. If so, coverage for such services in any new scheme would be critical.

Another issue in the financing of care for AIDS and other HIV-related conditions is the question of balance between public and private coverage. A sizable proportion of AIDS patients appears to have conventional private health insurance through employment-based groups, and this seems likely to continue, as is appropriate. (It is not the purpose of new mechanisms to transfer the costs of AIDS patients from existing private insurance schemes.) With 40 percent or more of AIDS patients currently covered under Medicaid, it appears likely that future financing of AIDS care will necessarily involve substantial public programs and funds. The scheme could be designed to shift the current balance in either direction or to maintain the status quo; the relative merits of these shifts need to be considered.

The issue of equity also needs consideration. Although HIV infection and AIDS are spreading throughout the United States, the major burden of cases is likely to be in urban centers and in particular states for the near future. To what extent the financial burden should be spread locally, within states, regionally, or nationally needs to be addressed.

Conclusions and Recommendations

In its review the committee found a number of causes for concern with the present financing of care for patients with AIDS and HIV-related conditions. Some of these reflect generic problems with health care financing. There also exists the potential for high-risk individuals to be apprehensive about discrimination in employment or in access to health care insurance, which could adversely affect efforts to stem the spread of HIV infection.

The committee believes that society has an ethical obligation to ensure that all individuals receive adequate medical care. This implies the opportunity to make provision for or otherwise be assured that their future health care costs will be covered. Those who can afford it should pay premiums so that they are insured, but those who cannot have a right to expect public provision.

• The committee recommends that the commission on financing of health care recommended in the *PHS Plan for the Prevention and Control of AIDS and the AIDS Virus* (Appendix G) take as its first order of business the evaluation of ways to ensure that all persons at risk of infection, seropositive, or already ill could make provision for or otherwise be assured that their potential health care costs will be covered. It suggests that the options considered include state pools for medically high-risk individuals and federal catastrophic health insurance. (These would supplement existing private and public insurance schemes.)

Private and public insurance coverage should be modified to provide effective incentives for the appropriate treatment of HIV-related conditions such as AIDS. To this end, more needs to be known about the most cost-effective means of treating the various manifestations of the disease and about shortcomings in the present systems in relation to the optimal approaches to care.

• Carefully designed studies should be made of medical expenditures for AIDS patients under different models of care. Similar studies of persons with other manifestations of HIV infection, such as ARC, are also required. Managed approaches to care should be included in these evaluations.

• Current financing mechanisms should be immediately and periodically examined to determine the extent to which they meet the costs of care for AIDS and ARC patients and their effect on incentives to provide care. Areas for attention should include the adequacy of hospital reimbursements by Medicaid for AIDS patient care; the appropriateness of eligibility periods; reimbursement for out-of-hospital care, hospice care, and home care; the use of diagnosis-related groups in reimbursement decisions; and coverage for home care not provided by nursing professionals.

REFERENCES

Abrams, D. I., J. W. Dilley, L. M. Maxey, and P. A. Volberding. 1986. Routine care and psychosocial support of the patient with AIDS. Med. Clin. North Am. 70:707-720.

American College of Physicians and Infectious Diseases Society of America. 1986. Acquired immunodeficiency syndrome. Ann. Intern. Med. 104:575-581.

Arno, P., and P. Lee. 1986. The economic aspects of AIDS. Unpublished paper. University of California, San Francisco.

Belmont, M. F. 1985. St. Luke's-Roosevelt Hospital Center Study: Resource Utilization by AIDS Patients in the Acute Care Hospital. New York: Health Services Improvement Fund.

Boufford, J. 1985. Testimony before the Subcommittee on Health and the Environment, U.S. House of Representatives, November 1, 1985.

Bowen, O. R. 1986. Memorandum from the Secretary of Health and Human Services to Alfred H. Kingon, Cabinet Secretary, March 25, 1986.

California Department of Health Services. 1986. Acquired Immune Deficiency Syndrome in California: A Prescription for Meeting the Needs of 1990. Sacramento: California Department of Health Services.

Cassens, B. J. 1985. Social consequences of the acquired immunodeficiency syndrome. Ann. Intern. Med. 103:768-770.

Christ, G. H., L. S. Wiener, and R. T. Moynihan. 1986. Psychosocial issues in AIDS. Psychiatr. Ann. 4:173-179.

Congressional Research Service. 1986. Health Insurance: Proposals in the 99th Congress, 2/1/86. Washington, D.C.: The Library of Congress.

Curran, J. W., W. M. Morgan, A. M. Hardy, H. W. Jaffe, W. W. Darrow, and W. R. Dowdle. 1985. The epidemiology of AIDS: Current status and future prospects. Science 229:1352-1357.

Douglas, C. J., C. M. Kalman, and T. P. Kalman. 1985. Homophobia among physicians and nurses: An empirical study. Hosp. Comm. Psychiatry 36:1309-1311.

Eggers, P., R. Connerton, and M. McCullan. 1984. The Medicare experience with end-stage renal disease: Trends in incidence, prevalence, and survival. Health Care Financing Rev. 5:69-88.

Greater New York Hospital Association. 1986. Executive Summary of the Study of Routine Costs of Treating Hospitalized AIDS Patients. New York: Greater New York Hospital Association.

Green, J., M. Singer, and N. Wintfeld. 1986. The AIDS epidemic: A projection of its impact on hospitals, 1986-1991. Background paper. Washington, D.C.: Committee on a National Strategy for AIDS.

Hardy, A., K. Rauch, D. F. Echenberg, W. M. Morgan, and J. W. Curran. 1986. The economic impact of the first 10,000 cases of AIDS in the United States. JAMA 225:209-211.

Holland, J. C., and S. Tross. 1985. The psychosocial and neuropsychiatric sequelae of the acquired immunodeficiency syndrome. Ann. Intern. Med. 103:760-764.

Intergovernmental Health Policy Project. 1986. A Summary of AIDS Laws from the 1986 Legislative Sessions. Washington, D.C.: The George Washington University.

Jonsen, A., M. Cooke, and B. Koenig. 1986. Ethics and AIDS. Issues Sci. Technol. 2:56-65.

Kizer, K. W., J. Rodriguez, G. F. McHolland, and W. Weller. 1986. A Qualitative Analysis of AIDS in California. Sacramento, Calif.: California Department of Health Services.

LaCamera, D. J., H. Masur, and D. K. Henderson. 1985. The acquired immunodeficiency syndrome. Nurs. Clin. North Am. 20:241-256.

Lifson, A., and P. Lierberman. 1986. Insurance coverage and AIDS. Background paper. Washington, D.C.: Committee on a National Strategy for AIDS.

Lo, B., T. A. Raffin, N. H. Cohen, R. M. Wachter, J. M. Luce, and P. C. Hopewell. 1986. Ethical dilemmas about intensive care in patients with AIDS. Background paper. Washington, D.C.: Committee on a National Strategy for AIDS.

Martin, J. P. 1986. The AIDS home care and hospice program. A multidisciplinary approach to caring for persons with AIDS. Am. J. Hosp. Care 3:35-37.

McHolland, G. F., and W. Weller. 1985. Summary Report on California AIDS Victims: Quantitative Analysis. Sacramento, Calif.: California Department of Health Services.

Meskin, S., and J. Klemm. 1986. Preliminary estimate of the impact of AIDS on the Medicaid program. Unpublished draft paper. Baltimore, Md.: Health Care Financing Administration.

Morin, S. F., K. A. Charles, and A. K. Malyon. 1984. Psychological impact of AIDS on gay men. Am. Psychol. 39:1288-1293.

Navia, B. A., B. D. Jordan, and R. W. Price. 1986. The AIDS dementia complex: I. Clinical features. Ann. Neurol. 19:517-524.

Nichols, S. E. 1985. Psychosocial reactions of persons with the acquired immunodeficiency syndrome. Ann. Intern. Med. 103:765-767.

Perry, S. W., and P. Jacobsen. 1986. Neuropsychiatric manifestations of AIDS spectrum disorders. Hosp. Comm. Psychiatry 37:135-142.

Perry, S. W., and J. Markowitz. In press. Psychiatric intervention for AIDS spectrum disorders. Hosp. Comm. Psychiatry.

Pindyck, J., J. Avorn, P. Cleary, et al. 1986. Notification of anti-HTLV-III/LAV positive blood donors: Psychosocial, counseling and care issues. World Health Organization Report on AIDS. Geneva: World Health Organization.

Polan, H. J., D. Hellerstein, and J. Amchin. 1985. Impact of AIDS-related cases on an inpatient therapeutic milieu. Hosp. Comm. Psychiatry 36:173-176.

President's Commission for the Study of Ethical Problems in Medicine and Biomedical and Behavioral Research. 1983a. Deciding to Forgo Life Sustaining Technology. Washington, D.C.: U.S. Government Printing Office.

President's Commission for the Study of Ethical Problems in Medicine and Biomedical and

Behavioral Research. 1983b. Securing Access to Health Care. Washington, D.C.: U.S. Government Printing Office.

Public Health Service. 1985. PHS recommendations for preventing transmission of infections with HTLV-III/LAV in the workplace. Morbid. Mortal. Weekly Rep. 34:681-695.

Raffin, T. A., B. Lo, R. M. Wachter, J. M. Luce, and N. H. Cohen. 1986. Intensive care for patients with the acquired immunodeficiency syndrome. Background paper. Washington, D.C.: Committee on a National Strategy for AIDS.

Rettig, R. A. 1980. The politics of health cost containment: End stage renal disease. Bull. N.Y. Acad. Med. 56:115-138.

Scitovsky, A. A., D. P. Rice, J. Showstack, and P. R. Lee. 1986. Estimating the Direct and Indirect Economic Costs of the Acquired Immune Deficiency Syndrome, 1985, 1986, and 1990. Task order 282-85-0061, #2. Atlanta, Ga.: Centers for Disease Control.

Smith, E. 1986. Testimony before the Subcommittee on Health and the Environment, U.S. House of Representatives, March 5, 1986.

Snider, W. D., D. M. Simpson, G. Nielsen, J. W. M. Gold, C. Metroka, and J. B. Posner. 1983. Neurological complications of acquired immunodeficiency syndrome: Analysis of 50 patients. Ann. Neurol. 14:403-418.

Steinbrook, R., B. Lo, J. Moulton, H. Hollander, and P. A. Volberding. 1986. Preference of homosexual men with the acquired immunodeficiency syndrome for life-sustaining treatment. N. Engl. J. Med. 314:457-460.

Stoller, B. 1986. Impact of AIDS on the well child. Paper presented at the public meeting of the Committee on a National Strategy for AIDS. New York, May 15, 1986.

Tross, S. 1985. Psychological and neuropsychological functions in AIDS patients. Paper presented at the International Conference on AIDS, Atlanta, Ga., April 14-17, 1985.

U.S. Congress. 1986. Consolidated Omnibus Budget Reconciliation Act, P.L. 99-272. Washington, D.C.: U.S. Government Printing Office.

Volberding, P. A. 1985. The clinical spectrum of the acquired immunodeficiency syndrome: Implications for comprehensive patient care. Ann. Intern. Med. 103:729-733.

Volberding, P. A. 1986. Variation in AIDS related illnesses: Impact on clinical research. P. 5 in Abstracts of the Second International Conference on AIDS, Paris, June 23-25, 1986.

6

Future Research Needs

In the brief period since the first descriptions of HIV and its unambiguous identification as the cause of AIDS, a tremendous amount has been learned about the genetic structure and transmission of the virus. Much less is known, however, about how it initiates infection, how it maintains infection, and what determines the progression and diversity of the resulting illness.

Research has been very effective in discovering the routes of viral transmission, enabling public health and education programs to be designed that incorporate increasingly accurate and specific information. Research has also been particularly effective in elucidating the complete genomic structure of the virus, allowing definition of many, if not all, of the virus's genes.

Such insights, however impressive, are only the beginning of what promises to be a long and difficult path toward effective therapeutic interventions to minimize or eliminate the debilitating effects of HIV infection and toward limiting the spread of the virus by means of safe and effective vaccines.

This chapter summarizes some of the opportunities and obstacles that will be encountered along that path. In many areas, predictions of progress are difficult to make. It is easier, however, to specify the mechanisms that will facilitate that progress. Successful development of vaccines or drugs to modify the prevalence or consequences of HIV infection will be greatly aided by a substantially improved basic understanding of the virus, of the functioning of the healthy and impaired human immune system, and of their interaction in the progression from infection to disease.

The progress achieved to date in identifying and characterizing the causative agent of AIDS would not have been possible without the scientific and medical knowledge achieved over the years through the pursuit of basic biomedical research. In that pursuit, the investigator is rarely certain of when or if research findings will be applicable to a disease. The instance of AIDS exemplifies the value of basic research, however, in that the current understanding of AIDS is based on knowledge derived largely from studies carried out before AIDS was even recognized as a disease. The unusual speed with which the etiologic agent of AIDS was isolated and remarkably well characterized was heavily dependent upon 20 years of investment in molecular biology and virology.

Continued support of the medical and scientific communities in their pursuit of basic knowledge related to HIV infection and AIDS will provide an essential adjunct to the necessary applied studies. These basic and applied studies can be expected to prove mutually beneficial as increased understanding of the mechanisms and consequences of HIV infection is translated into effective interventions to limit the virus's impact.

THE STRUCTURE AND REPLICATION OF HIV

Retroviral Structure

The molecular cloning and nucleotide analysis of a number of independent isolates of HIV have completely defined a retroviral genomic structure (see Figure 6-1) of unprecedented complexity and marked diversity (Meusing et al., 1985; Ratner et al., 1985; Sanchez-Pescador et al., 1985; Wain-Hobson et al., 1985). While HIV shares some genetic and structural elements with other known retroviruses, it possesses distinctive features that have not been observed previously.

The replication cycles of all previously known retroviruses depend on the functions of the protein products encoded by three viral genes termed *gag, pol,* and *env* (Weiss et al., 1985). These genes specify the structural and enzymatic functions required for viral infection and transmission and are situated in a common left-to-right (5' to 3') configuration in the retroviral genome. The *gag* gene encodes the proteins that constitute the internal core of the virion particle. The *pol* gene specifies the viral enzyme known as reverse transcriptase, which is responsible for synthesizing a DNA copy of the retroviral RNA genome early after infection. The gag and pol proteins are first synthesized as a large precursor, which is then cleaved by a virus-encoded protease to give the final proteins. The *env* gene codes for the surface envelope proteins of the retrovirus, which mediate the process of

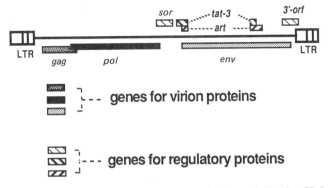

genes for virion proteins

genes for regulatory proteins

FIGURE 6-1 HIV genome. Source: Courtesy of Howard Temin, University of Wisconsin School of Medicine, Madison.

virus binding to the surface membranes of host target cells. The termini of the DNA form of the retroviral genome are provided by repetitive sequences known as long terminal repeats (LTRs), which contain the essential genetic regulatory elements controlling viral expression and integration.

With these three genes and the additional regulatory sequences in their LTRs, many animal retroviruses are fully competent to replicate in an appropriate host target cell. HIV, however, contains a minimum of four additional genes (see Figure 6-1), at least two of which are also functionally required in its replication cycle. Because they have been independently described in a number of laboratories, these novel genes carry a multitude of designations. A gene known as *tat*-III serves a necessary function in HIV replication by controlling, in a *trans*-acting fashion (i.e., at a distance by means of a diffusible product), the level of expression of the other viral genes (Arya et al., 1985; Sodroski et al., 1984). The most recently discovered HIV gene, variously known as *art* or *trs,* is thought to control, in a *trans*-acting manner, the differential expression of viral structural and regulatory functions; it is also necessary for viral replication (Feinberg et al., in press; Sodroski et al., 1986b). Two other viral genes, named *sor* (also known as *orf*-1, *P'*, or *Q*) and 3'-*orf* (also known as *orf*-2, *E'*, or *F*), serve unknown functions in the life-cycle of HIV, although they are known to be expressed. They are apparently not needed for replication in tissue culture cells (Allan et al., 1985; Fisher et al., 1986b; Kan et al., 1986; Lee et al., 1985; Sodroski et al., 1986a).

Retroviral Replication

Retroviral infection (see Figure 6-2) is initiated by the binding of a virus particle to a specific receptor molecule expressed on the surface of an

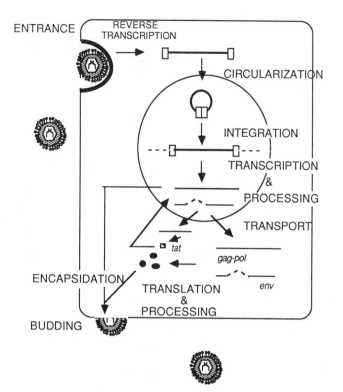

FIGURE 6-2 Life-cycle of HIV. Source: Courtesy of Howard Temin, University of Wisconsin School of Medicine, Madison.

appropriate target cell (Weiss et al., 1985). After binding takes place, the retrovirus enters the cell and uncoats in the host cell's cytoplasm. The retroviral genetic information contained in its single-stranded RNA genome is then transferred to a full-length linear duplex DNA intermediate by the synthetic activities of the reverse transcriptase enzyme, which accompanied it in the virion particle. This linear DNA intermediate is transported to the nucleus, where it is circularized before becoming stably integrated into the DNA of the host cell. The process of integration is thought to involve the specific interaction between retroviral sequences at the edges of the LTRs and an additional enzymatic function known as the integrase encoded by the *pol* gene.

Once integrated into the host chromosome, the retroviral genome is termed a provirus. There it serves as a template for RNA transcription, the primary product of which is a full-length viral RNA molecule. The gag and pol products are translated from the full-length transcript, while a portion of the viral transcript undergoes RNA splicing to yield an envelope-coding mRNA from which the *gag* and *pol* sequences have been deleted. The mRNAs encoding the sor, tat-III, art, and 3'-orf proteins of HIV are derived from the genomic RNA transcript via complex splicing events (Arya et al., 1985; Muesing et al., 1985; Rabson et al., 1985). The virus's structural and regulatory proteins are then synthesized in the cytoplasm. Following secondary processing, the constituents of the virions (gag, pol, and envelope proteins) proceed to assemble in the proximity of the cellular plasma membrane into virus particles that have incorporated the full-length viral RNA genome. The retroviral membrane is derived directly from the cellular plasma membrane as the virion is released from the cell by a process known as budding.

The development of specific antiviral therapies for HIV infection will depend upon identifying and interfering with critical stages of the retroviral life-cycle. Although the replicative mechanisms of HIV have not yet been studied in great detail, many of its essential processes may be understood through analogy with other, more thoroughly analyzed examples of retroviruses. It should not be assumed, however, that HIV follows a pattern of replication identical to those previously elucidated in other retroviral systems. Indeed, some significant differences have already been identified. As discussed below, these may provide additional targets for future antiviral strategies.

Definition of the Structural and Functional Constituents of HIV

The protein products from all seven of the genes so far identified in HIV isolates have been recognized by antibodies from persons infected with HIV. This has permitted the initial identification of these proteins and has demonstrated their expression *in vivo*. Some of these protein products have also been expressed in bacteria, yeast, or mammalian cells *in vitro*.

The production of large quantities of all of the virus's genes in a biologically active form will provide necessary substrates for structural and functional analyses. In addition to the study of such recombinant DNA products, it will be important to directly study the native proteins as they exist in the virion and in infected cells. Their directly determined amino acid sequences (as opposed to computer translations from the DNA sequence), and the nature and location of posttranslational modifications (e.g., glycosylation, phosphorylation, myristylation), should be ascertained. The nature of the proteolytic cleavages and other posttranslational processing involved in the synthesis of the virus's structural or functional components may thus be established, perhaps indicating new approaches for antiviral interventions.

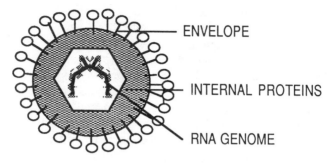

FIGURE 6-3 Structure of the HIV virion. Source: Courtesy of Howard Temin, University of Wisconsin School of Medicine, Madison.

Determination of the Structure of the HIV Virion

Figure 6-3 shows a model of the structure of the HIV virion. Electron microscopic examinations of HIV particles show that it possesses an envelope with protruding spikes surrounding a central electron-dense core. The virion's spikes are formed by collections of the viral envelope glycoprotein, gp120, which is anchored in the cell-derived plasma membrane through an attachment to the HIV transmembrane protein, gp41. The retroviral core is composed of collections of the gag proteins in association with the genomic RNA molecules, the reverse transcriptase, and other enzymes.

Although there are generally accepted models for the structure of the interior of retrovirus virions, the models are conceptual in character and lack experimental validation (Weiss et al., 1982, 1985). Thus, the detailed structure of the potentially analogous virion of HIV is not clearly understood. Specifically, the locations and amounts of the various internal proteins and the nature of their interactions are not known. Knowledge of these locations and interactions will be of great utility in drug design. For example, drugs that inhibit the formation of any of these complexes could block HIV replication.

High-resolution structural determinations of the viral proteins, separately and in complexes, need to be performed; important candidates include the external portion of gp120, the gp120-gp41 complex, and the gp120-gp41-internal protein complex. Similar structural studies have been performed with the hemagglutinin molecule of influenza virus and with the virions of rhinovirus 14 and poliovirus (Hogle et al., 1985; Rossman et al., 1985; Wilson et al., 1981) and have provided an important foundation for understanding the interaction between infecting viruses and host cells and between viruses and neutralizing antibodies.

Interrupting Infection by HIV

The progressive stages in the life-cycle of HIV present a number of opportunities for specific interruption. Much basic knowledge must be attained, however, before a rational approach to the development of prophylactic and therapeutic measures for HIV infection and AIDS will be feasible.

A critical and early event in HIV infection involves the virus's attachment, via its envelope glycoprotein, to a receptor on the surface of a susceptible cell. The primary, if not exclusive, cellular receptor for HIV appears to be provided by the CD4 molecule (Dalgleish et al., 1984; Klatzmann et al., 1984). The CD4 molecule is expressed by helper/inducer T lymphocytes and by certain types of cells of the macrophage/monocyte lineage, a distribution that parallels the target cells for HIV infection. The expression of the CD4 molecule may completely explain the tissue tropism of HIV, although further documentation of the complete repertoire of the cell types that express the molecule is necessary (see section on "Natural History of HIV Infection," below).

The interaction of the HIV envelope protein with the CD4 receptor can be inhibited by antibodies directed at specific determinants on either molecule (Robert-Guroff et al., 1985; Weiss et al., 1985). The structural definition of the molecular components involved in this specific recognition process will be of central importance in the development of vaccines or other prophylactic measures to prevent HIV infection. The HIV envelope protein, through its specific interaction with the CD4 molecule, plays an important role in the cytopathic effect of viral infection on T lymphocytes (Lifson et al., 1986, in press; Sodroski et al., 1986a). The specific inhibition of this interaction, if attainable, may ameliorate the immune deficiency that follows HIV infection.

The HIV envelope glycoprotein is unlike the similar components of most other retroviruses, both in its large size and in the extent and pattern of its sequence variability (Coffin, 1986). The primary translation product of the HIV envelope gene is heavily glycosylated during the course of its maturation. The extensive variation that has been observed in the nucleotides (and thus in the predicted amino acid sequences) among independent isolates of HIV is of important theoretical and practical concern in understanding the processes of viral replication and in developing an effective vaccine. Such variation, though striking, is not unexpected in a virus whose genome is composed of a single strand of nucleic acid. High mutation rates may be an unavoidable consequence of the replication of such genomes.

In addition, genomic variation in retroviruses can be affected by the insertion, duplication, and deletion of genetic sequences. HIV isolates show significant sequence divergence within the *env* gene by these mechanisms while their other genes are considerably better conserved between different viral isolates. The variability in the *env* gene is concentrated within several "hypervariable" domains, which are interspersed between regions that are better conserved (Coffin, 1986). The mechanisms that generate this pattern of variability and conservation of envelope sequences will be important to elucidate, as will the functions of the variable and relatively constant regions.

Because all HIV isolates apparently infect cells through the binding of the envelope protein to CD4, the domain of the viral envelope protein that facilitates binding to the cell surface receptor is presumably conserved between viral isolates. Inhibiting this recognition process through immunization or other approaches could in principle block infection by all viral isolates. It has been postulated, however, that the variable regions mask the essential constant regions from immunologic attack. Success in developing an HIV vaccine may thus be predicated on understanding and overcoming the problems presented by the genetic mutability and variation of HIV.

Following attachment to its cellular receptor, HIV enters the cell by a mechanism as yet poorly defined. The virus is internalized and uncoated, most probably through the normal absorptive endocytosis pathway used by animal cells to internalize cell surface receptors that have bound their respective ligand. As with other animal viruses, a low pH-mediated structural change in the gp120 molecule in the endocytotic vesicles probably results in the actual uncoating and entrance of the viral genome into the cytoplasm. In the case of HIV, this process may or may not involve a membrane fusion event. Increased understanding of this process may allow the derivation of drugs that inhibit these early stages of infection in a virus-specific manner.

Once the retroviral particle has uncoated in the cytoplasm, the critical and characteristic process of reverse transcription of the viral RNA genome into a double-stranded DNA copy ensues. The enzyme that catalyzes this process, reverse transcriptase, provides a specific and potentially very effective target for antiviral therapy. Inhibitors of HIV's reverse transcriptase comprise a number of the candidate drugs under current clinical and laboratory evaluation (see section on "Antiviral Agents," below). The protein components and processing pathways for the synthesis of HIV's reverse transcriptase are receiving substantial analytical attention. The forces that govern the HIV genome's migration to the nucleus and subsequent circularization are not known. The virus-specific integrase encoded by the *pol* gene is thought to be involved in the process of retroviral integration in other retroviruses. Unlike most retroviruses, HIV shares with the other lentiviruses a pronounced tendency to accumulate unintegrated viral DNA in the course of infection *in vitro* and *in vivo*. It is thus possible that HIV does not always require integration for virus production to ensue. With the related lentivirus visna virus, dividing cells are reportedly not required for productive infection, although many other retroviruses demonstrate an obligate linkage between cell division and viral integration (Haase, 1986). Whether cell division is required for HIV infection has not been established, but studies of viral production in macrophage cultures *in vitro* suggest that it may not be necessary (Gartner et al., 1986).

The significance and origin of unintegrated HIV DNA are unclear, but they may have significant implications for understanding the cytopathic effects of the virus and for the potential of therapeutic agents to limit infection. Improved understanding of the requirements for and mechanisms of HIV integration, increasing availability of enzymatically active viral proteins involved in the process, and the development of cell-free systems for their assay will help in drug design and screening.

Following integration into the host cell chromosome—a mechanism that needs to be studied further—the HIV proviral genome is transcribed into RNA by the cellular RNA polymerase. The potential host or viral factors that control the level of HIV expression are very poorly defined, but they may play a critical role in the persistence of HIV in the infected human host and the rate of immunologic compromise. It has been suggested that immunologic activation of infected T cells stimulates virus production (Hoxie et al., 1985; Zagury et al., 1986). The factors that activate provirus also need to be studied further. Subsequent to transcription, the processing of the HIV RNA transcripts also uses the host cell's machinery for capping, polyadenylation, and splicing. The *tat*-III gene is known to be essential for viral replication (Dayton et al., 1986; Fisher et al., 1986a), but there is much uncertainty about its precise mechanism of action. It appears to control the efficiency of translation of viral messages (Feinberg et al., in press; Rosen et al., 1986) and their stability, although effects on viral transcription have also been described. This gene operates through specific sequences contained in HIV mRNAs, and as there are no known host activities of similar character it may provide a specific target for drug attack.

A second HIV gene has been described that appears to operate subsequent to the transcription of viral RNA. This gene, variously known as *art* (Sodroski et al., 1986b) or *trs* (Feinberg et al., in press), effectively modulates the specific viral mRNAs available for translation. The art (trs) product regulates the pattern of viral RNA expressed, either through differential splicing or specific message stabilization, and is essential for HIV replication. Its exact role in the *in vivo* infectious process or pathology of HIV is unknown, but because it also appears to be an essential and virus-specific activity it is an important potential candidate for antiviral therapy.

As with the other viral components, the large-scale preparation and widespread availability of the tat-III and art (trs) proteins would aid in the design of inhibitors for their essential viral functions. Presently, the limiting factors are understanding their actions and developing *in vitro* assays for their functions.

The products of the HIV genes known as *sor* (*orf*-1, *P'*, and *Q*) and 3'-*orf* (*orf*-2, *E'*, and *F*) may not always be essential for virus replication in cell culture (Fisher et al., 1986b; Sodroski et al., 1986c). However, the continued presence of these open reading frames in HIV in the face of the high rate of mutation of retroviruses in general, and of HIV in particular, indicates that there has been strong selection for these genes in the virus infecting the human population. (With an estimated mutation rate of 1 alteration per 10,000 nucleotides per virus replication cycle, mutations would have appeared following only a few rounds of virus replication.) The importance of these genes is also suggested by the presence of antibodies against them in the sera of many HIV-infected persons. Their preservation and serologic recognition suggest that they serve an essential role in the *in vivo* expression of HIV.

Improved understanding of the *in vivo* role of these novel open reading frames of HIV is extremely important, especially if they are involved in the biological processes underlying the persistent nature or cytopathic consequences of HIV infection. Identifying their functions and developing *in vitro* assays for their measurement will be of great value in evaluating their candidacy as effective targets for pharmacologic inhibition. If their functions are only evident in infected hosts, the development of animal models will be central to progress in this area (see section on "Animal Models," below).

Viral precursor proteins are translated from viral mRNAs by use of host cell ribosomes and translation factors. The *gag* gene is translated through the synthesis of a protein precursor, Pr55, which is subsequently proteolytically processed into p17, p24, p9, and p7. The *pol* gene, which encodes the HIV reverse transcriptase, integrase, and probably protease, is thought to be initially translated into a polyprotein precursor, Pr150, which is then processed into p64/53, p22, and p34, respectively.

The proteolytic cleavage of the gag and pol precursor proteins may be carried out by the virally encoded protease enzyme. If so, this cleavage might be subject to specific inhibition. The derivation and production of enzymatically active p22 protease would provide a very useful substrate for drug screening and drug design.

The primary translation product of the *env* mRNA is a protein of approximately 90 kilodaltons (kd). During its transit to the cellular membrane, the envelope precursor is heavily glycosylated, which increases its apparent molecular weight to about 160 kd. The extent of this glycosylation of the HIV envelope protein is unprecedented among retroviruses. The observed relative conservation of glycosylation sites between divergent viral isolates suggests that glycosylation of the envelope protein plays an important biological role. Unlike that of many other retroviruses, the transmembrane protein (gp41) of HIV is also glycosylated. Glycosylation could conceivably be an important determinant of the structure of the envelope, it could mask functionally important antigenic sites from human immune responses, or it could do both.

The mature form of the viral envelope is achieved by the proteolytic cleavage of the gp160 precursor to gp120 and gp41. After the gp120-gp41 complex is inserted in the plasma membrane by cellular processes, there is probably an aggregation of gp120-gp41 molecules that excludes other cellular membrane proteins. The nature of the chemical bonds maintaining the stable interaction between the gp120 and gp41 molecules should be determined as a possible specific target for drugs. Likewise, the orientation of these proteins in the cell membrane and the virion particle has not been directly determined, but such information is important for drug design.

HIV is formed by budding from a modified portion of the cell plasma membrane, during which the viral nucleoid assembles and organizes the gag proteins in association with copies of the genomic RNA and polymerase components. The formation of the nucleoid involves the aggregation of p24 gag molecules in a virus-specific process. There may be further protein cleavages after budding, a process referred to as maturation in the life-cycle of other retroviruses.

As with other viruses the process of HIV assembly depends upon protein-protein interactions. The protein interactions in assembling virions have to be virus specific, otherwise virion production would be exceptionally inefficient or absent. As such, the process of HIV assembly may be subject to chemotherapeutic interference and hence merits further study. Interferons and related molecules have been demonstrated to inhibit the assembly and budding process in other retroviruses, including certain lentiviruses, and similar molecules may have relevance in combating HIV infection and spread (Narayan, 1986).

Conclusions and Recommendations

In the past few years the techniques of molecular biology have provided the starting materials for a detailed evaluation of the replicative pathways of HIV and for the development of therapeutic strategies to inhibit those pathways. Although HIV was only discovered in 1983-1984, research has been so rapid and so successful that almost as much is now known about its molecular virology as about any other retrovirus. However, less is presently known about HIV-cell interactions than for many other retroviruses. As the pathogenesis of AIDS is clearly related to the interaction of the causative virus with the susceptible host, at the levels of both the target cell and the host organism, much more must be learned about the biology of HIV infection.

Although an empirical approach to the development of prophylactic and therapeutic measures for HIV infection and AIDS may work, rational strategies are more likely to succeed, and these will require a good knowledge base. Thus, most of the basic information on HIV and the consequences of its infection may be relevant to the prevention, control, and treatment of AIDS. Furthermore, much of the research on HIV will not only be relevant to AIDS but will increase understanding of the human immune system in health and disease, of pathogenic infections and cancers, and of the basic mechanisms controlling gene expression.

• Success in the development of vaccines or drugs to prevent and treat AIDS will be facilitated by a greatly improved understanding of the basic biological processes and consequences of HIV infection. Rational approaches to interfering with the mechanisms of HIV replication and spread present the most hopeful path to the development of effective antiviral agents but will require a substantial increase in the knowledge base concerning the genetic, structural, and biological characteristics of HIV and viruses apparently related to it, such as LAV-2 and HTLV-IV (see Chapter 2). Continuing efforts to fully determine the life-cycle and structure of HIV should be expanded and actively encouraged. The characterization of all viral proteins and their interactions with cellular proteins and processes should have a high priority. These studies should include structural (X-ray crystallographic) studies of HIV, reverse transcriptase, protease, integrase, glycoproteins, and regulatory proteins.

• Strategies dedicated to prevention of the clinical manifestations of HIV infection and AIDS must also be predicated on a greatly improved understanding of the normal functioning of the human immune system (see section on "Natural History of HIV Infection," below).

• Expansion of the research base on HIV is limited by the availability and adequacy of biological containment facilities, especially for virus production. Adequate financial support should be made available for expansion and creation of appropriate facilities. Coordinated and shared use of containment facilities should be a concern in the minimization of costs and maximization of access.

• An extremely important aspect of the entire future AIDS research effort is the wide and free distribution among scientists of various viruses, DNA clones, proteins, cell lines, and other reagents as they are created. This availability will speed the entry of researchers into the field and ensure compatibility and quick dissemination of results.

• To facilitate the most productive pursuit of AIDS-related research, it is important to widen the pool of investigators and laboratories engaged in the analysis of HIV. Efforts must be undertaken to encourage an ever-increasing breadth and expertise in the area of AIDS research.

• The benefits of the United States' traditional commitment to basic biomedical research are clearly demonstrated in the expeditious identification of the causative agent of AIDS, the derivation of a test to detect its presence, and the rapidly evolving understanding of its genetic constitution and replicative requirements. The types of basic studies that permitted these impressive accomplishments may also be expected to yield valuable insights into therapeutic approaches to limit the establishment and progression of HIV infection. Thus, basic research studies in virology and immunology should be considered an important part of the AIDS research effort and should be fortified in the years ahead (see section on "Funding for Research Related to AIDS and HIV," below).

• Given the current and expected level of public interest and anxiety relating to AIDS, scientists must recognize their special obligation in this situation to communicate their results in an accurate, responsible fashion. Biomedical scientists have an important role to play in the public educational efforts related to AIDS. However, the all too prevalent tendency toward simplistic interpretation or sensationalization of AIDS-related research in the media should actively be discouraged. Significant harm to the public's perception of the AIDS threat and to the credibility of the scientific community will also accrue if laboratory, clinical, or epidemiologic results are presented with exaggerated significance.

NATURAL HISTORY OF HIV INFECTION

Transmission of HIV

For an HIV infection to become established, infectious virus must be delivered to a susceptible host. The presence of HIV has been reported in samples of peripheral blood, cell-free plasma, lymph nodes, bone marrow cells, cerebrospinal fluid, brain tissues, semen, cervical and vaginal secretions, lung tissue, saliva, and tears (Gartner et al., 1986; Ho et al., 1985c; Salahuddin et al., 1985; Shaw et al., 1985). Although termed "isolations," some of these reports have, in fact, been based only on transient measurements of reverse-transcriptase-like activities in a tissue culture sample. As such, they have not definitively documented the presence of infectious HIV. It is important to validate each of these reported sources of HIV isolation and to attempt to meaningfully estimate the resident viral load and the frequency with which the virus can be detected.

Exposure to any fluid containing HIV could, in theory, present a risk for viral transmission. However, a substantial body of epidemiologic data indicates that the virus is spread only from a limited number of sources and received through a limited number of routes (see Chapter 2). These are sexual intercourse with an infected individual involving the exchange of semen or cervical/vaginal secretions, exposure to infected blood or blood products through therapeutic transfusion or the sharing of needles and other equipment that allow the passage of blood from one individual to another, and the perinatal passage of virus from infected mothers to their infants.

The relative efficiencies of transmission of HIV from different sources and through different routes are not known in detail, but these are important questions for future epidemiologic and laboratory analyses. Levels of the dose of HIV needed for establishment of an infection may also vary with the mode of spread and the portal of entry. Such differences presumably underlie the apparent discrepancies that exist between the sources of viral isolations and the common routes of transmission that have been defined through epidemiologic studies.

Certain host behaviors or factors have been suggested to enhance the transmission of HIV infection, although the presently available data are inadequate to allow certainty. For instance, studies of the risk of infection among African heterosexual populations have suggested that an increased efficiency of HIV spread is associated with the presence of other sexually transmitted diseases (see Chapter 2). It is not known if there are important interactions occurring in a host during infection with different infectious agents, if local compromise or inflammation of the genital mucosa may be the factors that enhance the viral infection, or if these processes are coincidental.

So-called "traumatic" sexual behaviors such as receptive anal intercourse have also been postulated to enhance HIV transmission by permitting the virus to enter the bloodstream through locally damaged blood vessels. While epidemiologic studies clearly show that receptive anal intercourse is associated with an increased risk of HIV infection, interpretation of this observation is difficult in light of the high prevalence of viral infection in the sexual partners of persons engaging in this practice. Recent reports of seroconversion in women who were artificially inseminated by an asymptomatic virus carrier argue against a requirement for "traumatic" sexual intercourse in the transmission of HIV (Stewart et al., 1985). Furthermore, in experimental animal systems, chimpanzees can readily be infected by atraumatic vaginal inoculation with HIV (Fultz et al., 1986a). Thus, trauma may have no biological relevance in HIV transmission, and emphasizing it may obscure the demonstrated potential for both heterosexual and homosexual spread of the virus. However, this issue requires clarification. The relative efficiency of male-to-female compared with female-to-male transmission of HIV is not known, but these efficiencies will be crucial determinants of the rate of spread of HIV infection within the heterosexual population.

The state of HIV actually involved in viral transmission, whether cell-free or cell-associated, has not been determined. It is a critical concern, however, for understanding HIV infection and for the development of an antiviral vaccine. Research on other lentiviruses suggests that viral transmission by cell-to-cell contact provides the major route of exposure for the previously uninfected host (Haase, 1986; Narayan, 1986). Moreover, very little, if any, cell-free virus can be detected in chronically infected animals. Unfortunately, a similar situation may prevail in the transmission of HIV, but this remains to be established. HIV infection of hemophiliacs by virally contaminated clotting-factor concentrates (see Chapter 2) suggests that cell-associated virus may not always be necessary, yet it may still provide the most frequent vehicle for transmission.

The cell types that provide the earliest targets for HIV replication in the initiation of an infection are not known. Their location at the time of infection is also unknown, but both of these variables may depend on the route of initial exposure. Both T lymphocytes and macrophages that express the CD4 molecule provide susceptible host cells for HIV infection *in vitro,* and these may also be the initial *in vivo* targets for infection. Given the relative longevity and mobility of these cells, the HIV infection may then spread throughout the host. Systematic studies need to be conducted to determine the frequency with which virus can be isolated from various cells and tissues of persons who show antibodies to HIV.

The Immune System Response to HIV Infection

As described in Chapter 2, the earliest and most easily detectable marker for viral infection is the presence of antibodies reactive with HIV in the serum of an infected individual. However, a very small subset of infected individuals have been reported to remain seronegative for prolonged periods of time (Salahuddin et al., 1984). The available studies cannot establish the length of time that such a virus-positive antibody-negative state exists in those individuals, nor can they estimate the prevalence of such individuals in the population. Future studies must address these questions, especially since clarification of this problem is necessary for better protection of the blood supply (see Appendix C).

Unlike many other viral infections of humans, antibody synthesis against HIV does not herald the clearing of the infection. With HIV, the virus can continue to be isolated from seropositive persons long after their initial exposure (Feorino et al., 1985; Jaffe et al., 1985). The lentiviruses of other animals are known to cause infections that persist throughout the lifetime of the infected host. Unfortunately, it appears that HIV may similarly establish a lifelong infection in humans. The presence of antibodies against HIV in the serum is thus not a marker of immunity but rather, in most instances, an indication of ongoing infection.

It is not yet known if the immune response of some individuals, although unable to eliminate HIV infection, may protect them from the development of immunologic damage and disease. While there may be some change in the pattern of serologic reactivity with specific HIV protein components during the progression from infection to disease (see Appendix B), so far no specific patterns have been found to correlate with protection of health or development of disease.

One aspect of the immune response critical to vaccine development efforts is the possible existence of specific antibodies to HIV that could prevent, limit, or eliminate infection by the virus. Such antibodies are referred to as neutralizing antibodies, and an important goal for candidate vaccine immunogens is to elicit these types of antibodies. Neutralizing antibodies have been found in some individuals over the course of their infection with HIV, but they are present in rather low concentrations (Robert-Guroff et al., 1985; Weiss et al., 1985) and appear incapable of curing an individual's infection.

With HIV, neutralizing antibodies have been measured using *in vitro* assays that involve mixing the cell-free virus with a test serum and then evaluating the continued infectivity of the virus preparation by exposing susceptible target cells to it. If, as with other lentiviruses, HIV is spread by transmission from an infected cell to a normal cell, then the presently employed neutralization assays may have little relevance to the immunologic mechanisms that would effectively prevent viral infection. In humans infected with HIV, as in other animals infected with lentiviruses, the viral infection persists in the face of a neutralizing antibody response. Whether the currently used assays for HIV neutralization bear any correlation with disease progression remains to be established, but this is an important area for further evaluation.

In addition to the antibody response generated by the humoral components of the host immune system, a protective response to a viral infection can also be mediated through the cellular immune system. With many other types of viruses, the host's cellular immune system is the critical determinant of protection from and cure of viral infection. This system consists of specifically immune cytotoxic T cells and a variety of other effector cells, including natural killer cells, macrophages, and other constitutive killer cells. The disruptive effects inflicted on the human immune system by HIV are well documented with respect to the obvious clinical manifestation of disease. However, the more subtle interactions concerning the specific cellular immune response to HIV and the determinants of that response's success or failure are almost a complete mystery. Many questions remain to be answered, including the specific types of cellular immune responses that might afford some protection from HIV infection, potential means of enhancing their antiviral efficacy, and the reasons for their apparent failure in the course of a natural infection (Weissman, 1986).

The Immunologic Consequences of HIV Infection

Once an HIV infection becomes established, compromise of the immune system can be detected in most, if not all, infected persons. The severity of this compromise may range from abnormalities detectable only by sophisticated immunologic analyses to the virtual collapse of the immune system seen in AIDS. The factors that determine the initiation of this immunologic decline, the rate of its progression, and its ultimate outcome are unknown. While it is possible that specific strains of HIV may be particularly pathogenic or have proclivities to induce specific types of immunologic or neurologic pathology, such correlations have yet to become evident.

The possible existence of endogenous (e.g., genetic) or exogenous (e.g., environmental) exposures that modulate the course of HIV-induced immunocompromise is a topic of great interest. Generally referred to as "cofactors," these secondary factors could provide a target for limiting disease development in persons infected with HIV. *In vitro* studies of HIV expression have suggested that virus production and cytopathic effects are enhanced by the immunologic stimulation of infected T lymphocytes (Hoxie et al., 1985; Zagury et al., 1986). However, it is not known if an *in vivo* analogy exists for this observation, and epidemiologic analyses have so far failed to identify any environmental cofactors that strongly correlate with disease development (see Chapter 2). Nevertheless, the relevance of cofactors to disease development remains of exceptional theoretical and practical importance. Well-controlled epidemiologic and laboratory evaluations are needed to assess this issue.

The range of cells that harbor virus *in vivo* during the course of an HIV infection has yet to be completely elucidated. Infection can be documented in T cells and macrophages in the lymphatic tissues, peripheral bloodstream, and extralymphatic organs (e.g., the lung). The central nervous system also provides a common target for viral infection and pathology, although the identity of the infected target cells within the brain is controversial (see section on "Neurologic Complications" in Appendix A). The number, type, and location of all cells infected by HIV within an infected person need to be documented from the earliest stages of infection and throughout the development of immunosuppression.

Very little is known about the ability of HIV to infect or damage organs critical for T-lymphoid maturation—namely the bone marrow, where T-lymphoid precursors originate, or the thymus, where they are thought to assume antigenic specificity and functional competence. For any potential antiviral drug to have clinical benefit in a highly immunocompromised AIDS patient, it is essential that the immune system remain able to regenerate numerically adequate and functionally active lymphocytes. Should the T-lymphoid progenitor pool in the marrow be exhausted or the thymic environment be irrevocably damaged, this might not be possible.

Only a very small percentage (less than 0.01 percent) of peripheral blood and lymph node cells in an HIV-infected person appear to express viral proteins and nucleic acids (Harper et al., 1986b). It is not known whether virus-expressing cells constitute all of the cells infected *in vivo* or whether HIV infection can assume a latent state wherein the virus, although present in a cell, is not expressed. Latent states in which virus expression is variously restricted at the levels of transcription and translation of viral RNA have been described for other lentiviruses and are thought to play an essential role in the maintenance of their characteristic persistent viral infection (Haase, 1986; Narayan, 1986). A latent state of HIV infection has been produced *in vitro* using a leukemia T-cell line (Folks et al., 1986), but it is not clear if an *in vivo* parallel exists. A truly latent infection of normal CD4 T cells has not yet been definitively established *in vitro;* reports of persistent infections of peripheral blood lymphocytes may actually represent smoldering cytopathic processes (Hoxie et al., 1985; Zagury et al., 1986). This may not be surprising, for in the case of certain animal lentiviruses and human and animal herpesviruses the maintenance of viral persistence appears to rely on an interplay of viral and host regulatory contributions (Haase, 1986).

Since latent states might facilitate continued viral persistence and host infectiousness, as well as provide a mechanism of escape from antiviral therapies predicated upon the inhibition of HIV replication, their possible existence remains a critical unresolved research issue. It is very important to determine what fraction of cells in an infected person might be latently infected, what state the virus genome assumes in latently infected cells, how viral expression is maintained in a silent state, and how virus production may be reactivated.

As previously described, HIV has a rapid and obvious cytopathic effect on infected CD4 lymphocytes *in vitro*. Although the identical population of T lymphocytes is also depleted *in vivo*, a number of questions remain to be resolved before the mechanism and range of cytopathic consequences manifest in an infected person will be understood. Because HIV expression is only detectable in rare cells *in vivo*, it remains to be established whether direct virus-induced damage adequately explains the decline in CD4 cells, or whether indirect mechanisms are also involved. Postulated indirect effects include autoimmune destruction of T lymphocytes somehow selected by viral infection (Klatzmann and Montagnier, 1986; Williams et al., 1984), the liberation of immunocytotoxic substances from infected cells, or lymphoid inhibition secondary to the infection of cells with critical supporting roles in the immune response (e.g., macrophages). While indirect effects may play a critical role in the CD4 T-cell depletion, little experimental support is available for their existence. The slowly progressive tempo of immunologic decline may alternatively result from the persistent direct effects of viral infection resulting in slow but cumulative infliction of damage.

The exact mechanism of cell killing by HIV has not been established. In the few other retrovirus systems that have been studied in detail (Temin, 1986), cell killing upon viral infection is correlated with the expression of envelope proteins of particular antigenic type and the accumulation of quantities of unintegrated viral DNA resulting from a continuing process of reinfection. The cytopathic effect of the viral envelope and the presence of unintegrated DNA are also demonstrable in the course of HIV infection, and both may be intimately related to the ability of the virus to bind to the CD4 surface molecule. One of the most obvious cytopathic manifestations of HIV infection *in vitro* is the formation of multinucleated giant cells arising from the fusion of susceptible T lymphocytes, which results in their death (Klatzmann et al., 1984; Popovic et al., 1984). The formation of multinucleated cells, known as syncytia, is known to be a direct consequence of the interaction between the HIV envelope glycoprotein and the CD4 T-cell surface molecule (Lifson et al., in press; Lifson et al., 1986; Sodroski et al., 1986a). This interaction can readily be blocked by specific antibodies directed against the CD4 molecule, but it is only weakly inhibited by sera from infected persons (Lifson et al., in press; Lifson et al., 1986). The relative inability of sera from persons infected with HIV to prevent virus-induced T-lymphocyte cell fusion may allow both the continued spread of viral infection and the cytopathic consequences of viral expression. Also, the ability of one HIV-expressing cell to recruit other uninfected CD4-expressing T lymphocytes into syncytia may greatly amplify the extent of T-lymphocyte depletion, given only a few virus-expressing cells.

Cell fusion is an obvious manifestation of HIV-induced cytopathology, but it is not necessarily the only one. Furthermore, the mechanisms accounting for the depletion of CD4-positive T cells *in vivo* may also involve cell fusion, but essentially nothing is known about the specific processes of cell killing in an HIV-infected host. Determination of the mechanisms of cell death both *in vitro* and *in vivo* will be necessary in future efforts to understand and prevent the pathology of AIDS.

The cytopathic consequences of HIV infection may correlate with the level of expression of CD4 on susceptible target cells. This may underlie the ability of certain T lymphocytes and macrophages to support continued virus production (also known as a chronic infection) *in vitro* (De Rossi et al., 1986; Gartner et al., 1986; Lifson et al., in press; Popovic et al., 1984). It is not known if chronically infected cells can be maintained *in vivo* and if so how they differ from cells that die upon infection. The cytopathic effects of HIV infection have been attenuated *in vitro* by artificially constructed viral mutants that compromise envelope expression (Fisher et al., 1986b). The important and as yet unexplored possibility exists that different viral isolates vary in their ability to kill or infect cells and induce immunosuppressive disease. Because the interaction between the HIV envelope protein and the CD4 molecule plays an important role in both viral infectivity and pathogenicity, development of ways to interfere with it may afford valuable strategies for disease prevention.

As discussed in Chapter 2, the opportunistic infections and unusual malignancies that characterize AIDS are the most obvious manifestations of a severe underlying state of immunodeficiency. The broad spectrum and serious magnitude of the medical complications seen in HIV-infected persons have emphasized the central regulatory role that T lymphocytes play in the functioning of the immune system and in the preservation of health. However, there remain tremendous gaps in our understanding of the pathogenesis of the immunologic compromise of AIDS. Although apparent in *in vitro* assays and clinical manifestations, the nature and origin of the relevant immune deficits are not well established. The nature of the damage to the immune system that results from infection is not known, and the mechanisms and cellular targets by which the immunologic damage is manifest remain to be delineated. Similarly, the processes by which these specific defects in immune responsiveness and regulation are translated into specific susceptibility to opportunistic infections and malignancies are poorly defined. Much of this uncertainty reflects the limited basic knowledge about the functioning of the healthy human immune system. Future insights and interventions into the state of immunologic compromise in AIDS may necessarily depend on improved understanding of these basic processes.

Just as the mechanisms of HIV-induced cytopathology remain unresolved, the precise processes that account for the often profound immunologic impairment following viral infection await elucidation. A direct cytopathic insult to the CD4 T lymphocytes that results in their depletion is an attractive hypothesis. However, the simplicity of this hypothesis fails to adequately explain the complexity and pervasiveness of HIV-induced immunopathology. As discussed in Chapter 2, virtually all T-cell functions for which there exist *in vivo* or *in vitro* assays are markedly compromised or absent in persons with AIDS. These include delayed cutaneous hypersensitivity reactions, mitogen- and antigen-induced proliferative responses, generation of allogenic and autologous mixed lymphocyte reactions, cytotoxicity, lymphokine production, available help for B-cell antibody synthesis, and expression of interleukin-2 and interleukin-2 receptors (Seligmann et al., 1984). The specific defect accounting for most of these manifestations of immunodeficiency can be explained by the paucity of CD4 helper/inducer T cells, since most of these abnormalities are not measurable when the assay systems are corrected for CD4 T-cell number (Lane et al., 1985). However, an intrinsic defect has been observed in the ability of residual CD4 T cells derived from AIDS patients to recognize and respond to soluble antigens, irrespective of numerical correction (Lane et al., 1985). A measurable defect in reactivity to soluble antigens can also be identified in HIV-infected persons who possess near-normal levels of CD4 T cells. In one study this defect correlated more highly with the progression from persistent generalized lymphadenopathy to clinical AIDS within a one-year period than did the absolute numbers of CD4 T cells (Murray et al., 1985b). It is not known if this specific insensitivity to antigens among CD4 T cells from AIDS patients reflects the preferential depletion of an antigen-responsive population or indirect immunosuppressive factors resulting from HIV infection. The direct inhibitory effects of HIV components themselves have been found *in vitro,* although their *in vivo* relevance is unclear (Pahwa et al., 1985).

A number of the above-noted immunologic deficits in AIDS patients can be corrected *in vitro* through the provision of lymphokines that are normally produced by the CD4 T-cell population. Defective specific cytotoxic activity of CD8-positive T cells derived from AIDS patients and nonspecific natural-killer cell function can be partially corrected by exogenous interleukin-2 (Rook et al., 1983). Similarly, many aspects of the observed monocyte defect of AIDS, specifically the compromised intracellular killing of *Toxoplasma gondii,* the reduced hydrogen peroxide release, and the low expression of HLA class II antigens, can largely be corrected through the provision of gamma interferon (Heagy et al., 1984; Murray et al., 1985a). The lymphokine-mediated correction of these abnormalities suggests that they, too, derive from an inadequate inductive influence produced by the numerically limited CD4 T cells. It also suggests that, with greatly increased knowledge, immunoregulatory therapy of AIDS may one day be possible.

B-cell function is also abnormal in patients with AIDS, marked by the frequent presence of hypergammaglobulinemia and the production of autoantibodies occurring in the absence of an ability to generate specific antibodies upon challenge by novel or recall antigens (Ammann et al., 1984; Lane et al., 1983). It is not known whether failure of appropriate B-cell function derives from the decline of normal regulatory control by CD4 cells, from the proliferative effects of Epstein-Barr virus infections resident in almost all AIDS patients (Quinnan et al., 1984), or from the reported stimulatory potential of HIV virion components (Pahwa et al., 1985). Since many of the opportunistic infections of AIDS patients may result from disrupted humoral immunity, improved understanding of its pathogenesis is needed. Indeed, the increased frequency of aggressive B lymphomas in HIV-infected persons may also result from the aberrant regulation of B-lymphocyte reactivity.

The relationship of the appearance of Kaposi's sarcoma to HIV infection is also not understood. Because Kaposi's sarcoma appears with increased frequency in homosexual AIDS patients, it may result from the oncogenic influences of another agent with which they are infected. The lesions of Kaposi's sarcoma seen in AIDS patients appear to arise in a nonclonal, multifocal manner and as such are not conventional malignancies.

As discussed in Chapter 2, the appearance of Kaposi's sarcoma in HIV-infected persons does not correlate with the degree of observed immunodeficiency, and it is unclear whether it derives from an absence of normal direct or indirect regulatory influences exerted on the Kaposi's target cell by a specific subpopulation of CD4 T cells or from the failure of immune surveillance against incipient tumors. Since the manifestations of Kaposi's sarcoma may not predict the extent of underlying immunosuppression, it may be a poor determinant of which patient population to use in the evaluation of the efficacy of antiviral drugs (see section on "Antiviral Agents," below). However, study of these unusual lesions could contribute greatly to the understanding of AIDS, of the normal interactions between lymphoid and endothelial cell elements, and of the immune response to cancer.

Recommendations

• Continued study of HIV infections in human beings should include an intensified effort to define the introduction and spread of HIV *in vivo,* to identify the *in vivo* reservoirs of infected cells, and to determine the effects of HIV on the lymphoid and central nervous systems throughout the course of infection.

• The CD4 molecule has been directly implicated as the receptor for HIV infection of cells. Although it was first discussed as a T-lymphocyte marker, several other cell types throughout the body have been found that express the CD4 molecule or the mRNA that potentially encodes it. Because AIDS involves pathologic alteration in several organs previously not thought to contain CD4-expressing cells, and because the whole-body reservoir of HIV-infected cells is unknown, more needs to be learned about the molecule and the full extent of cells expressing it. The developmental biology, function, and lifespan of all cells that express CD4 at some stage in their life history should be studied.

• Future evaluations of potential drug therapies for HIV infection and AIDS will require more comprehensive immunologic and virologic analyses than are presently practical. Improved analytical techniques in these areas are also of critical importance for future epidemiologic studies of the natural history of infection and the existence of possible cofactors in the development of AIDS. Similarly, a number of presently unresolved issues of tremendous importance to public health will remain inadequately explored until such techniques are developed and widely available. These issues include the definition of the infectious state, the existence and extent of a virus-positive antibody-negative population, the relevance of host or environmental cofactors in the development of AIDS, and the efficiency of heterosexual transmission.

EPIDEMIOLOGIC APPROACHES TO UNDERSTANDING THE TRANSMISSION AND NATURAL HISTORY OF HIV INFECTION

The current understanding of the natural history and transmission of HIV infection and AIDS is reviewed in Chapter 2. Much, perhaps most, of the available knowledge about the disease derives from epidemiologic research for two reasons: there are presently no entirely suitable animal models in which to study the disease, and certain sorts of experimentation with human beings are precluded by the ethics of research. Much has been learned from epidemiologic research during the first five years of the AIDS epidemic, but future research needs remain great. (The background to the recommendations below is presented in Chapters 2 and 3.)

Recommendations on Surveillance

• The accuracy and completeness of the reporting of AIDS and ARC should be evaluated periodically; this should be done in several different areas because the prevalence of AIDS in those areas may affect that reporting. Such evaluations should be carried out according to a standardized protocol to ensure consistency. These studies should be coordinated and supported by the Centers for Disease Control.

• Surveillance of AIDS should be augmented by selective reporting of other stages of HIV infection, e.g., ARC, as determined by the Association of State and Territorial Health Officials in conjunction with the Centers for Disease Control, and by enhanced use of data from serologic testing of potential recruits to the armed forces.

• Additional surveillance of HIV infection and AIDS is needed in groups of particular epidemiologic importance (not necessarily high risk), such as heterosexuals, non-IV drug users in high-incidence areas, IV drug users and homosexual men in low-incidence cities, spouses of infected individuals, pregnant women, newborn children of infected mothers, prostitutes throughout the country, and recipients of blood products.

• Surveillance efforts for HIV infection and AIDS should not be at the expense of control efforts for other sexually transmitted diseases.

• In general, better information is needed to quantify the number of persons infected with HIV. Extensive and repeated surveys of seropositivity rates are needed to determine the incidence and prevalence of infection by age, race/ethnicity, geographic area, and sex. Such studies should be supported on a national basis, and standardized protocols should be developed to ensure comparability of the collected data.

• There is an urgent need to incorporate capabilities for virus isolation in ongoing and future epidemiologic studies. Basic needs—such as improving the efficacy of isolating virus from frozen samples, the ability to reproduce isolate virus from the same patient on multiple occasions, and the provision of adequate personnel and resources to isolate virus from large numbers of samples quickly—all need to be addressed.

• Some critical epidemiologic studies have both surveillance and basic science components and hence do not fall neatly within the ambit of either the Centers for Disease Control or the National Institutes of Health. The broad epidemiologic research program must be coordinated so that important proposals are not allowed to "fall through the cracks." A separate study section for AIDS epidemiology should be temporarily established within the National Institutes of Health.

Recommendations on Natural History of HIV Infection

• There is a need to determine what proportion of HIV-infected persons will become sick and to define many other features of the disease's natural history.

• Additional information is needed on the natural history of HIV in infected persons of all AIDS risk groups. The NIH-funded cohort studies of homosexual men should be continued and extended, and new studies should be developed for other current or potential high-risk populations, such as IV drug users and heterosexually active populations. Special attention should be directed to bisexual men and women with multiple sex partners. These studies should be geographically distributed, of sufficient duration (5 to 10 years), and coupled with studies of HIV molecular virology. Careful attention should also be given to the definition and assessment of important predictive parameters of the human immune response.

• Prospective studies of individuals with HIV infections should be initiated in order to better assess the incidence of various manifestations and complications of infection with time. Presently, most data concerning clinical manifestations of the infection are limited to those listed at presentation or are derived retrospectively from small series of hospitalized patients. Such data will be invaluable in assessing the effects of various therapeutic interventions.

• Prospective cohort studies should develop standard classification schemes for disease manifestations or use those previously developed by others, such as the Centers for Disease Control or the Walter Reed Army Institute for Research. These schemes should be evaluated for their predictive value. Case-control studies of rare or uncommon findings in AIDS and ARC patients should be developed and supported by the Centers for Disease Control and/or the National Institutes of Health. Such studies are relatively inexpensive and may provide valuable information on the pathogenesis of HIV and point the way toward additional clinical or laboratory studies.

• Studies to determine differences in the presentation, manifestations, and rate of progression of disease between subgroups of AIDS patients based on route of transmission (parenteral versus sexual), age (adult versus pediatric), or area of residence (United States versus Africa) should be started in an attempt to better understand the pathogenesis of the disease.

• Possible cofactors should be clinically studied. Possible factors for investigation include coinfection with cytomegalovirus or other agents, stress modification, nutritional intervention, genital ulcers, and HIV superinfection.

• Very little is known about the full extent of the introduction, spread, and pathogenic consequences of HIV infection throughout the course of human disease. Every effort should therefore be made to develop means to identify HIV-infected volunteers from whom tissue samples can be obtained in an ethical manner. For instance, logistics and funding should be developed for identifying and carrying out immediate and sterile autopsies on HIV-infected individuals who have previously volunteered for such research and who die as a result of some other cause (e.g., accidents, homicide, suicide, myocardial infarction).

Recommendations on Transmission of HIV

- The range of individual variability in levels of infectious HIV should be quantified, including the levels of virus shed into semen and other potentially infectious body fluids.
- Present education programs designed to limit the spread of HIV infection are hampered by the lack of a meaningful definition of "safer sex" practices. There is a tremendous need for the epidemiologic evaluation of how various protective measures influence the transmission of the virus. The effectiveness of barriers, such as condoms, in preventing sexual transmission of HIV should be evaluated epidemiologically. Data on this issue should become available from the current prospective studies of homosexually active men and the spouses of infected hemophiliacs. Complementary laboratory and epidemiologic research on viricidal lubricants for vaginal and anal use is also desirable, since these could be useful adjuncts to condom use (but almost certainly are not an acceptable primary mode of protection).
- The risk of HIV transmission from men to women through vaginal intercourse should be estimated. Factors that affect this risk need to be identified.
- The risk of HIV transmission from women to men through vaginal intercourse should likewise be estimated. It is not known if data from central Africa will be directly applicable in this regard to Western countries. Therefore, studies of heterosexual couples in which the female is the initial source of infection are needed to identify possible routes of transmission and factors related to the risk. Such data would also be critical for assessing the possibility that HIV transmission will be perpetuated among heterosexuals, as are many other sexually transmitted diseases. The ideal subjects for this type of study are the male sexual partners of women who acquired HIV infections through transfusion.
- The relative importance of various routes of transmission in central Africa should be determined. It is of particular interest that accurate data be obtained on heterosexual transmission, including risk factors related to sexual activity that may be unique to Africa or quantitatively different from Western countries. Parallel studies should be conducted in Africa and in the United States as far as possible.
- Studies to monitor the risk of transmission through accidental needlesticks should continue to be supported. Such data are important in

assessing the risk of infection in health care settings and may be relevant to the design of intervention trials.

• The current risk of HIV infection among the hemophiliac recipients of clotting-factor concentrates in which the plasma donors have all been screened for HIV antibodies and the product has been treated to inactivate residual virus should be monitored.

• The risk of HIV transmission within hemodialysis settings should be assessed.

• The time and route of maternal-infant transmission and the factors related to the risk of HIV infection in infants should be identified. Data also are needed to confirm the detection of virus in breast milk and to determine whether it can be transmitted orally to infants through breast feeding.

In assessing responsibility for the various studies recommended above, policymakers should take account of the fact that certain agencies have traditional strength in certain types of activity and others may be situated to take advantage of unique opportunities. For example, the Department of the Army has the capacity to follow infected individuals over time more readily than other groups. Agencies and policymakers should recognize that collaboration in some project will be essential—for example, in follow-up of seropositive military applicants.

Recommendations on the Need for Improved Serologic and Virologic Tests

Much evidence suggests that the serologic tests now available are generally accurate and useful (see Appendix B). However, there are some obvious needs for their improvement and for other techniques in virus detection and isolation. Improved or new techniques would greatly facilitate studies of the natural history and epidemiology of HIV infection and AIDS. The areas of greatest need are as follows:

• Improved tests for antibodies to HIV, particularly tests having greater specificity. (In this area, competitive assays and possibly tests using antigens derived through recombinant DNA techniques appear to hold the greatest promise.)

• New and improved methods for the detection of virus, both through the identification of viral antigens and through the detection of infectious viral particles.

• Standardized procedures for virus isolation that maximize recovery and that could be used to evaluate other techniques.

These areas of work are no less important than others mentioned in this chapter, and policymakers may need to consider special arrangements to ensure that work in some of them—e.g., viral isolation techniques—is not neglected.

ANIMAL MODELS

New methods have allowed rapid progress to be made in understanding the molecular biology of HIV. However, because AIDS is a uniquely human disease, the biologically relevant aspects of the infection and disease will be far more difficult to unravel. The sequence of cells initially infected; the sites of latency and persistence; the host determinants and cofactors in disease development; the timing, incidence, and sites of nervous system infection; and similar questions cannot be answered in cell cultures and cannot be solved solely by epidemiologic observations. Animal models of immunosuppressive retroviral infections will be crucial in addressing and resolving these biological questions.

Similarly, studies of methods to control HIV infection—whether by blocking transmission, by chemotherapy of the infected, or by immunization of the uninfected—will ultimately have to be done in human populations. Such studies must conform to ethical standards and thus raise problems of research design. In patients with clinical AIDS, the evaluation of potentially dangerous drugs can be justified. But the testing of vaccines in uninfected populations or the testing of potentially dangerous drugs in seropositive yet healthy persons will pose major practical and ethical problems. Again, animal models are needed.

Animal models of HIV infection will be critical components of both vaccine and antiviral development programs. These models provide an important intermediate level of drug evaluation between *in vitro* studies and testing in humans. Many agents active against HIV *in vitro* will never have been used on humans, so drug evaluation in other animals will provide essential information about efficacy, pharmacology, penetration of the central nervous system, and toxicity.

In the search for experimental counterparts of human diseases, two strategies have been used (Johnson, 1985). One involves the infection of experimental animals with the human agent in hopes of simulating the human disease. The other involves studying analogous diseases in their natural hosts, such as the classic studies of the pathogenesis of ectromelia virus in mice that illuminated the pathogenesis of smallpox. Both approaches have their value.

There is no entirely satisfactory animal model for human HIV infection and disease. However, several experimental approaches are being taken that may shed light on the infection process.

HIV Infection of Chimpanzees

The only host thus far found to be susceptible to chronic infection with HIV is the chimpanzee. To date, infected chimpanzees have been shown to develop antiviral antibodies, viremia, and an occasional transient adenopathy but no disease (Alter et al., 1984; Francis et al., 1984; Fultz et al., 1986b; Gajdusek, 1985). This model is therefore of little use in studying the later stages of disease pathogenesis, but it will be indispensable in the development of HIV vaccines. Chimpanzees are the only animals now known in which HIV vaccines can be tested before clinical application. They can be immunized with a candidate vaccine and subsequently challenged with the human virus to determine if the vaccine provides safe, effective prevention of infection. For example, an envelope protein subunit vaccine could be given and the animals then monitored following challenge with infectious HIV for seropositivity to core proteins as well as for recoverable virus in the blood. Chimpanzees may also play a critical role in the evaluation of the ability of antiviral drugs to prevent, limit, or cure HIV infections.

Only about 1,400 chimpanzees are now available for all biomedical research. Housing and maintaining these long-lived animals require major expense. There is also convention among researchers against sacrificing chimpanzees for complete pathologic or virologic studies, which impedes the progress of animal research related to human disease. Increasing the number of chimpanzees available through breeding is a slow process, and their importation is presently not legal because they are designated as an endangered species.

A transient HIV viremia has been found occasionally in inoculated macaques, but this would be of very limited experimental value.

HIV-Related Viruses in Old World Primates

Retroviruses resembling HIV have been isolated from rhesus macaques, African green monkeys, sooty mangabeys, and pig-tail macaques (Desrosiers and Letvin, 1986). These agents (collectively termed STLV-III or SIV) have tropism for T4 cells similar to that of HIV; they also have a similar morphology, antigenic relatedness, and distant sequence homology (less than 75 percent).

SIV was initially isolated from captive rhesus monkeys (*Macaca mulatta*) suffering from a disease resembling AIDS (Daniel et al., 1985; Kanki et al., 1985). Later, it was found in a large number of healthy African green monkeys (*Cercopithecus aethiops*) in the wild (Kanki et al., 1985). Although the viruses isolated from the different monkeys appear similar if not identical, they have clearly different effects on their infected hosts. Understanding why SIV-infected African green monkeys remain healthy while rhesus monkeys develop profound immunosuppression may provide very useful insights into the pathogenesis of AIDS.

Two patterns of disease have been observed in rhesus monkeys inoculated with SIV. In an initial study, four monkeys developed low titers of antibody, hypogammaglobulinemia, inversion of CD4/CD8 cell ratios, and death with opportunistic infections and an encephalitis resembling the subacute encephalitis of AIDS. In the initial study two animals developed a good antibody titer, a persistent viremia, a decline in CD4 cells, and lymphadenopathy, but they did not die (Letvin et al., 1985). Subsequent rhesus monkeys have shown a second pattern of nonlethal disease, with wasting, diarrhea, and decreased CD4 cells (N. Letvin, New England Primate Center, personal communication, 1986; Yanagihara et al., 1986). When the mangabey SIV isolate was inoculated into the juvenile rhesus macaques, it induced antibody and viremia with diarrhea and lymphadenopathy (M. Gardner, University of California at Davis, personal communication, 1986). However, a subsequent similar study described additional isolates that did not cause clinical immunodeficiency in either their natural hosts or rhesus macaques (Fultz et al., 1986a).

In general, SIV induces a disease in monkeys remarkably similar to human AIDS, making it suitable for studies of pathogenesis, drug trials, and vaccine development. This could be an extremely useful animal model. A detailed description of SIV's character and relevance to HIV infection and AIDS is presented in the background paper prepared for the committee by Letvin and Desrosiers (1986).

The recently identified novel human viruses HTLV-IV and LAV-2 demonstrate similarities to SIV. Although HTLV-IV is reported to be apathogenic, LAV-2 was isolated from persons with AIDS. These viruses need better molecular and genetic, as well as biologic, characterization. The variables influencing pathogenicity of these agents may provide important insights into the mechanisms of disease causation and evolutionary origins of the immunosuppressive retroviruses related to HIV.

Lentiviruses of Ungulates

Lentiviruses distantly related to HIV include equine infectious anemia virus (of horses), ovine visna virus (of sheep), and caprine arthritis-encephalitis virus (of goats). HIV shares structural and biologic similarities with these other lentiviruses (Gonda et al., 1985; Sonigo et al., 1985). Although the different animal lentiviruses demonstrate a variety of different pathogenic effects and strategies for evasion of the host immune system during the course of an infection, they provide a wealth of opportunities for understanding or anticipating the complexities of HIV infection. The animal lentiviruses and their relevance to HIV infection and AIDS are discussed in the section on "Vaccines" later in this chapter and in the accompanying background papers by Haase (1986) and Narayan (1986).

The animal lentiviruses show epidemiologic features similar to those of HIV, being transferred by blood or mononuclear cells in secretions. These infections largely involve the macrophages, and none of the ungulate viruses directly affect T helper lymphocytes to cause the severe immunosuppression seen in AIDS. These diseases have long incubation periods, persistent viremia, development of weak neutralizing antibody responses, a tendency for the virus to undergo extensive antigenic mutation and antigenic drift, neurotropism, and lytic virus infection of selected leukocyte cell populations. Because lentiviruses are the nearest known relatives of HIV, are partially related in sequence, and have similar biological properties, they can be very useful in understanding HIV-induced disease. Studies of pathogenesis, drug trials, and vaccine strategies could be explored first in these ungulate hosts (Haase, 1986; Narayan, 1986).

Conclusions and Recommendations

The committee is particularly concerned about the nurturing and preservation of primate animal model resources, which will be essential for drug and vaccine development and for basic investigation of disease pathogenesis and natural history. There are approximately 1,400 chimpanzees in the United States today available for all biomedical research. About 800 of these are outside federal control, and a significant proportion of the approximately 600 under federal control (or possibly otherwise available—e.g., not in private ownership) are not available for AIDS-related research because they are reserved for breeding programs or are in reserve for use with other emergent diseases. In addition, only those chimpanzees who have already been exposed to non-A, non-B hepatitis virus, making them unsuitable for breeding purposes, are currently being approved for use in AIDS-related research. This leaves a very small number, approximately 200, potentially available for research on AIDS and HIV.

An NIH committee following commonly agreed standards of research with animals approves experiments on chimpanzees under federal control. The use of approximately 85 chimpanzees for AIDS-related research has already been approved.

As of August 1986, $4.5 million of discretionary funds have been allocated to the NIH Division of Research Resources for a chimpanzee breeding program (Barnes, 1986).

The committee is gravely concerned that chimpanzees have been and might be used for experiments for which the rationale is not compelling in light of the scarcity and irreplaceable nature of these animals; extreme caution must be exercised in their use. Chimpanzees must be treated as an endangered national resource that will be irreplaceable if squandered. Mechanisms must be found to ensure that AIDS-related experiments with these animals are conducted only if there is a broad consensus among the interested scientific community that the experiment proposed is critically important to development of vaccines or antiviral agents and cannot be conducted in any other species or by any other means. These considerations apply equally to animals not under federal control.

• Animal models that reproduce or mimic the consequences of HIV infection will play a crucial role in improving our understanding of disease pathogenesis and the development and testing of antiviral drugs and vaccines. Available animal models of HIV infection and the immunocompromised state must be vigorously supported, and efforts must be made to develop and validate new animal models. Because the most relevant and promising animal models are provided by nonhuman primates, the nation's primate centers should be strengthened to permit the expansion of the primate populations available for AIDS-related research, the development of appropriate biocontainment facilities, and the education of appropriately trained investigators.

• For fiscal and ecological reasons, studies that can be done with relatively well-defined disease models in domestic animals should be carried out in sheep, goats, and horses rather than in primates.

• Available supplies of primates will probably be inadequate for future research needs, and the plans for their conservation, expansion, and optimal use appear inadequate. Funding for the systematic evaluation of additional model systems and the validation of existing ones should be a top research priority. Presently available animal resources should be expanded as rapidly as possible to meet expected future demands. Also, a national system should be installed to facilitate appropriate access to test animals for valid experimentation by qualified investigators, regardless of institutional affiliation.

• Naturally occurring retroviral infections leading to significant acquired immunodeficiencies have been found in several vertebrate species. Although only a few potentially produce a syndrome quite similar to human AIDS, none has been studied sufficiently to elucidate mechanisms of pathogenesis, so that one could know whether the different types of immunodeficiency result from similar or different basic mechanisms. Therefore, support of known animal systems of retrovirus-induced immunodeficiency, including murine, feline, and especially simian models, should be increased and broadened.

• A virus related to HIV that has been isolated from nonhuman primates, SIV, has great potential as a model system to study immunocompromise resulting from a retroviral infection. However, the generalizability of conclusions derived from SIV must be evaluated with respect to similarities with and differences from HIV infections. Further studies need to be carried out with SIV in rhesus and other breeds of monkeys. If the rhesus model is to be widely used, more biocontainment space must be made available.

• A completely analogous animal model of HIV-induced human AIDS has not yet been found. Most of what has been learned about the fundamental aspects of animal virology, immunology, lymphocyte biology, and, to a lesser extent, neurobiology, has come from extensive investigations with genetically defined inbred strains of rodents. In these times of recombinant DNA manipulations of retroviruses, of tissue culture cells, and of transgenic mouse strains, it is possible that a completely analogous animal model of HIV-induced human diseases might be developed. Therefore, development of possible animal models should be considered that would include both natural models and the deliberate modification of existing species to render them susceptible to AIDS by HIV infection. At the same time the possible biohazards of this type of research need careful consideration.

ANTIVIRAL AGENTS

Infectious viral agents remain a major threat to human health both in the United States and around the world. Recent years have therefore seen considerable effort directed toward the development of new antiviral agents for the treatment of acute viral infections. However, even though there are now many examples of successful chemotherapeutic conquests of bacterial infections, there are only a few examples of drugs that are effective in the treatment of viral diseases.

Much of the difficulty in treating viral infections is a consequence of their nature as intracellular pathogens—that is, they replicate within the cells of their chosen host. Because viruses use many of the host cell's synthetic pathways in their reproductive processes, specifically inhibiting their replication without also severely compromising the metabolic activities and health of their hosts is difficult.

As a virus that appears to cause persistent lifelong infection, HIV must be approached as a member of the class of viruses for which successful treatment may be most difficult to find. Furthermore, as a member of the family of retroviruses, HIV represents a type of viral pathogen whose therapy has never before been attempted in humans. Because the contemplated development of drugs to treat HIV infection and AIDS represents such a novel and difficult challenge, predictions of ultimate success are presently impossible to offer. Likewise, the timing of the development and availability of potential drugs cannot be accurately forecast.

These notes of caution and even pessimism must be tempered by an appreciation of the remarkable scientific advances that have been made to date in understanding HIV. Similarly, recent developments in molecular biology, virology, immunology, structural chemistry, and drug design have initiated what may be a new era in the treatment of previously intractable human viral infections. In many ways the problems of HIV infection and AIDS may provide the first and most substantial test of these emerging capabilities. Rational drug design based on the specific characteristics of viral processes is still a long-term prospect, but with the impressive skills and commitment of the biomedical research community, this theoretical approach could become a reality.

The basic objective of antiviral therapies for AIDS and its related conditions is to effectively inhibit the replication of HIV. Underlying this objective is the belief that continued viral replication is involved in the development and progression of the disease. This belief is corroborated, up to a point, by the limited available studies of the natural history of HIV infection. As discussed in the section on "Natural History of HIV Infection," above, at any given time only a small proportion of cells in an infected person actively express HIV (Harper et al., 1986a). The decline in CD4 T cells, which is thought to account for much of the immunologic compromise of AIDS, appears to be a slowly progressive one. Recent *in vitro* analyses suggest that the cytopathic effects that HIV exerts on CD4 T lymphocytes result from the active expression of viral gene products. The exact mechanisms of CD4 T cell depletion *in vivo* are not known, but they have been postulated to include a direct cytopathic effect of the viral envelope protein (Lifson et al., in press; Sodroski et al., 1986a) as well as potential indirect, possibly autoimmune processes (Klatzmann and Montagnier, 1986).

The persistent, although low-level, expression of the cytopathic determinants of HIV may explain the progressive immunologic deficit seen in infected persons. Thus, a chemotherapeutic approach designed to limit viral expression or treat HIV infection may be reasonably expected to minimize the resulting damage to the immune system. However, clinical improvement as a result of antiviral therapy can only be expected if the host immune system has not been irrevocably damaged and maintains regenerative potential. Antiviral therapies may thus have limited utility in persons whose immunologic damage has progressed beyond the point of recovery. Because the regenerative capacities of the adult human immune system are not well understood, the existence or designation of this point is presently impossible to evaluate. Regardless, antiviral therapies might be expected to be most useful in persons infected with HIV but not yet clinically ill. Attention is being focused on potential immunoregulatory and restorative therapies for end-stage HIV infection, yet a great deal must be learned before their practicality can be assessed.

A related and important consideration is the potential ability of antiviral agents to beneficially affect the neurologic manifestations of HIV infection. While the consequences of viral infection in the central nervous system are well documented, their potential for reversal is unknown (see section on "Neurologic Complications" in Appendix A).

The development of antiviral drugs for HIV infection must also take into account a number of problematic aspects of the behavior of the virus *in vivo*. HIV is known to establish an infection that persists in the face of a host immune response, probably for the lifetime of the infected individual. This behavior, referred to as viral latency, is typical of the lentiretroviruses. The mechanisms that permit the establishment and maintenance of viral latency are not known, but determining them will be extremely important as drug therapies are considered. Should a candidate drug limit, but not eliminate, HIV expression, lifelong therapy may be necessary to achieve the desired protection. If lifelong therapy is required, the already difficult challenge of devising drugs of acceptable toxicity will prove even more severe. In addition to the predictable mechanisms of drug toxicity, AIDS patients have demonstrated unusual toxic reactions upon treatment with anti-infectious or anticancer chemotherapies (Jaffe et al., 1983). Similar problems not anticipated in drug development may arise during long-term therapy in persons with AIDS. Prolonged administration of an antiviral agent may also result in the selection of drug-resistant viral variants. However, it is possible that if a drug effectively limits replication, the host viral load will progressively decline and ultimately vanish.

Successful development of antiviral therapies for HIV must also consider the cellular reservoirs that are involved in viral persistence. Cells of the macrophage/monocyte lineage are known to be susceptible to viral infection *in vitro* and may also serve as *in vivo* hosts for viral replication (Gartner et al., 1986). Given their relative longevity, wideranging migration, and apparent relative resistance to the cytopathic effects of viral infection, protracted systemic antiviral therapy may be required for cure or even stabilization. Similarly, the central nervous system is known to be an early and common target of HIV infection (Ho et al., 1985c; Resnick et al., 1985). Because the brain may carry a substantial viral load (Shaw et al., 1985), it may provide a sanctuary for viral persistence. The presence of a reservoir of HIV within the central nervous system requires that antiviral drugs that cross the blood-brain barrier be developed if total viral elimination is to be achieved.

A number of possible targets exist for a rational approach to designing drugs to specifically inhibit HIV replication. These include such viral processes as assembly and uncoating, integration, reverse transcription, and proteolysis.

Drug Evaluation *in Vitro*

Candidate drugs for the treatment of HIV infection must fulfill criteria of antiviral efficacy and acceptable toxicity. Certain parameters of these criteria can be measured *in vitro,* and innovative assay systems have been established to permit the screening of potential candidate drugs. The HIV reverse transcriptase plays an essential role in the viral life-cycle and is presently a primary target of antiviral agents. Its activity can easily be measured *in vitro.* Also, as discussed earlier in this chapter, the production of large amounts of active reverse transcriptase by recombinant DNA methodologies is an important goal.

Many substances may successfully inhibit purified HIV reverse transcriptase *in vitro* yet prove unacceptably toxic. Screening methods to simultaneously measure effective inhibition of viral replication and *in vitro* drug toxicity have recently been described (Mitsuya and Broder, 1986; Mitsuya et al., 1985). Additional assay systems to evaluate agents that inhibit HIV replication need to be developed and validated, as do methods to measure the specific inhibition of the novel viral gene products, as described earlier.

Drug Evaluation in Humans

Evaluation of the efficacy of antiviral therapies in persons infected by HIV is a critical but difficult task. In contrast to the direct determination of antiviral effects that may be measurable *in vitro,* it may prove extremely challenging to accurately evaluate the benefit of candidate drugs in infected persons. As opposed to many other viral diseases in humans, where the immediate clinical symptoms directly relate to ongoing replication of the causative virus, many of the clinical symptoms of AIDS represent indirect manifestations of prior viral damage. For instance, the diagnostic opportunistic infections or typical malignancies of AIDS are the presumed consequences of HIV-induced damage to helper/inducer lymphocyte populations. Even if a drug could effectively halt HIV replication, it might not resolve these immediate clinical signs and symptoms. Once established, certain clinical diseases may be independent of HIV regulation. By the same token, failure of an antiviral drug to halt the progression of established opportunistic infections or Kaposi's sarcoma may not de facto indicate lack of efficacy.

Protection of healthy individuals infected with HIV but showing no AIDS-related infections or malignancies may be the most useful measure of antiviral effects. But the evaluation of this protection requires large populations and long time periods. There are also ethical constraints involved in the administration of potentially toxic agents to persons who are not overtly ill. Drugs that may show no beneficial effects in AIDS patients may, in fact, be beneficial in forestalling the immunologic compromise that follows HIV infection. These may, however, be difficult to identify.

The clinical and laboratory measures presently in use to evaluate candidate drugs for antiviral activity against HIV involve virologic, immunologic, and clinical parameters. Virologic measures attempt to measure virus load, but at present they do so rather poorly. Measurements of HIV expression *in vivo* are not generally applicable, and given the low levels of viral expression they currently detect, they may be at the limits of their resolution (Harper et al., 1986a). Recent advances in the detection of HIV antigens *in vivo* have suggested that such an approach would be very useful, but it is presently not known to provide adequate sensitivity of viral detection. Current methodologies of viral isolation from infected persons are only semiquantitative, are of limited sensitivity, and require expertise that is not now widely available. Measurement of drug efficacy using *in vitro* methods for viral isolation is further limited by an inability to identify viral production *in vivo,* and by the documented variability in the ease of isolation of various HIV strains (Gartner et al., 1986).

Measurements of immunologic competence in AIDS patients generally involve determinations of CD4 T-lymphocyte levels, cutaneous hypersensitivity testing, and *in vitro* measures of T-cell responsiveness (see Chapter 2). It is not yet known which, if any, of these factors provide accurate insights into the most clinically relevant immunologic consequences of HIV infection or can act as usable barometers of the extent of viral replication.

The clinical impact of antiviral therapy is ultimately the most important measure of efficacy. As discussed above, however, it also may be the most difficult to quantify meaningfully. Prolonged survival, amelioration of the frequency or severity of opportunistic infections, and freedom from malignant diseases or neurologic sequelae provide the most important guideposts. However, the natural history of HIV infection has not yet been defined completely, so the efficacy of antiviral agents will have to be determined as this definition is being established.

Current Antiviral Agents Under Clinical Study

The major candidate drugs undergoing preclinical and clinical evaluation for efficacy against HIV infection have been identified empirically in studies of other viruses. Although the mechanisms of action of many of them are unknown, some are thought to exert their antiviral effects through inhibition of reverse transcriptase. Following *in vitro* evaluation of their ability to inhibit HIV reverse transcriptase, replication, or cytopathology, these drugs have progressed through subsequent levels of pharmacologic and toxicologic tests before being administered to infected humans.

Some agents have demonstrated an antiviral activity *in vitro* but have yielded disappointing results when tested in AIDS patients. For instance, suramin treatment, besides failing to improve the immunologic impairment seen in AIDS, caused serious toxicity. Thus, agents that appear promising *in vitro* may yield no benefit, and perhaps even serious toxicities, when administered to humans.

There are currently no drugs with documented efficacy in the treatment of HIV infection. The drugs described below have shown variable degrees of initial promise *in vitro* and are undergoing clinical evaluation in HIV-infected persons. As previously discussed, dramatic breakthroughs in this pursuit are unlikely, but therapeutic benefits could aid in the increased understanding of the basic mechanisms responsible for the clinical development of AIDS.

Suramin

Suramin was the first drug reported to have *in vitro* inhibitory effects on HIV replication (Mitsuya et al., 1984). Suramin is used to treat trypanosomiasis and onchocerciasis (Hawking, 1981). It has also been noted to inhibit the reverse transcriptase activities of a number of murine and avian retroviruses (de Clercq, 1979). Although it is a potent inhibitor of HIV reverse transcriptase, it also significantly inhibits mammalian DNA polymerase alpha (Chandra et al., 1985) and lymphocyte proliferation, thus limiting its therapeutic index.

Clinical evaluation of suramin in AIDS patients resulted in a transient inability to recover virus from treated individuals, but it produced little or no evidence of clinical improvement or immunologic recovery (Broder et al., 1985; Levine et al., 1985; Rouvroy et al., 1985; Stein et al., 1986). Suramin therapy was complicated by fever, rash, renal and liver function abnormalities, and serious adrenal compromise. In addition, the effects of suramin on lymphocyte proliferation may exert a counterproductive immunosuppressive influence at higher doses. Finally, suramin could not be a viable single-drug modality because the drug does not penetrate into the central nervous system.

HPA-23

Ammonium 21-tungsto-9-antimoniate, or HPA-23, inhibits the reverse transcriptase activity of a number of murine oncornaviruses *in vitro* and protects against the leukemogenic consequences of their replication *in vivo* (Chermann et al., 1975; Jasmin et al., 1974). Although HPA-23 is reported to act as a competitive inhibitor of reverse transcriptase, the mechanism of its antiviral activity against HIV is not known.

Initial limited clinical evaluations indicated that HPA-23 could exert a transient virustatic effect in patients with AIDS or ARC as measured by failure to isolate HIV following a two-week course of treatment (Rozenbaum et al., 1985). Following cessation of treatment, HIV could again be isolated, and there was no indication of beneficial immunologic effects. Toxicities included thrombocytopenia and transient liver function abnormalities.

Although clinical evaluation is continuing in the United States and France, no therapeutic benefit of HPA-23 for persons infected by HIV has been documented.

Azidothymidine (AZT)

3'-Azido-3'-deoxythymidine (AZT), which has been previously referred to as "compound S" and BW A509U, is a thymidine analog modified so that it acts as a chain terminator during DNA synthesis. Although not an inhibitor of reverse transcriptase *per se,* it can effectively prevent the synthesis of proviral DNA by HIV reverse transcriptase by frequently interrupting the growing viral template. Following conversion to a triphosphate form by cellular enzymes, AZT effectively inhibits the *in vitro* infectivity and cytopathic effects of HIV (Mitsuya and Broder, 1986; Mitsuya et al., 1985). The drug is well absorbed following oral administration and effectively penetrates into the central nervous system (Yarchoan et al., 1986).

Initial phase I clinical trials defined a relatively short half-life for the drug, with dose-dependent toxicities involving suppression of certain hematologic measures and headaches (Yarchoan et al., 1986). However, it was generally well tolerated. A virustatic effect against HIV was documented at higher doses of AZT. Some patients experienced increases in their levels of CD4 T cells during the course of therapy, and there were occasional indications of partial immunologic improvement involving amelioration of cutaneous anergy, clearing of infections, improvement in neurologic symptoms, and weight gain. Surprisingly, clinical and immunologic improvements were seen in individuals receiving doses that permitted the continued isolation of HIV. Some patients developed episodes of opportunistic infections during the treatment course. With prolonged administration of AZT, declines in CD4 T-cell levels were seen in some patients, perhaps reflecting pharmacologic suppression of the bone marrow.

The AZT-induced suppression of hematopoiesis and immune reactivity is correlated with drug-related pyrimidine starvation that accrues with continued administration. These side effects may limit both the acceptable dose of AZT that can be administered and the permissible length of therapy.

Shortly before the publication of this report, data were released by the National Institutes of Health and the Burroughs Wellcome Company from a study of azidothymidine administered for 20 weeks to a group of approximately 140 AIDS patients while a similar group received a placebo. The patients were selected for having had no more than one bout of *Pneumocystis carinii* pneumonia. There was 1 death in the AZT group compared with 16 deaths in the placebo group.

Because of the time at which this information became available, the committee was not able to analyze the data from this study in enough detail to judge the risks and benefits of this drug. Further evaluation will be needed to fully determine the side effects of AZT treatment and its long-term efficacy and safety for various categories of patients.

More recent analyses of other nucleoside analogs that function as terminators during DNA synthesis have uncovered a variety of compounds that are very potent inhibitors of HIV replication and cytopathology *in vitro* (Mitsuya and Broder, 1986). Of these agents, 2′,3′-dideoxyadenosine and 2′,3′-dideoxycytidine have shown the most promise and are currently undergoing toxicity testing in animals in preparation for their evaluation in HIV-infected persons.

Ribavirin

Ribavirin is a nucleoside that has demonstrated *in vitro* activity against a number of RNA viruses *in vitro* and clinical utility in the treatment of influenza A (Knight et al., 1981), respiratory syncytial virus (Hall et al., 1983), and Lassa fever (McCormick et al., 1986). Ribavirin has been noted to exert *in vitro* antiviral effects against certain bovine and avian retroviruses (Jenkins and Chen, 1981; Sidwell and Smee, 1981) and has been shown to limit retroviral replication *in vivo* in mice infected with murine leukemia viruses (Shannon, 1977; Sidwell et al., 1975). It has also been reported to partially inhibit HIV replication as measured by a decreased level of viral reverse transcriptase activity produced following infection of lymphocytes with HIV (McCormick et al., 1984). *In vitro* suppression of reverse transcriptase activity, however, was not complete even at doses known to elicit toxic reactions *in vivo*.

Although ribavirin is thought to interfere with the capping of viral RNA transcripts in certain RNA viruses by inhibiting the activity of virally encoded guanylyl transferases, HIV uses cellular capping activities and thus would not be subject to this mechanism. Ribavirin also results in the synthesis of poorly translatable viral mRNAs in specific RNA viruses, but it is not yet known if this involves mechanisms independent of compromised cap formation (Toltzis and Huang, 1986).

In previously reported clinical applications, ribavirin has demonstrated dose-dependent toxicities expressed mainly as nomocytic anemia. The potential *in vivo* efficacy of ribavirin against HIV infection was suggested in recent phase I clinical studies, where decreased viral replication and enhanced immune function were noted (Roberts et al., 1986). Should ribavirin prove to be an inadequate single-agent therapy, it may still be of use in combination with a drug acting by a presumably distinct mechanism, such as an inhibitor of HIV reverse transcriptase.

An independent safety and evaluation committee has reviewed the first 12 weeks of a 24-week clinical trial of ribavirin with 373 patients at eight clinical centers in the United States. The committee found that ribavirin's safety profile through 12 weeks is acceptable and that the drug has been well tolerated by the patient groups (ICN Pharmaceuticals, 1986).

Foscarnet

Trisodium phosphonoformate, also know as foscarnet, is a drug with noncompetitive inhibitory activity against the reverse transcriptases of certain avian and murine oncornaviruses (Sundquist and Oberg, 1979). Also able to inhibit the DNA polymerases of a number of human herpes viruses (Helgstrand et al., 1978), foscarnet has been used to treat cytomegalovirus infection in immunocompromised patients. Recent studies have documented an *in vitro* inhibition in HIV reverse transcriptase activity at levels pharmacologically acceptable *in vivo* (Sandstrom et al., 1985; Sarin et al., 1985). Administration of foscarnet is occasionally complicated by acute renal failure.

Although the results of clinical evaluation of foscarnet in HIV-infected persons have yet to be reported, clinical trials are in progress.

Alpha Interferon

Alpha interferon is a member of a rapidly expanding category of naturally occurring proteins, referred to as biological response modifiers, that are finding clinical application. Before HIV was identified as the cause of AIDS, alpha interferon was administered to patients with Kaposi's sarcoma in the hope of exploiting its known activity against certain tumors. The earliest attempts to isolate retroviruses from AIDS patients were, in fact, facilitated by the depletion of alpha interferon from the cell cultures (Gallo et al., 1984), and alpha interferon has recently been shown to exert a virustatic effect against HIV *in vitro* (Ho et al., 1985a).

Although it is not known whether alpha interferon exerts similar antiviral action *in vivo,* clinical studies have demonstrated potentially beneficial effects against Kaposi's sarcoma. In early clinical studies of alpha interferon in AIDS patients, no enhancement of immunologic function was detected, but a percentage of persons with Kaposi's sarcoma (especially those with early disease restricted to the skin) achieved a complete remission (Gelmann et al., 1985; Groopman et al., 1984; Krown et al., 1983).

Continuing clinical analyses are in progress to evaluate the potential therapeutic efficacy of alpha interferon in the treatment of HIV infection and Kaposi's sarcoma.

New Antiviral Agents Against AIDS

Although NIH, largely through the National Cancer Institute (NCI), has started a program to test *in vitro* for agents active against HIV, the program has to date been limited largely to in-house selection of compounds collected over the years by NCI for evaluation against cancer in animal models. The program has so far tested approximately 250 compounds. There is presently no satisfactory program whereby scientists from academic institutions, research institutes, or the pharmaceutical industry may send significant numbers of candidate antiviral agents for evaluation against HIV *in vitro*. The problems related to safe handling of the virus have greatly restricted its use in most laboratory settings.

It is absolutely essential to future drug development in this area that the NIH testing program be substantially enlarged to serve industrial and academic research and research institutes outside of NIH, under a confidentiality agreement if necessary. These testing results must be readily available to recruit the scientific talent from both the academic community and the private sector. This *in vitro* testing program must be supported by adequate animal models to determine those agents that are unique candidates for clinical evaluation against HIV. (While the NIH effort should be of adequate size, it should not be turned into a mass screening program as these tend to be inefficient at finding useful drugs.)

The NIH drug development program for contract proposals from cooperative multidisciplinary groups is woefully inadequate in funding to meet the stated needs. Research efforts to synthesize and evaluate new agents potentially active against AIDS have been minimal to date. That new agents will be found active *in vitro* is unquestionable, but how the agents will be selected for clinical trials is presently not clear. Similarly, guidelines and animal testing protocols need to be established for new candidate drugs for potential clinical evaluation against AIDS.

Conclusions and Recommendations

Development of therapy for HIV infection will most likely be a difficult and long-term process with no presently available guarantees for success. The ideal AIDS antiviral drug must fulfill a number of requirements. It must be conveniently administered, preferably orally, and it must be sufficiently nontoxic to be used for prolonged periods—perhaps for a lifetime—by asymptomatic individuals. In addition, it must not only be active in peripheral lymphocytes but also in the central nervous system, as HIV may infect the nervous system early in the disease process. Clearly, the ideal AIDS antiviral drug has not yet been identified, but several drugs are under clinical evaluation. The testing of these agents may be of value in developing subsequent, more useful agents.

• The committee recognizes the urgent need to develop and test experimental agents for the treatment of HIV infection and resulting clinical disorders and the need to make active agents widely available as soon as possible. The committee believes that randomized clinical trials using a placebo control group are required until the first agent is identified that is both safe and effective. After an effective agent is identified, newer drugs can and should be compared to it rather than to a placebo. The committee agrees strongly with current practice whereby subjects participating in any controlled trial who have been in the placebo groups should be offered subsequent treatment with the more active agent if one is identified. The committee recognizes the desire of some to forgo use of placebo controls and immediately test experimental drugs against one another. A compelling argument against such a stratagem is the possibility that promising agents will turn out to be harmful to patients. This was, in fact, the unfortunate experience with suramin in patients with AIDS and ARC. When drugs may offer slight, yet clinically important, benefit or harm, it is especially important to establish that the benefits outweigh the risks in a placebo-controlled randomized trial. This is the quickest, most efficient, and least-biased way to ensure the most efficacious treatment possible for present and future AIDS patients. Many patients, including those with ARC as well as AIDS, have a good intermediate prognosis (up to several months), and these patients deserve to have access to drugs with documented benefits that outweigh toxicity.

• Decisions on the design of studies to test new drugs for HIV infection must be made on a case-by-case basis. Such decisions should take into account the results of further studies on the efficacy and toxicity of AZT, the category of patients to whom the drug under consideration would be given, and preliminary information on the safety and efficacy of the drug.

- The ethical aspects of the design of antiviral drug and vaccine trials should be kept under review by the National Commission on AIDS proposed in Chapter 1.

- Efforts should be undertaken now to ensure that appropriate levels of organizational and financial support are in place to permit the expeditious drug evaluation through phase I, II, and III clinical trials of promising therapeutic agents against HIV infection as they become available.

- A mechanism for providing equal patient access to clinical trial enrollment without regard to area of residence and patient demographics is most desirable. A system such as Physicians' Data Query, which provides on-line access to information about existing cancer chemotherapy trials, should be put in place. However, it may not be realistic to expect that all patients with AIDS or ARC can be accommodated in clinical trials. If such accommodation is impossible, policies providing access to trials should be as equitable as possible. In analogous situations, age, stage of disease, overall health, and absence of specific contraindications to the use of the experimental drugs have been used as entry criteria. This is a complex issue that should be addressed by ethicists and experts in the conduct of clinical trials.

- The magnitude and importance of the AIDS epidemic dictate that all of the potential technical research and development capabilities of governmental agencies, university researchers, pharmaceutical companies, research institutes, and other organizations from the private sector become active in the overall drug development effort as a major approach to the treatment of HIV infection.

- A conference should be convened as soon as possible to bring together researchers from industry, academia, and the Public Health Service to consider the key issues necessary for the development of antiviral drugs. Such a meeting could consider the unique capabilities of NIH—including its drug screening program, its treatment evaluation units, and its provision of special animal models—to facilitate industry's development efforts. Such a conference could also review the experience gained to date from clinical studies with antiviral drugs and strategies for development based on knowledge of the molecular biology of HIV.

- Cooperative and coordinated efforts should be undertaken in the realms of basic and applied research to provide a solid experimental foundation for future drug development efforts.

- Government-sponsored *in vitro* and *in vivo* testing and evaluation programs for potential agents active against HIV should be established. These programs should include antiviral agents from all sources, including the private sector.

• Mass screening approaches to identifying drugs have in the past not been very productive. The committee favors a more rational approach based on the selection of unique viral processes or proteins as drug targets.

• NIH-sponsored drug development involving multidisciplinary efforts should continue to be strongly supported for the discovery of new agents active against HIV.

• Guidelines should be established regarding the acceptability of new antiviral agents for clinical evaluation against AIDS. These should include the efficacy of *in vitro* and *in vivo* models, toxicology and preclinical pharmacology, and the effects of new agents on the immune system.

• Studies to establish, validate, and standardize measures of relevant parameters of the human immune response should be actively encouraged. Likewise, techniques and facilities to definitively detect HIV infection and improve the isolation of viruses from infected persons should be developed. In the absence of such improvements, the therapeutic efficacy of novel agents (drugs and vaccines) may be difficult to establish, validate, or compare with alternative treatments.

VACCINES

Development of an effective vaccine to prevent HIV infection must be a prominent goal in any program designed to halt the continuing spread of the AIDS epidemic. However, it is also likely to be one of the most difficult to realize. Active immunization has proved to be an extremely effective means to limit or eliminate the exceptional morbidity and mortality inflicted upon human populations by many types of viruses, but the derivation of an effective vaccine against a human retrovirus has never been seriously attempted, much less achieved. Similarly, experience in the production of vaccines for retroviruses of other animals has been rather limited and often disappointing.

Programs to develop an HIV vaccine face many difficult challenges. Biologically, the characteristic genomic diversity and persistence of infection by HIV may present serious obstacles to the generation of broadly effective immunity. Vaccine development is also constrained by the presently limited basic understanding of the immune response to HIV infection, its apparent impotence in clearing the viral load, and the ways it might be bolstered through protective immunization.

Should the biological and scientific obstacles be surmounted, there remain a number of other factors that may delay or limit the availability of an HIV vaccine. As discussed earlier in this chapter, the scarcity of available chimpanzees to test the safety and efficacy of candidate vaccines may compromise or delay adequate preclinical evaluation. Initiation of testing in human populations will also present serious ethical and practical considerations, which will undoubtedly affect the clinical evaluation of an HIV vaccine.

Traditionally, vaccine manufacturers have looked to the federal government to develop the basic understanding of the pathogen and disease before they become actively involved in vaccine development. Their decision to become involved often depends on a balance of economic and social factors. Given the extremely high cost of vaccine development programs and the present concerns over liability for vaccine-related injuries, many manufacturers may be unwilling to initiate or pursue the derivation or distribution of a vaccine to prevent AIDS.

Animal Retrovirus Vaccines

In the course of natural infections, certain retroviruses establish transient infections that are eventually cleared by the host immune system through the development of protective immunity. Other retroviruses establish infections that persist in the face of the host's active but ineffective immune response. Viruses of the former category include members of the oncornavirus subfamily, as may be typified by feline leukemia virus, while retroviruses of the latter category include all known members of the lentivirus subfamily, including HIV. (Classification schemes for retroviruses may, in the near future, be undergoing revision based on better knowledge of their genetic relationships.)

Feline leukemia virus (FeLV) is a naturally occurring retrovirus that is relatively common in domestic cats and causes a spectrum of pathologic consequences, ranging from inapparent infections to immunosuppression and leukemia. Many naturally infected cats recover and are immune from subsequent reinfection. Various approaches have been pursued in the development of an effective vaccine against FeLV, and some have achieved a high level of efficacy. Although early vaccines against FeLV infection were not completely protective (Jarrett et al., 1975; Yohn et al., 1976) and some actually enhanced the process of infection (Olsen et al., 1977), recent preparations induce protection from laboratory or experimental challenges (Lewis et al., 1981; Olsen et al., 1980; Osterhaus et al., 1985). Effective vaccines have been formulated consisting of prepared aggregates of the viral envelope glycoproteins shed from infected cells and combined with immunostimulatory adjuvants. Protection from FeLV infection has been found to correlate with the presence of virus-neutralizing antibodies directed against the viral envelope glycoprotein (Hardy et al., 1976; Lutz et al., 1980). Similar approaches have been pursued in mouse model systems, in which vaccines have been developed that effectively prevent infection and pathology induced by certain murine leukemia viruses (Hunsmann et al., 1981). In the murine retrovirus systems as well, protection from infection can be induced by immunization with preparations of viral envelope glycoproteins designed to elicit neutralizing antibodies.

In contrast to the feline and murine oncornaviruses, the development of effective vaccines against other types of retroviral infections has been very difficult, although such efforts have been under way largely in just the last few years. The most elusive category includes the viruses that, like HIV, cause chronic lifelong infections. Consideration of these viruses highlights some of the practical and theoretical difficulties in preparing an HIV vaccine. For instance, bovine leukemia virus (BLV) is a retrovirus that results in chronic latent infections of cattle. It is thought to spread among animals by the transmission of virus-infected cells. Although not phylogenetically related to HIV, it is related to the other T-lymphotropic retroviruses of humans, HTLV-I and HTLV-II. Attempts to protect cattle from BLV infection through use of vaccines have had mixed, but disappointing, results. Immunization with purified inactivated virus induced antibodies that neutralized the infectivity of BLV *in vitro* and reportedly could protect from low levels (Patrascu et al., 1980) but not higher levels (Miller et al., 1985) of challenge with virally infected cells. Thus, neutralizing antibodies alone may not be sufficient to protect against retroviral infections transmitted through cellular intermediates. A similar situation may prevail in humans infected with HTLV-I, where high titers of neutralizing antibodies are detectable using sera from infected persons in *in vitro* assays, but the infection persists *in vivo* (Ho et al., 1985b; Robert-Guroff et al., 1985; Weiss et al., 1985).

Experiences with protection from lentiviral infection through immunization are extremely limited. Preliminary attempts involving immunization of goats with caprine arthritis-encephalitis virus have failed to produce protective immunity (McGuire et al., 1986). Although disappointing, this result is too limited in scope and in its demonstrated relevance to HIV to draw conclusions about the feasibility of an AIDS vaccine. As discussed above in the section on "Animal Models," the ungulate lentiviruses may provide valuable model systems for basic studies concerning an AIDS vaccine. Given appropriate experimental support, increased activity can reasonably be expected in this area.

Recent advances in the isolation and characterization of a number of previously unknown primate retroviruses offer potential avenues for explorations of biological issues relevant to an HIV vaccine. Although not closely related to HIV, a type D primate retrovirus has been isolated that causes severe syndromes of immunosuppression and chronic wasting (Desrosiers and Letvin, 1986). Viral infection and disease resulting from inoculation with this virus can be successfully prevented by active immunization (M. Gardner, University of California at Davis, personal communication, 1986).

In addition, simian immunodeficiency viruses may provide excellent animal models for HIV infection and AIDS. Attempts to prevent SIV infection and disease in rhesus macaques are currently in progress (N. Letvin, New England Primate Center, personal communication, 1986).

Study of the natural history, virology, and immunobiology of the recently discovered human retroviruses HTLV-IV and LAV-2 may also yield important insights to further the HIV developmental efforts (Kanki et al., 1986). For instance, because infection with HTLV-IV reportedly does not cause any obvious disease, epidemiologic studies of its distribution in Africa may indicate whether prior HTLV-IV infection protects against superinfection with HIV.

The mechanisms by which the lentiviruses evade the immune response of their hosts appear rather diverse, and it is not clear which of these lentiviruses, if any, employ tactics similar to HIV (Haase, 1986; Narayan, 1986). The visna-maedi virus causes chronic progressive interstitial pneumonia and a severe demylinating encephalomyelitis in sheep. Persistent infection of sheep is accompanied by the progressive accumulation of mutations in the envelope glycoprotein, resulting in a process of antigenic drift wherein novel viral variants emerge that can escape neutralization by previously existing antiviral antibodies (Narayan et al., 1978; Thormar et al., 1983). Although new antigenic viral variants arise in the course of infection by visna viruses, the original viral strain is not replaced by them, suggesting that antigenic variation is not necessary for the maintenance of a persistent infection. Rather, the low titers and low affinity of virus-neutralizing antibodies seen following visna virus infection appear unable to prevent viral infection and spread (Kennedy-Stoskopf and Narayan, 1986).

Equine infectious anemia virus, which can maintain a chronic infection in horses and results in intermittent episodes of acute fever, weight loss, and anemia, appears to employ a different mechanism of persistence. Antigenic variation in the envelope gene of this virus also occurs, but unlike with visna the new variants that emerge in a cyclic fashion during the course of an infection escape the host immune response while previous types are replaced (Montelaro et al., 1984). However, between cycles of viremia and neutralization, viral persistence is maintained by latent infection of macrophages (Cheevers and McGuire, 1985).

Caprine arthritis-encephalitis virus, which causes a progressive leukoencephalomyelitis in goats, appears to use yet another mechanism. In this case, infection of susceptible animals fails to elicit detectable neutralizing antibodies, and, in the absence of an effective immunity, viral infection may persist unabated (Narayan et al., 1984).

Vaccines Against HIV

Virus-neutralizing antibodies are detectable in persons infected with HIV, although they are present in rather low titers (Ho et al., 1985b; Robert-Guroff et al., 1985; Weiss et al., 1985). As discussed above in the section on "Natural History of HIV Infection," these antibodies are most frequently detected using *in vitro* assays of the inhibition of free-virus infectivity. Should HIV be transmitted via infected cells, as appears likely, the relevance of the presently used neutralization assays is unclear. Similar assays are poor predictors of protection or immunity from lentivirus systems (Haase, 1986; Narayan, 1986). The developmental effort for an HIV vaccine is handicapped by the lack of a meaningful *in vitro* measure of immunologic protection from infection.

The extent of antigenic variation generated during lentivirus replication presents a major concern for development of an HIV vaccine. Isolates of HIV derived from different individuals demonstrate substantial variation in the nucleotide sequences of their envelope glycoprotein genes, although it is not yet known if these are translated into biologically significant antigenic variations (Coffin, 1986). Preliminary studies indicate that detectable immunologic differences do exist between HIV isolates; antibodies raised in animals and directed against the envelope glycoprotein purified from virions (Matthews et al., in press) or produced by recombinant DNA methods (Berman et al., 1986) will neutralize the virus type used for immunization but not divergent isolates. Independent isolates from single infected humans also demonstrate genomic variation of a similar type, but to a lesser extent (Hahn et al., 1986). It is not yet known if the observed genomic variation of HIV is involved in the virus's resistance to immune clearance, but the existence of many different strains of HIV creates a major potential difficulty for the generation of a broadly cross-reactive and protective vaccine. The regions of the viral envelope gene that are well conserved between isolates may provide targets for protective immunization, although their immunologic significance has not yet been established.

Similarly, there seems to be less variation in HIV's internal structural and regulatory proteins. The internal proteins probably have functions that do not allow so much variation in protein sequence. Unfortunately, these proteins may not be readily available to neutralizing antibodies because they are localized within cells or virions.

Preliminary reports suggest that sera from HIV-infected persons are able to neutralize variant isolates *in vitro* (Robert-Guroff et al., 1985; Weiss et al., 1985), but this result requires more extensive survey and exploration to establish its *in vivo* relevance. Evaluation of the spectrum of protection provided by vaccine candidates will require testing in relevant animal models, primarily chimpanzees.

Although most attention has focused on the antibody response against HIV as a potential agent of protection from infection, evaluation of the cellular response to virally infected cells has not been explored in detail. Since the cellular arm of the immune response is thought to be most relevant to the elimination of virally infected cells, its recruitment may be the most effective target for vaccination strategies (Weissman, 1986). The cellular immune response is known to be involved in the immune clearance of a number of types of viruses. In several of these instances, including certain retroviruses, cytotoxic T cells recognize conserved viral internal proteins expressed on the surfaces of infected cells (Holt et al., 1986; Pillemer et al., 1986; Townsend et al., 1985). If a similar reactivity exists to the conserved core proteins in HIV-infected cells, the problems posed by envelope sequence variation may be less significant.

Models of Vaccine Delivery

If antigens capable of inducing immunity to HIV infection can be identified, possible systems for vaccine delivery must be considered. The vaccines currently in use in humans generally fall into the broad categories of live or killed vaccines. Killed-virus vaccines may consist of either inactivated whole virus or viral subunits. Live vaccines against HIV would fall into two categories: those using attenuated live HIV or HIV-related viruses and those using attenuated live viral vectors into which the genes coding for appropriate HIV antigens have been inserted.

Because retroviruses in general and HIV in particular have a pronounced tendency for recombination and mutation, live attenuated retroviruses may be likely to revert to virulent forms. Problems of reversion have been overcome in the development of other live vaccines—for example, poliomyelitis. Although the problems of ensuring the safety of a live HIV vaccine would be very difficult, they should not be assumed to be insurmountable. However, other candidates, if promising, might be more attractive.

Live viral vaccines, such as vaccinia virus, carrying inserted genetic sequences encoding HIV antigens have been considered for use (Chakrabarti et al., 1986; Hu et al., 1986). Even if excellent expression of appropriate viral antigens were obtained, there are concerns about the use of these antigens that might require extensive research, development, and testing to resolve. Vaccinia vaccination with most strains may itself cause rare but serious complications, especially when given to persons who are immunocompromised. These concerns may be compounded if the effective immunogen (e.g., the envelope glycoproteins) exerts additional cytopathic effects on exposed cells.

Killed-virus vaccines may consist of inactivated viruses, of antigens extracted from the whole virus, or of antigens produced in the laboratory through recombinant DNA technologies or chemical synthesis. Killed whole HIV might not be effective against the antigenically diverse spectrum of HIVs unless an appropriate mixture of viral strains could be identified and included. This approach seems unlikely at present, given the lack of a clear definition of the extent or significance of viral heterogeneity.

As noted above, the most likely approach to an HIV vaccine is through the discovery of meaningful, broadly protective immunizing antigens and epitopes and their expression by recombinant DNA technology. Chemically synthesized peptide antigens, which are most useful in defining epitopes that are related to immunity, suffer from poor immunizing capability and are less ready for practical application than are more complex antigens made by recombinant DNA technologies. The systems presently used for the production of recombinant proteins employ bacteria, yeast, or mammalian cells. However, the candidate immunogens, including the external glycoproteins of HIV, are heavily glycosylated, which may influence the choice of organism used to produce antigens. Bacteria do not glycosylate recombinant proteins, and yeast do so quite differently than do mammalian cells. If glycosylation of an HIV antigen is necessary for appropriate immunogenicity, then production in mammalian cells may be required. Recently, the production of a large segment of the HIV envelope glycoprotein has been achieved in mammalian tissue culture cells (Berman et al., 1986). But antigen production in mammalian cells, however useful, is plagued by continuing concerns over safety. The Food and Drug Administration has approved Chinese hamster ovary cells for the production of an investigational hepatitis B vaccine. These cells have also provided usable substrates for HIV envelope production (Berman et al., 1986).

Anti-idiotype antibodies, which are produced by immunization against the variable region of specific antibodies and present an image of the original antigen, have also been explored for vaccine potential, because it is possible that the important epitopes of HIV may be discontinuous and require close proximity of more than a single continuous amino acid sequence. In the practical sense, however, there is no present example of a human anti-idiotype vaccine, just as there is no example of an adequate synthetic peptide vaccine for human use.

Any killed-virus or subunit vaccine against HIV would probably require, or at least benefit from, immunopotentiation (optimal antigen presentation) by being combined with adjuvants. Although alum is accepted as a safe adjuvant, if it proves insufficient other approaches will require evaluation and approval.

Approaches to HIV Vaccine Development and Evaluation

Testing of an HIV vaccine in human populations will present a number of difficult logistical challenges. Initial vaccine evaluation must address issues of safety and immunogenicity and is traditionally carried out in volunteer populations not at risk of infection so as to avoid confusion with immune responses that would accompany infection. This is particularly a problem when the immune response to the vaccine would be difficult to distinguish from that to a natural infection, as would likely be the case with inactivated- or attenuated-virus vaccines. With subunit vaccines, probably derived from recombinant DNA technology, the immune response would be distinguishable from natural infection. Some have argued that it might be possible for this reason to compress the usual evaluation schedule to use those at risk of infection in early safety and immunogenicity trials. This issue needs further and early discussions as actual vaccine candidates appear more promising. The selection of populations for subsequent testing for vaccine efficacy will require even more careful advance planning.

To permit trials of manageable size, populations must be identified that demonstrate a significant rate of incident HIV infections. These test populations should at the same time be representative of other target populations if the results obtained in them are to be broadly relevant. Rigorous determinations of the immunologic and virologic status of participants will be necessary at the outset to ensure that they have not already been exposed to HIV. Persons who are infected with HIV but not yet seropositive may present a difficult confounding variable.

Testing of vaccine efficacy will require double-blind, randomized, placebo-controlled trials. However, the nature and severity of HIV infection may make it difficult to design such trials so that they meet the standards of ethics commonly accepted or required for research. It can be argued that allowing susceptible persons at high risk of HIV infection to persevere in their high-risk behaviors is distinctly unethical when health education could lessen their likelihood of HIV infection and disease. Participation in the vaccine trials may also positively or negatively affect the frequency of high-risk behaviors practiced by test subjects, influencing their rate of incident infection independent of vaccine effectiveness. These difficulties must begin to be addressed now.

Another difficulty involves the unwillingness of many pharmaceutical companies to commit to a significant financial and scientific investment in vaccine development in the face of present liability threats and insurance considerations. Concerns exist over liability both during the testing phase of vaccine development and after a vaccine is licensed but are perhaps greater during the latter period. Unless problems of vaccine liability are dealt with swiftly and effectively, no manufacturer may be willing to produce HIV vaccine for use in the American market.

The liability issue is critical, but the degree of its impact will depend on the proposed approaches and target populations for vaccine development. Should a vaccine be targeted solely at defined groups at high risk, specific statements of risk-benefit analysis might serve to lessen liability concerns. Perhaps a vaccine candidate, once proven useful, could be made available to significant numbers of individuals as a subsidized, semipermanent, investigational product. However, any proposed strategy of general use—whether for adolescents or for the general public—immediately raises the multitude of problems experienced during the mass immunization initiative for swine influenza. Most notably, the temporal coincidence of diseases of unknown etiology with mass immunization programs predictably raises the level of litigiousness to a point where even federal resources for compensation of perceived vaccine-related injuries can be strained. In addition, the real or imagined risk of administration of an HIV vaccine might be considered much greater than for other vaccines. Similarly, the consequences of failure of vaccine protection might be considered more severe in the case of an HIV vaccine. These issues must be addressed in advance of any such efforts with respect to HIV vaccination.

Conclusions and Recommendations

Developing a vaccine to prevent HIV infection and AIDS presents a number of scientific challenges that have never before been responded to successfully. As a result, an effective vaccine may be very difficult, if not impossible, to produce. Should an effective vaccine candidate become available, there are significant social concerns that may limit or prevent its testing and use. Therefore, a vaccine may not be reasonably expected to be available in less than 5 years. Even for the next 5 to 10 years, the committee generally believes that the probability of a licensed vaccine becoming available is low.

• An aggressive basic and applied research endeavor is essential to evaluate the possibilities and prospects for effective vaccines. It is clear that a successful vaccine development program will depend on a greatly expanded foundation of basic research knowledge concerning HIV. Because of the long developmental process for vaccines, basic and applied studies should be adequately supported and effectively organized.

• Vaccine development programs will benefit from the active and interactive participation of government, academia, and industry. New methods to encourage the interchange of information and minimize proprietary considerations should be evaluated.

• The committee finds that there has been inadequate federal coordination of vaccine development. The NIH has recently reorganized its efforts on AIDS, and the committee encourages the appointment of strong leadership to the vaccine program, with authority and responsibility to develop a strategy for a broad-ranging vaccine development program. This program should take advantage of the strengths available within NIH, in the external scientific community, and in industry.

• Industry is fearful of involvement in the development of vaccines because of the potential liability it must accept in distributing them. Creative options for the governmental support of industrial research, guarantees of vaccine purchase, and assumption of reasonable liability should therefore be explored. (The only alternative to commercial production is the establishment of government production facilities and total assumption of liability.) For instance, states could enact malpractice and product liability reform laws that would encourage programs of HIV vaccine development. The enactment of a reasonable financial limitation or "cap" on court and jury awards in personal injury and product liability cases arising out of the clinical testing of an HIV vaccine or out of the use of a licensed vaccine on the market may provide one reasonable approach.

• It is imperative that ethical and pragmatic problems be addressed simultaneously with scientific ones, so that possible success in developing a vaccine candidate can be exploited expeditiously in a way that meets ethical and legal criteria. The committee therefore recommends that its proposed National Commission on AIDS consider establishing a special subcommittee on the ethical, legal, and social issues involved in the testing of HIV vaccines.

SOCIAL SCIENCE RESEARCH NEEDS

As much as AIDS is a medical and biological issue, it also has important social dimensions. HIV infection is spread through particular types of behavior, and presently the best hope for stopping the epidemic spread of the virus is through changes in the types of behavior responsible for its continued transmission. Yet the forces that shape human behavior, and the best approaches to influencing behavior to protect health, are among the most complex and poorly understood aspects of society's response to the AIDS epidemic. It is instructive to note that virologic research, having received reasonable levels of funding over the years, was well poised to begin addressing the many biological problems posed by HIV. In contrast, the knowledge base in the behavioral and social sciences needed to design approaches to encouraging behavioral change is more rudimentary because of chronic inadequate funding. This lack of behavioral and social science research generates some of the most important and immediate research questions surrounding the epidemic.

Social science research can play a number of valuable roles in meeting the challenge of AIDS. It can help in the development of effective education programs to encourage changes in behavior that will break the chain of HIV transmission. It can contribute to the development of informed public policies that reduce the public's fear of AIDS and discriminatory practices toward AIDS sufferers. And it can guide the establishment of improved health care and social services that further the ability to treat AIDS patients effectively, humanely, and at reasonable cost.

To date, there has been little social science research specifically focusing on HIV infection and AIDS, but there have been studies of the factors influencing behavior change, risk perception, attitudes toward civil liberties, tolerance and discrimination, communication, and the organization of health care that are relevant to the AIDS epidemic. These studies suggest avenues for research more directly related to AIDS. Such research can be useful in guiding short-term administrative and social responses to the epidemic and in providing the clarification necessary for developing longer-term measures for coping with AIDS and, more generally, with future health crises.

Breaking the Chain of Transmission

As discussed in Chapter 4, educational efforts aimed at providing accurate information to persons at risk of infection are currently the best available public health measures to stop the spread of HIV infection. However, a great deal must be learned before the optimal educational approaches can be derived, accurately targeted, and effectively transmitted. The literature on behavioral risk modification generally concedes the extraordinary difficulty of modifying behavior, even when there is clear demonstration of risk (Leventhal and Cleary, 1980). Much of this research focuses on alcoholism, cigarette smoking, and dietary risks; it is therefore only indirectly related to the risks of infectious disease. Even research on other sexually transmitted diseases is not entirely analogous to AIDS, because of AIDS' exceptionally dire consequences and the lack of effective medical therapies.

In all of these areas, a common assumption (and a common assumption in discussions of AIDS) is that repetitive media information will induce people to change their behavior to avoid risk. While research on this hypothesis is scattered and results are inconclusive, several useful points emerge. There are areas where extensive media reports (for example, those relating cholesterol-producing foods with heart disease) have contributed to positive changes in consumer behavior over a long time period. Similarly, media publicity about the possible adverse effects of birth control pills and intrauterine devices (IUDs) also resulted in a significant decline in their use (Jones et al., 1980). However, these and other examples of behavioral responses to information are all in areas where alternatives are easily available. By the same token, the risks may be lower and less poorly defined in many of these areas as compared with the risks associated with HIV infection.

Deliberate efforts to use the media to influence behavior have not necessarily achieved their desired result. Despite extensive public information about the Salk polio vaccine in the late 1950s when it was first available, relatively few individuals agreed to be vaccinated at that time (Robinson, 1963). Similarly, media coverage of the 1964 Surgeon General's report on smoking and cancer had little direct effect on smoking habits in the short term (Troyer and Markle, 1983). Although people seek information to guide even the most personal decisions, they use this information mainly when it corresponds to prior inclinations or when it is reinforced by their social situation and the beliefs and attitudes of their reference groups.

Review of the literature on the effect of risk information on smoking behavior shows that communication is generally ineffective unless it is directed to specifically defined target populations, contains an "action plan," comes from credible sources, and is combined with community and peer support (Leventhal and Cleary, 1980). Other analyses (Lichtenstein, 1982) emphasize the importance of peer leaders and social support networks in effecting behavior change. Studies of drug treatment and rehabilitation programs confirm these findings. For example, a study of narcotics treatment programs by Caloff (1967) identified different types of narcotics users and stressed the need to adapt information and rehabilitation programs appropriately. In a study of methadone mainte-nance programs, Nelkin (1973) indicated that without an adequate social support system and appropriate changes in the environment, the effect of methadone on the behavior of heroin addicts has been limited. The importance of group support and pressure has been evident in the relative success of groups and programs such as Alcoholics Anonymous in changing life-styles (Roman and Trice, 1972).

Research in other social science areas yields similar results. Persuasion research (often performed in laboratory settings) offers compelling evidence of the importance of group pressure and credible sources as variables in influencing behavior (Bostrom, 1983; Roloff and Miller, 1980). Similarly, research on the diffusion of innovation finds that acceptance of new ideas depends on the role of personal networks and opinion leaders who are trusted, especially when innovation requires changes in social or cultural norms (Rogers, 1983).

This research consistently emphasizes, first, the importance of shaping information appropriately for specific groups and distributing it through credible and trusted sources within the target community. Second, it points to the need for providing social reinforcement to maintain behavior change.

Enough is known to suggest that education and other techniques of persuasion may achieve success in inducing behavior change if pursued intensively and systematically (Farquhar et al., 1984), but it is also necessary to strive to improve these intervention strategies. Several directions for social science research specifically relevant to AIDS and HIV transmission need to be pursued, in addition to the evaluation of the effectiveness of various education programs described in Chapter 4. Knowledge acquired through this research will enable interventions to be better designed and directed.

A first necessary task would be to develop a demography of HIV infection that would identify not only high-risk groups but also spouses, sexual partners, children of infected parents, family members, and so on. In essence, a more detailed, representative, and contemporary evaluation of sexual behavior analogous to the Kinsey Report is needed to assess the range and varieties of sexual behaviors in both the homosexual and heterosexual communities. Increased knowledge of sexual behaviors and the factors that affect those behaviors will be necessary to design improved approaches to inducing behavior change. Areas for study include the development of sexual orientation, the selection of sexual partners and practices, and choices about methods for safeguarding health or preventing pregnancy in various groups. It is desirable to gather information on these topics not only for adults but also for adolescents. Additionally, it is essential to know the size of those groups that engage in various sexual practices. It would then be essential to map out the existing and potential sources of health information available to these groups and to target credible sources (i.e., ex-addicts, organizations within the homosexual community, churches, social networks, neighborhood groups) that will be trusted as conveyers of information and that can offer social support.

Similarly, more needs to be known about the reasons why people begin using drugs, especially IV drugs, about the influences on choice of drugs and routes of administration, about what motivates cessation of drug use, about the factors that can reinforce choices to quit, and about the variation of these in various groups of drug users. Influences on behavior in adolescents as well as adults should be studied. International comparisons will be necessary to ascertain the best methods for combating drug use and the efforts of various interventions (e.g., needle availability) in reducing HIV transmission, since the full range of methods cannot be tried in any one country.

It will also be very important to study the social dynamics, rituals, and practices of various risk populations. The point of such studies would be to analyze and develop effective means to reach people at risk, delineate the obstacles to behavior change (for example, rituals concerning the sharing of needles and syringes among IV drug users), and determine an effective language and style of communication. The use of appropriate language is particularly critical given the diverse background of the populations at risk. What is meaningful to the gay community may be quite irrelevant for IV drug users. Just as AIDS clearly affects certain high-risk groups, it also has the potential to affect the whole of society. It is necessary to reach individuals in groups where the prevalence of HIV infection is presently high, but it is also imperative to reach individuals in lower-prevalence communities, many of whom do not consider themselves at risk of infection or AIDS. Information aimed at high-risk groups may in delivery and content miss other persons potentially at risk, such as men who consider their bisexual behavior as safe, sexual partners of IV drug users or bisexual men, heterosexually active persons in high-risk areas, or the clientele of prostitutes. Specifically targeted information will not be enough to stop the spread of AIDS. Novel approaches must be evaluated to reach and inform all individuals and social groups.

Another type of research should monitor the adoption of safer sex practices and other positive changes in behavior by those at risk. Similarly, studies of sex education programs should be under way to evaluate the means of communicating information about sex, the effectiveness of various approaches in fostering protective behavioral change, and the factors that make such programs politically viable as well as effective. Finally, social experiments could be devised to develop strategies for intervention (e.g., information campaigns, distribution of free sterile needles and syringes to IV drug users) to evaluate their effectiveness and to better understand the variables that encourage safe behavior.

Reducing Public Fear and Its Effects

The public response to AIDS has been one of fear, often reflected in excessive caution, discriminatory behavior, and recommendations for drastic policy measures that are unwarranted in terms of what is known about the actual risk. As described in Chapter 4, national polls of public attitudes about AIDS indicate that most people are highly attentive to news about AIDS and that many are inclined to overestimate risks (Singer and Rogers, 1986).

Important dimensions of the public response to AIDS are suggested in a study by McClosky and Brell (1983) of tolerance in the United States. The study addresses the fragility of tolerance; most Americans voice support of civil liberties, but they often reject concrete applications. The study found persistent intolerance and fear of homosexuals and only fragile respect for their rights, a fact that certain groups concerned about "moral erosion" are able to exploit politically. Finally, the study suggests that opinion leaders—clergy, media, community leaders—are likely to be more tolerant and protective of civil liberties than is the public at large.

An important research question involves the dynamics of discriminatory practices and behavior relating to HIV infection and AIDS. For instance, why do some schools or workplaces exclude AIDS sufferers, while others accept and help them? Because factors other than the actual extent of risk enter into public perceptions, studies of the response to AIDS should probe well beyond people's factual understanding. How and by whom were employers or colleagues informed? How do the backgrounds of the persons involved in a dispute influence their perceptions? What were their prior relations in the work setting? Do different responses reflect the structure of the social setting or the mode of disseminating information? The object of such research is to develop effective means of public communication that will counter discriminatory practices and lead to workable decision-making procedures predicated on the most accurate scientific understanding available rather than prejudice resulting from inadequate or inaccurate information.

Public attitudes that tend to overestimate the risks surrounding AIDS are consistent with research findings about public perceptions. Studies of risk perception suggest that the public underestimates familiar risks and overestimates those that are unfamiliar, involuntary, invisible, and potentially catastrophic (Fischoff et al., 1981). Fear is often attributed to people's inability to deal with uncertainty. However, this generalization has been questioned by those who observe the considerable ability to deal in a probabilistic manner with uncertain variables in many occupations (Douglas, 1986). AIDS appears to be a new problem, one of uncertain origin and rapid but silent spread. It thus presents enormous challenges regarding the adjustment of public perceptions to the accumulating medical and scientific understanding of AIDS and HIV transmission.

Sociological studies also suggest that perceptions of risk are heavily influenced by political and social attitudes. Thus, different cultures or social groups will emphasize certain risks and minimize others (Douglas and Wildavsky, 1982). Perceptions of risk are also closely connected to legitimizing moral principles (Berger and Luckman, 1966). In the United States, the strength of religious feeling and morality has turned issues of abortion, animal welfare, evolution, and reproductive technologies into major policy disputes and has of course influenced the public response to AIDS as well. (It should also be noted that some churches have been in the forefront of promoting a positive, constructive, and compassionate attitude toward AIDS sufferers. They can play an important role in educating their members, as mentioned in Chapter 4.) Finally, risk research indicates that political factors, in particular trust in authority and expertise, also shape perceptions and fears (Nelkin and Brown, 1984). Mistrust of experts and failure to distribute information through locally available and respected community leaders have contributed to public fear of AIDS—for instance, in the exacerbation of disputes over allowing children with AIDS to attend public schools (Nelkin and Hilgartner, 1986).

A rhetoric of accountability and blame often pervades the discourse about risks. Many have observed the tendency to blame the victim as a means of silencing indictments of the social order. The sick are often blamed for their ill health, the poor for their economic plight (Navarro, 1977; Donzelot, 1979). For instance, there has been a striking contrast between media accounts of AIDS patients in pediatric and transfusion-associated cases, who are often portrayed as "innocent victims," as opposed to the depiction of implicit responsibility in cases among homosexual men and IV drug users.

Efforts to influence risk perception usually begin with proposals to improve public education (Kunreuther, 1978). Yet many studies suggest that educational measures alone do little to change public attitudes (Slovic et al., 1981). People interpret information in highly selective ways, a fact well documented in the studies of the effect of media information on attitudes (Klapper, 1960). Information from the media is absorbed and assimilated in different ways depending on the predispositions of the reader, the influence of peers and opinion leaders, and the trust in the credibility of sources (Cohen, 1964). However, the press does help to establish a framework of expectations, so that isolated events take on meaning as public issues. By widening the base of public information, the press defines a context for public policy and forces a policy response (Lang and Kurt, 1983; Tuchman, 1978).

A major challenge is to provide information in a way that will create the sense of urgency necessary without causing undue panic. The communication literature suggests that effective information campaigns must distribute the judgments of experts through credible and trusted opinion leaders who can effectively channel information to various targeted communities.

Organizing Health and Social Services

There are several important directions for research on providing services to AIDS patients. A necessary first step will be to map the now poorly defined multiplicity of state, federal, and local agencies and private and public institutions involved in health and social policies relating to AIDS. Goals of such a project would be to identify areas where institutional fragmentation or professional specialization are counterproductive, to understand the effects of the present system of financing medical care and social services, and to develop better and more cost-effective means of coordination. Similarly, there is a need to document and evaluate the various types of services that are presently available to persons infected with HIV in different communities, ranging from hospitals to terminal care facilities and home services. It will be important to evaluate their effectiveness, their acceptability to patients and the community, their cost, and their distribution of costs.

Comparative studies of hospital management practices—for example, the allocation of beds, the distribution of resources within a hospital, and the ways in which the staff copes with the stress of working with patients with a fatal and intractable disease—could be useful in improving the effectiveness of hospital practices. Social experiments based on different models of patient care developed in high-incidence areas (see Chapter 5) will permit evaluation of their applicability to other areas and will provide a foundation on which to build locally relevant programs.

Studies are also needed that recognize the difficulties HIV-infected patients have in gaining access to services, the effects of homophobia and negative attitudes toward drug users, and the conflicts that may arise between individuals in high-risk groups over access to care. The problem of providing treatment and care to IV drug users is especially intractable but has been virtually ignored as a focus of research since the development of methadone and other treatment programs.

Finally, understanding the policy and social service response to AIDS would be enriched by comparative international studies that could provide alternative models and new ideas. What legal, social, fiscal, and administrative structures have been instituted in response to AIDS in different countries? How do those countries provide services for patients; report, contain, or restrict high-risk groups; try to protect the general population; or deal with testing, blood donation, employment, and the allocation of resources for health services and research? How do their national policies and practices reflect the legal context; the cultural and social definitions of disease, the cultural biases about homosexuality and drug abuse, concepts of civil liberties, and the general structure of their social and medical services? If not alternative models, such comparative studies could at least provide new ideas for approaching AIDS within the United States and fostering international cooperation.

Conclusions and Recommendations

Because effective drugs or vaccines to counter HIV infection are not now available, effective educational interventions are essential to limit the spread of the virus. However, previous experience with educational programs to promote behavioral change for disease prevention is rather discouraging. There is a great need to explore novel approaches in AIDS-related education and to vigorously examine the relative efficacy of various approaches.

Social science research should be directed toward the following goals:

- Establishing the demography of heterosexual, homosexual, and IV drug use behaviors and the characteristics of the groups that practice different patterns of behavior;
- Identifying credible information sources for various groups and opinion leaders;
- Conducting experiments and demonstration projects on approaches to behavior change to understand what does or does not work;
- Tracking discriminatory practices and their dynamics (Why is discrimination a problem in some areas and situations and not in others?);
- Evaluating treatment, social service programs, and hospital management practices to understand what works and is cost-effective;
- Studying the special problems of caring for addicted individuals and preventing transmission among IV drug users;
- Linking experimental educational programs with epidemiologic evaluation of their effectiveness in reducing the rate of seroconversion across the spectrum of populations at risk;
- Making comparative studies of international responses to the epidemic;
- Studying the public's understanding of and attitudes toward AIDS and related issues in order to better design interventions to promote accurate awareness;
- Studying and analyzing the ethical and legal aspects of the AIDS epidemic.

FUNDING FOR RESEARCH RELATED TO AIDS AND HIV

The current national commitment to AIDS and HIV research must be considered in light of the nation's overall commitment to biomedical research. In 1985 the United States spent an estimated $13.5 billion for health research and development (Wyngaarden, 1985). The federal government contributed $6.8 billion—about one half of the total. The National Institutes of Health alone provided $4.8 billion, or 70 percent of the total federal investment in biomedical research. Thus, the NIH was responsible for over 35 percent of the funding from all sources in the nation.

In 1985, industry spent about $5 billion on health research and development, or 37 percent of the national total. About $3.3 billion of industry's expenses were for biomedical research and development for human health. Large pharmaceutical firms contributed the major portion of this investment in biomedical research. A number of large firms have emphasized the new biotechnologies by creating new institutional arrangements. A variety of novel and innovative partnerships have been formed between industrial firms, private research institutes, and the academic research community. In addition, a number of relatively small research-intensive companies have arisen in recent years and have invested significant energies and funds in the new biotechnologies.

Foundations and other private sources contributed about 8 percent of the total national effort in biomedical research. An important component of this contribution is research and training grants.

Current Levels of and Mechanisms for Funding

The total amount spent on research on AIDS and HIV is a very small portion of the overall national effort for biomedical research and development. The largest commitment has been made by the federal government through the Public Health Service (PHS), which includes the National Institutes of Health, the Centers for Disease Control (CDC), the Food and Drug Administration (FDA), the Alcohol, Drug Abuse, and Mental Health Administration (ADAMHA), and the Health Resources and Services Administration. The actual PHS expenditure in 1985 was about $108 million. Out of this, the NIH spent $63 million, the CDC $33 million, FDA $9 million, and ADAMHA $2.6 million. For 1986, Congress appropriated the following amounts to PHS agencies: CDC, $64.9 million; NIH, $140.7 million; FDA, $10 million; and ADAMHA, $12.7 million, for a total of $244.3 million (including expenditures in the Office of the Secretary of Health and Human Services).

Centers for Disease Control

Funds allocated to the CDC are used for many purposes, including research. Most research is applied, reflecting the CDC's primary role in disease detection, surveillance, and education. Each CDC grant for demonstration projects aimed at AIDS prevention must contain an evaluation research component, but the size and scope of these research components are difficult to assess.

A number of cooperative agreements have been made between the CDC and various states and localities for specific epidemiologic studies of AIDS. Considerable central direction and protocol development are involved in these studies, but ideas for the studies may originate from persons outside the CDC's staff. The cooperative agreements are awarded after open competition based on published requests for proposals.

National Institutes of Health

Funds assigned to the NIH are distributed through institutes. Most AIDS-related funding is provided by the National Institute of Allergy and Infectious Diseases (NIAID) and the National Cancer Institute. Funds are distributed in the form of peer-reviewed research grants, contracts, and cooperative agreements and to NIH staff scientists.

Other Federal and State Agencies

The Food and Drug Administration has a key responsibility in the development of new therapeutics and devices such as the HIV antibody test. Recent changes in the agency are facilitating the investigation of new therapeutics for AIDS. In addition, the Alcohol, Drug Abuse, and Mental Health Administration will be handling social sciences research in all three of its institutes.

The Department of Defense has a significant effort under way in monitoring military personnel who have been identified as being infected with HIV. Significant research capacity resides in military institutes such as the Walter Reed Army Institute for Research, some of which is being focused on AIDS. In FY 1986, approximately $37 million has been allocated to the Department of the Army for the support of AIDS-related research. However, the committee is not aware of projections for AIDS-related research funding in the military budget for future years.

Some state governments have also become directly involved in the support of AIDS-related research activities, including those of California, Massachusetts, and New York. Other states are also considering the support of AIDS research, either as it relates to specific issues within their jurisdictions or as it relates to broader basic or applied research questions.

Industry

It is not possible to estimate the contribution by industry to AIDS research and development, but the amount must be only a small portion of industry's total biomedical research and development expenses. The smaller biotechnology firms have the manpower and capabilities to contribute much to this effort. A number of these companies have programs to develop AIDS vaccines or new diagnostic tests. Other small biotechnology firms have ongoing programs of research on interleukin-2, interferon, and various immunomodulators.

The commitment of pharmaceutical and biotechnology companies to AIDS research must be considered in terms of the research and development investment risks involved. In a number of these areas, the developmental costs are quite high and must be weighed against the anticipated commercial returns of new products.

A number of large pharmaceutical firms also have research and development programs for diagnostic tests and new treatment and prevention strategies for AIDS. Some of these companies have been able to redirect their existing research capabilities to address the AIDS problem. Among the areas under investigation are possible antiviral drugs for individuals already infected with HIV, drugs for treating opportunistic infections, and new kinds of diagnostic tests.

The creation, testing, and distribution of new drugs and vaccines require numerous and diverse types of expertise. Strategies for the development of agents to treat or prevent HIV infection and AIDS will greatly benefit from the most effective use of all of these needed resources. Large pharmaceutical firms can make a tremendous contribution by investment of their demonstrated skill toward the evaluation, production, distribution, and marketing of candidate AIDS drugs or vaccines. Many smaller companies could also provide innovative contributions to the derivation of such agents. Thus, the involvement of commercial companies in vaccine and treatment efforts is highly desirable and may well be essential in the nation's response to the AIDS epidemic. In addition, a commitment to AIDS-related research is not understood fully by the management of most companies; usually, the motivation comes from the scientific staff. The effort is usually viewed as a public service, and the therapeutics being developed are perceived to have a limited orphan drug status. However, the development of new therapeutics for AIDS, ARC, and HIV infection, such as safe and effective antiviral drugs for seropositive individuals, would have an exceptionally large national and international market potential (see Chapters 3 and 7).

Current NIH Funding Mechanisms

A detailed analysis of the history and evolution of NIH AIDS funding was commissioned by the committee (Stoto et al., 1986). In FY 1982, 47 percent of NIH AIDS funds went to intramural research, and 39 percent went to extramural research grants. Since then, there has been an increasing emphasis on contracts and cooperative agreements, as work in more applied areas, such as clinical trials of new drugs, increases. Most of the extra congressional appropriation for AIDS in FY 1986 ($70 million) was for contracts or cooperative agreements. In FY 1986, $22.7 million (19 percent) of NIH AIDS funds went for support of new or continuing research grants (including some cooperative agreements); $28.1 million (23 percent) went for intramural research; and $64.1 million went for research contracts, not counting an additional $13.9 million still in the NIH director's office that will probably also go to contracts. It is thus apparent that, as a proportion of the total amount allocated, distribution by the contract mechanism has proportionally grown by the greatest amount, and well over 50 percent of NIH AIDS funds are now used to support contracts. Some of this increase is represented by the advent of funding of clinical testing programs for the evaluation of AIDS therapeutics, but this represents only a part of the total growth in this category. Between FY 1983 and 1986, there was a steady decline in the proportion of NIH funds spent for investigator-initiated research grants and an increasing proportion expended for NIH-designed contracts.

This changing emphasis on the distribution of research funding is cause for some concern. Much of the most important research that needs to be addressed is of a basic nature. The major NIH support for basic research is provided through investigator-initiated, peer-reviewed grants. This system traditionally has been used to evaluate the scientific merit of a research proposal and, by comparing it with competing grants, to prioritize the allocation of funds. It has been widely acknowledged as an effective means of promoting innovative, novel, and important work. This mechanism stimulates the broadest possible involvement of high-caliber nonfederal researchers in the development and evaluation of projects. With contract funding, the scope of work and approaches used tend to be specified by federal scientists, and the critique and prioritization of applications tend to involve scientists from the nonfederal sector to a lesser extent.

Emphasis on the contract mechanism for the channeling of funds for AIDS and HIV research means that a lower proportion of the total funding is available for investigator-initiated proposals. Hence, fewer proposals and less interest are generated in the nonfederal research community. Additionally, the influence of that community—an acknowledged major source of scientific expertise—in setting the national research agenda is substantially diminished.

Notwithstanding the quality of researchers and policymakers in federal agencies, the problem of AIDS demands that the broadest range of expertise be involved. A more balanced growth of support is desirable in coming funding cycles to promote the involvement of the nonfederal research community to a greater extent.

Reliance on centrally planned studies is advantageous in certain situations, particularly where many federal agencies are involved and where the problem clearly requires a well-coordinated effort. A central organization can be expected to be particularly useful when studies require many different types of expertise and where needed actions can be clearly defined. However, an overcommitment to centrally planned studies may prove detrimental to the nation's broader research effort and potential. If the tendency toward centralized research studies continues to the exclusion of the creative scientific input from researchers outside of the NIH, or if it results in the compromise of research funding for investigator-initiated, peer-reviewed grants, extremely deleterious consequences may result. The intramural and extramural NIH efforts must be mutually interactive and beneficial if the nation's research on AIDS and HIV is to be optimally productive.

An additional problem with NIH's funding for AIDS research in recent years is that it has been derived largely through reprogramming of funds from other health areas (Krause, 1986; Stoto et al., 1986). These funds were diverted from ongoing NIH activities, in the form of personnel positions and research support, to satisfy expectations of progress on AIDS in the absence of a commensurate provision of adequate funding. As a result, many of the NIH's non-AIDS programs have been detrimentally affected. However, these areas have not diminished in importance or urgency. Hence, reprogramming of funds is not an appropriate response to research funding for AIDS and HIV, because it delays progress toward controlling other health problems and toward establishing the knowledge base needed to deal with AIDS. It is important that funds and personnel positions be restored to these areas. The current situation at the NIH and its resultant ability to respond to the AIDS epidemic are further constrained by a hiring freeze that affects the recruitment of new investigators.

The essential point in this regard is that HIV infection and its consequences are a new and additional problem. Other problems have not diminished, nor has the public expectation diminished that they will be pursued actively by the biomedical research community.

The ability to act flexibly to exploit new information and pursue new ideas is essential in this rapidly moving field. For the reasons noted above, future reprogramming of monies would damage the capacity to maintain stability of funding for other important areas. Congress and the administration should continue to be open to consideration of supplemental requests to ensure that research on prevention and treatment of HIV infection is not delayed or other areas penalized.

Decisions on the appropriate level of overall funding for research on AIDS and HIV need to take into account all of the criteria listed above, and no simple formula exists to assist this process. The National Commission on AIDS proposed by the committee could provide a useful service by monitoring the distribution and needs for research funding in these areas. Decision makers should keep these activities under review, and the total allocation of funds to research on AIDS and HIV should be reexamined periodically.

Distribution of Funds Among Agencies and to Specific Research Areas

The committee identified a number of research areas in need of support that fall under various agencies, but it did not attempt to assess the distribution of funds among agencies. Nor did it attempt to address in detail a variety of specific questions, such as the relative claims of research on vaccines versus drug development or research versus educational efforts (in each case both efforts are justifiable).

Although no comprehensive attempt was made to prioritize funding needs, some specific needs were thought to be particularly important. The committee noted a particular dearth of research in social science and behavioral research related to AIDS and HIV. It recommends that its assessment of research needs and funding levels act merely as a starting point for an extensive evaluation of these topics.

Some funding for research on AIDS and HIV has, in recent years, been provided by states, and this has been critically important in certain areas. An assessment is needed of the respective roles and responsibilities of federal agencies, states, and other funding sources in the support of this research.

Assessing Desirable Levels of Research Support

The task of determining the appropriate level of federal funding for any health research area is exceedingly complex. Consideration of the problem usually starts with an assessment of the impact of the disease, sometimes in comparison with other health problems. The numbers of cases can be tabulated in a variety of ways—mortality, morbidity, duration, severity, disability, type of complication, or sequelae. Such considerations can include not only the severest consequences but also the burden of milder cases. Some measures of burden address the age distribution of disease, including early deaths and years of life lost. Particular types of morbidity may be weighted particularly heavily—e.g., neuropsychiatric impairment. The burden of disease can also be calculated in terms of the health care costs or other impacts on the health system—e.g., the percentage of beds occupied by AIDS cases. To these considerations must be added some weighting related to knowledge about the trends and spread of the disease, including the uncertainty and public anxiety over these factors.

The total federal funding initially allocated for research on AIDS and HIV for FY 1986 (exclusive of the military allocation of $37 million) was about $192.8 million. This was later increased to approximately $240 million. This amount compares to research allocations of about $1,500 million in FY 1986 for cancer; $650 million for heart disease; $59 million for motor vehicle accidents; and $27 million for sickle cell disease. A research investment ratio can be calculated for these diseases, in which the present federal investment is compared to estimated deaths by each disease category during the next decade (Graham, 1986).

Such analytical measures are useful, but they provide only one factor to be considered in the overall decision processes determining the distribution and relative levels of research funding. Other factors include

• The strength of desire to ameliorate the problems;
• The perceived opportunities and likelihood that funding will result in applicable results;
• The spillover effect for basic research in which findings have applicability to other health problems (For example, the rapid progress on HIV was largely a result of funding for basic research in cancer virology in the late 1960s and 1970s.);
• The likely quality of research that will result if funds are allocated (In this area the question is whether additional funds can be effectively used. Peer review priority scores for NIH-funded grants related to AIDS are now equal to those in other areas and are likely to improve further if active recruitment of more high-caliber individuals to the area is attempted.);
• Inducements (or the lack of them) other than federal funding to conduct research, including the market size for potential products and their patent or liability protection (e.g., for vaccines).

A compelling reason for increasing AIDS funding is the nature of the uncertainty about the future course of the epidemic. It is clear that the problem will worsen considerably over the next 5 to 10 years, and without much question it will persist into the next century. The presently uncertain rate of spread of HIV infection further into the heterosexual population will determine the ultimate magnitude of the epidemic. Rather than waiting to see how bad the problem will become, all eventualities must be prepared for now by putting a very high priority on AIDS and HIV research. If the epidemic worsens dramatically, as is quite conceivable, it may be too late to mount the required effort.

The United States has a special responsibility to assist the rest of the world in handling disease problems. This country has the largest biomedical research community in the world, has been the main source of progress in biomedical research for the world since the 1950s, and is looked to as a major intellectual and financial resource for dealing with international health crises. As discussed in Chapter 7, AIDS is presently a health crisis of extraordinary magnitude in Africa and is rapidly spreading to many countries in the world. Much is expected of the United States, and U.S. efforts have the potential to be of great benefit in the world's struggle against AIDS.

Taking into account the projected impact of the disease and balancing the opportunities and implications of research on this and other diseases, research related to AIDS and HIV ranks high on all of the scales normally used to assess research funding levels. However, it is a new disease, recently added to the existing agenda for health research. The rapid accumulation of knowledge regarding the magnitude and nature of the problem has meant that unforeseen needs and opportunities have constantly been arising.

The committee was not able to identify any currently funded area that is not potentially useful. However, as noted earlier in this chapter, it did identify many areas of basic and applied biomedical, epidemiologic, and social science research that are urgently in need of extra emphasis. Because of the necessarily long lag time from basic research to the benefits of that research, and because of the increasing magnitude of the problem, investments in research on AIDS and HIV should be made immediately. Thus, the level of funding for such research should be increased substantially.

Those assessing the committee's proposed increase in research funds may question whether the base of scientific personnel and facilities in the United States is large enough to usefully absorb this extra funding. The answer is clearly yes. As discussed above, funds are needed for a variety of efforts and must be distributed to a diverse set of research questions. Furthermore, the money should not all be appropriated through the NIH. Some should go to the CDC; some should go to the ADAMHA; and some should go through the National Science Foundation to social science research.

The quality of institutional resources and facilities available for the job is another important question. The U.S. biomedical research establishment is physically in poor shape and cannot take full advantage of modern instrumentation because of policies that have limited funds to upgrade equipment in recent years. The ability to deal with the continuing problem of HIV infection and other existing and new health problems may be drastically impaired within the next decade if major investments are not made in facilities, equipment, and training programs.

It is apparent that AIDS is a multifaceted problem that will not be solved easily or quickly and that many of the areas requiring attention are fundamental, needing long-term research to yield any benefit. Thus, all groups funding research (e.g., the Public Health Service, the Department of Defense, states, foundations) need to recognize the desirability of a long-term commitment to substantial programs of research on AIDS and HIV. It is prudent to act as though the problem will escalate and to increase research funding accordingly.

The committee did not attempt to build a detailed budget that could be used, for example, in the appropriations process. Rather, it strove to assess the desirable overall magnitude of such a budget. The PHS request to the U.S. Department of Health and Human Services for AIDS-related research in FY 1988 was $471 million. If appropriated, this budget request would represent about a doubling of funds from FY 1986 to FY 1988. The NSF spends just over $50 million annually on social science research, but presently a very small amount of this is on studies related to AIDS.

The committee believes that there are sufficient areas of need and opportunity to double research funding again by 1990, leading to an approximately $1-billion budget in that year. The areas of clear need include the following:

- *High-Containment Facilities for Primate Research*   Upgrading primate centers will require millions of dollars for construction and increased support.
- *Better Containment Facilities for Universities and Research Institutes*   Improved containment facilities are needed to foster wider involvement of the non-NIH research community. Certain types of AIDS research cannot be carried out under normal laboratory conditions.
- *Training Funds*   Fewer biomedical scientists are being trained under federal programs every year, which will eventually result in fewer new biomedical investigators. The AIDS research program must have a strong training component to ensure that sufficient talent exists for future programs. Also, training in specific areas, such as primate physiology, will be needed.
- *Construction and Renovation Funds*   The facilities for biomedical research in the United States are in great need of renovation because of years of chronic underfunding of their maintenance.
- *Equipment*   Funding for equipment, which has been neglected by sponsors in recent years, also needs to be part of a balanced AIDS research program.
- *Social Science and Behavioral Research*   Funding for the various types of social science and behavioral research needed, especially that for mounting effective public education programs, is seriously deficient.
- *Vaccine and Drug Development*   Efforts to develop both vaccines and drugs will have to expand as new leads develop and new candidates are identified.

• *International Studies* Surveillance, epidemiologic research, and educational assistance are all needed to understand conditions abroad and to ameliorate the disease burden in affected countries.

• *Basic Research Efforts* A massive effort is needed to understand at the molecular level every aspect of HIV and a host's response to infection. This will involve characterizing the structure and function of each of the viral components and greatly expanded *in vivo* research efforts.

• *Epidemiologic Studies* Greatly expanded epidemiologic research will be needed to monitor the spread of the infection in various groups and to better understand its natural history.

• *Return of Reprogrammed Funds and Personnel* The AIDS program was initiated by borrowing funds and facilities from other ongoing extramural and intramural NIH research efforts (Krause, 1986). In FY 1986 this amounted to perhaps $70 million. Also, almost all of the intramural personnel working on AIDS were reprogrammed from other duties; there has been a net reduction in NIH personnel over the last few years (Krause, 1986). To maintain the strength of research efforts on other diseases and to ensure that knowledge gained from basic research is as extensive as possible, these reprogrammed funds and people should revert back to their original purposes.

The committee discussed amounts likely to be needed in specific research areas by 1990 and believes its estimate of an annual total of $1 billion to be realistic. However, it refrained from identifying specific amounts for particular research areas because others will be in a better position to assess relative needs and the agencies through which these should be channeled as the time to assign these funds approaches.

Recommendations

• The committee recommends that the federal appropriations for research on AIDS and HIV continue to increase toward a goal of at least $1 billion annually by 1990. These funds must be new appropriations, not a reprogramming of existing PHS funds. The PHS, through the diversity of its activities, is responsible for research and public health activities relating to a wide variety of important medical problems. The funding for these activities should not be compromised by increased expenditures on AIDS research. In addition, funds should be restored to the NIH programs that have suffered from the personnel and funding diversions to the ongoing intramural AIDS effort.

• The $1 billion cited above is needed to support ongoing efforts and to provide for additional research studies on AIDS and HIV. Necessary studies include those designed to improve the understanding of the natural history of HIV infection and those directed toward therapeutic interventions. There is a great need for applied research in the pursuit of effective drugs and vaccines, but, as previously discussed, much of the effort must focus on basic studies. The contributions of both the federal research effort and the extramural scientific communities should be actively supported. The potential input provided by independent investigator-initiated proposals in the elucidation of basic research questions has not yet been fully developed and should be emphasized in future funding. Necessary studies include, but are not limited to, increased epidemiologic surveillance and study, increased examination of multiple routes to vaccine or drug development, increased investigation of the nature of the virus and its effects on the immune system, increased study of the immune system itself, increased investigation of animal models, increased study of modes of human behavior modification, investigation of human sexuality, and analysis of ethical and legal options in responding to the AIDS epidemic. Many of these are expensive areas of research; $1 billion may prove to be insufficient. Ways are needed immediately to prevent the spread of HIV and to cure AIDS, and a very high priority must be given to finding them.

• The level of funding for investigator-initiated studies in all areas (including non-AIDS studies) must be adequate to continue to attract the most able younger scientists to clinical, social science, and basic biomedical research or the quality and productivity of the scientific enterprise will suffer.

• The development of new fundamental knowledge in the areas of immunology, virology, and developmental and cellular neurobiology has traditionally come primarily from investigator-initiated grants to laboratories. These laboratories are generally staffed by graduate students, medical students, and postdoctoral fellows. The trend in PHS funding for the past several years, and acutely in 1986, is to limit or decrease the numbers of fellowships for graduate students, M.D.-Ph.D. students, and postdoctoral fellows. Because they will play an important role in the future research effort on AIDS, new investigators should receive adequate support for their training and education.

REFERENCES

Allan, J. S., J. E. Coligan, T. H. Lee, M. F. McCane, P. J. Kanki, J. E. Groopman, and M. Essex. 1985. A new HTLV-III/LAV encoded antigen detected by antibodies from AIDS patients. Science 230:810-813.

Alter, H. J., J. W. Eichberg, H. Masur, W. C. Saxinger, R. Gallo, A. M. Macher, H. C. Lane, and A. S. Fauci. 1984. Transmission of HTLV-III infection from human plasma to chimpanzees: An animal model for AIDS. Science 226:549-552.

Ammann, A. J., G. Schiffman, D. Abrams, P. Volberding, J. Ziegler, and M. Conant. 1984. B-cell immunodeficiency in acquired immune deficiency syndrome. JAMA 251:1447-1449.

Arya, S. K., C. Guo, S. F. Joseph, and F. Wong-Staal. 1985. *Trans*-activator gene of human T-lymphotropic virus type III (HTLV-III). Science 229:69-73.

Barnes, D. M. 1986. The challenge of testing potential AIDS vaccines. Science 233:1151.

Berger, P., and T. Luckman. 1966. The Social Construction of Reality. New York: Doubleday.

Berman, P. W., W. Nunes, C. Fennie, and L. A. Lasky. 1986. Expression of recombinant AIDS retrovirus envelope protein analogues in genetically engineered cell lines. P. 15 in Abstracts of the Second International Conference on AIDS, Paris, June 23-25, 1986.

Bostrom, R. 1983. Persuasion. New Jersey: Prentice Hall.

Broder, S., R. Yarchoan, J. M. Collins, H. C. Lane, P. P. Markham, R. W. Klecker, R. R. Redfield, H. Mitsuya, D. F. Hoth, E. Gellman, J. E. Groopman, L. Resnick, R. C. Gallo, C. E. Myers, and A. S. Fauci. 1985. Effects of suramin on HTLV-III/LAV infection presenting Kaposi's sarcoma or AIDS-related complex: Clinical pharmacology and suppression of virus replication *in vivo*. Lancet II:627-630.

Caloff, J. 1967. A Study of Four Voluntary Treatment and Rehabilitation Programs for New York City's Narcotics Addicts. New York: Community Service Society.

Chakrabarti, S., M. Robert-Guroff, F. Wong-Staal, R. C. Gallo, and B. Moss. 1986. Expression of the HTLV-III envelope gene by a recombinant vaccinia virus. Nature 320: 535-537.

Chandra, P., A. Vogel, and T. Gerber. 1985. Inhibitors of retroviral DNA polymerase: Their implication in the treatment of AIDS. Cancer Res. 45(suppl.):4677s-4684s.

Cheevers, W. P., and T. C. McGuire. 1985. Equine infectious anemia virus: Immunopathogenesis and persistence. Rev. Infect. Dis. 7:83-88.

Chermann, J. C., F. Sinoussi, and C. Jasmin. 1975. Inhibition of RNA-dependent DNA polymerase of murine oncornaviruses by 5-tungsto-2-antimoniate. Biochem. Biophys. Res. Commun. 65:1229-1236.

Coffin, J. M. 1986. Genetic variation in AIDS viruses. Background paper. Washington, D.C.: Committee on a National Strategy for AIDS.

Cohen, A. 1964. Attitude Change: Social Influences. New York: Basic Books.

Dalgleish, A. G., P. C. L. Beverley, P. R. Clapham, D. H. Crawford, M. F. Greaves, and R. A. Weiss. 1984. The CD4 (T4) antigen is an essential component antigen of the receptor for the AIDS retrovirus. Nature 312:763-767.

Daniel, M. D., N. L. Letvin, N. W. King, M. Kannagi, P. K. Sehgal, R. D. Hunt, P. J. Kanki, M. Essex, and R. C. Desrosiers. 1985. Isolation of T-cell tropic HTLV-III-like retrovirus from macaques. Science 228:1201-1204.

Dayton, A. I., J. G. Sodroski, C. A. Rosen, W. C. Goh, and W. A. Haseltine. 1986. The *trans*-activator gene of the human T cell lymphotropic virus type III is required for replication. Cell 44:941-947. de Clercq, E. 1979. Suramin: A potent inhibitor of the reverse transcriptase of RNA tumor viruses. Cancer Lett. 8:9-22.

de Clercq, E. 1979. Suramin: A potent inhibitor of the reverse transcriptase of RNA tumor viruses. Cancer Lett. 8:9-22.

De Rossi, A., G. Franchini, A. Aldovini, A. DelMistro, L. Chreco-Bianchi, R. C. Gallo, and F. Wong-Staal. 1986. Differential response to the cytopathic effects of HTLV-III superinfection in T4+ (helper) and T8+ (suppressor) T-cell clones transformed by HTLV-I. Proc. Natl. Acad. Sci. USA 83:4297-4301.

Desrosiers, R., and N. L. Letvin. 1986. Animal models for AIDS and their use for vaccine and drug development. Background paper. Washington, D.C.: Committee on a National Strategy for AIDS.

Donzelot, V. J. 1979. The Policing of Families. New York: Pantheon Books.

Douglas, M. 1986. Risk Acceptability According to the Social Sciences. New York: Russell Sage.

Douglas, M., and A. Wildavsky. 1982. Risk and Culture. Berkeley: University of California Press.

Farquhar, J. M., N. Macoby, and D. S. Solomon. 1984. Community applications of behavioral medicine. Pp. 437-480 in Handbook of Behavioral Medicine, W. D. Gentry, ed. New York: Guildford Press.

Feinberg, M. B., R. F. Jarrett, A. Aldovini, R. C. Gallo, and F. Wong-Staal. In press. HTLV-III expression and production involve complex regulation at the levels of splicing and translation of viral RNA. Cell.

Feorino, P. M., H. W. Jaffe, E. Palmer, T. A. Peterman, D. P. Francis, V. S. Kalyanaraman, R. A. Weinstein, R. L. Stoneburner, W. J. Alexander, C. Raevsky, J. P. Getchell, D. Warfield, H. W. Haverkos, B. W. Kilbourne, J. K. A. Nicholson, and J. W. Curran. 1985. Transfusion-associated acquired immunodeficiency syndrome: Evidence for persistent infection in blood donors. N. Engl. J. Med. 312:1293-1296.

Fischoff, B., S. Lichtenstein, P. Slovic, S. Derby, and R. Keeney. 1981. Acceptable Risk. New York: Cambridge University Press.

Fisher, A. G., M. B. Feinberg, S. F. Josephs, M. E. Harper, I. M. Marselle, G. Reyes, M. A. Gonda, A. Aldovin, C. Debouk, R. C. Gallo, and F. Wong-Staal. 1986a. The trans-activator gene of HTLV-III is essential for a virus replication. Nature 320:367-371.

Fisher, A. G., L. Ratner, H. Mitsuya, L. M. Marselle, M. E. Harper, S. Broder, R. C. Gallo, and F. Wong-Staal. 1986b. Infectious mutants of HTLV-III with changes in the 3′ region and markedly reduced cytopathic effects. Science 233:655-659.

Folks, T., D. M. Powell, M. M. Lightfoote, S. Benn, M. A. Martin, and A. S. Fauci. 1986. Induction of HTLV-III/LAV from a nonvirus-producing T-cell line: Implications for latency. Science 231:600-602.

Francis, D. P., P. M. Feorino, J. R. Broderson, H. M. McClure, J. P. Getchell, C. R. McGrath, B. Swenson, J. S. McDougal, E. L. Palmer, A. K. Harrison, F. Barre-Sinoussi, J.-C. Chermann, L. Montagnier, J. W. Curran, C. D. Cabradilla, and V. S. Kalyanaraman. 1984. Infection of chimpanzees with lymphadenopathy-associated virus. Lancet II:1276-1277.

Fultz, P. N., H. M. McClure, D. C. Anderson, R. B. Swenson, R. Anand, and A. Srinivasan. 1986a. Isolation of a T-lymphotropic retrovirus from naturally infected sooty mangabay monkeys (Cerecocebus atys). Proc. Natl. Acad. Sci. USA 83:5286-5290.

Fultz, P. N., H. M. McClure, R. B. Swenson, C. R. McGrath, A. Brodie, J. P. Getchell, F. C. Jensen, D. C. Anderson, J. R. Broderson, and D. P. Francis. 1986b. Persistent infection of chimpanzees with human T-lymphocyte retrovirus in brains and other tissues from AIDS patients. Lancet I:55-56.

Gajdusek, D. C., H. L. Amyx, C. J. Gibbs, Jr., D. M. Asher, P. Rodgers-Johnson, L. G. Epstein, P. S. Sarin, R. C. Gallo, A. Maluish, L. O. Arthur, L. Montagnier, and D. Mildvan. 1985. Infection of chimpanzees by human T-lymphocyte retrovirus in brain and other tissues from AIDS patients. Lancet I:55-56.

Gallo, R. C., S. Z. Salahuddin, M. Popovic, G. M. Shearer, M. Kaplan, B. F. Haynes, T. J. Palker, R. Redfield, J. Oleske, B. Safai, G. White, P. Foster, and P. D. Markham. 1984. Frequent detection and isolation of cytopathic retroviruses (HTLV-III) from patients with AIDS and at risk for AIDS. Science 224:500-503.

Gartner, S., P. Markovitz, D. M. Markovitz, M. H. Kaplan, R. C. Gallo, and M. Popovic. 1986. The role of mononuclear phagocytes in HTLV-III/LAV infection. Science 233:215-219.

Gelmann, E. P., O. T. Preble, R. Steis, H. C. Lane, A. H. Rook, M. Wesley, J. Jacob, A. Fauci, H. Masur, and D. Longo. 1985. Human lymphoblastoid interferon treatment of

Kaposi's sarcoma in the acquired immunodeficiency syndrome: Clinical response and prognostic parameters. Am. J. Med. 78:737-741.

Gonda, M. A., F. Wong-Staal, and R. C. Gallo. 1985. Sequence homology and morphologic similarity of HTLV-III and visna virus, a pathogenic lentivirus. Science 227:173-177.

Graham, J. D. 1986. AIDS and biomedical research: A comparative analysis. Background paper. Washington, D.C.: Committee on a National Strategy for AIDS.

Groopman, J. E., M. S. Gottlieb, J. Goodman, R. T. Mitsuyasu, M. A. Conant, H. Prince, J. L. Fahey, M. Derezin, W. M. Weinstein, C. Casavante, J. Rothman, S. A. Rudnick, and P. A. Volberding. 1984. Recombinant alpha-2 interferon therapy for Kaposi's sarcoma associated with the acquired immunodeficiency syndrome. Ann. Intern. Med. 100:671-676.

Haase, A. T. 1986. Pathogenesis of lentivirus infection. Nature 322:130-136.

Hahn, B. H., G. M. Shaw, M. E. Taylor, P. D. McNeeley, W. P. Parks, S. Modrow, R. C. Gallo, and F. Wong-Staal. 1986. Nature and extent of genetic variation in HTLV-III/LAV. P. 16 in Abstracts of the Second International Conference on AIDS, Paris, June 23-25, 1986.

Hall, C. B., J. T. McBride, E. E. Walsh, D. M. Bell, C. L. Gala, S. Hildreth, L. G. Ten Eyck, and W. J. Hall. 1983. Aerosolized ribavirin treatment of infants with respiratory syncytial viral infection: A randomized double-blind study. N. Engl. J. Med. 308:1443-1447.

Hardy, W. D., P. W. Hess, E. MacEwen, E. McClelland, E. Zuckerman, M. Essex, S. M. Cotter, and O. Jarret. 1976. Biology of feline leukemia virus in the natural environment. Cancer Res. 36:466-847.

Harper, M. E., L. M. Marselle, K. J. Chayt, R. C. Gallo, M. H. Kaplan, and F. Wong-Staal. 1986a. Detection of concomitant infection of HTLV-I and HTLV-III in situ hybridization. J. Cell. Biochem. Suppl. 10A:189.

Harper, M. E., I. M. Marselle, R. C. Gallo, and F. Wong-Staal. 1986b. Detection of lymphocytes expressing human T-lymphotropic virus type III in lymph nodes and peripheral blood from infected individuals by in situ hybridization. Proc. Natl. Acad. Sci. USA 83:772-776.

Hawking, F. 1981. Chemotherapy of filariasis. Antibiot. Chemother. 30:135-162.

Heagy, W., V. E. Kelley, T. B. Strom, K. Mayer, H. M. Shapiro, R. Mandel, and R. Fineberg. 1984. Decreased expression of human class II antigens on monocytes from patients with the acquired immune deficiency syndrome: Increased expression with interferon gamma. J. Clin. Invest. 74:2089-2096.

Helgstrand, E., B. Eriksson, N. G. Johansson, B. Lannero, A. Larsson, A. Misiorny, J. O. Noren, B. Sjoberg, K. Stenberg, G. Stening, S. Stridh, B. Oberg, S. Alenius, and L. Philipson. 1978. Trisodium phosphonoformate, a new antiviral compound. Science 201:819-821.

Ho, D. D., K. L. Hartshorn, T. R. Rota, C. A. Andrews, J. C. Kaplan, R. T. Schooley, and M. S. Hirsch. 1985a. Recombinant human interferon alfa-A suppresses HTLV-III replication *in vitro*. Lancet I:602-604.

Ho, D. D., T. R. Rota, and M. S. Hirsch. 1985b. Antibody to lymphadenopathy-associated virus in AIDS. N. Engl. J. Med. 312:649-650.

Ho, D. D., T. R. Rota, R. T. Schooley, J. C. Kaplan, J. D. Allan, J. E. Groopman, L. Resnick, D. Felsenstein, C. A. Andrews, and M. S. Hirsch. 1985c. Isolation of HTLV-III from cerebrospinal fluid and neural tissues of patients with neurologic syndromes related to the acquired immunodeficiency syndrome. N. Engl. J. Med. 313:1493-1497.

Hogle, J. M., M. Chow, and D. J. Filman. 1985. Three-dimensional structure of poliovirus at 2.9 Å resolution. Science 229:1358-1365.

Holt, C. A., K. Osorio, and F. Lilly. 1986. Friend virus-specific cytotoxic T lymphocytes recognize both *gag* and *env* gene-encoded specificities. J. Exp. Med. 164:211-226.

Hoxie, J. A., B. S. Haggarty, J. L. Rackowski, N. Pillsbury, and J. A. Levy. 1985. Persistent noncytopathic infection of normal T lymphocytes with AIDS-associated retrovirus. Science 229:1400-1402.

Hu, S.-L., S. G. Kosowski, A. F. Purchio, and J. M. Dalrymple. 1986. Expression of AIDS virus envelope gene in recombinant vaccinia virus. P. 9 in Abstracts of the Second International Conference on AIDS, Paris, June 23-25, 1986.

Hunsmann, G., J. Schneider, and A. Schultz. 1981. Immunoprevention of Friend virus-induced erythroleukemia by vaccination with viral envelope glycoprotein complexes. Virology 113:602-612.

ICN Pharmaceuticals. 1986. Safety of Ribavirin. News Release, October 3, 1986, Costa Mesa, Calif.

Jaffe, H. W., D. J. Abrams, A. J. Amman, B. J. Lewis, and J. A. Golden. 1983. Complications of co-trimoxazole in treatment of AIDS-related *Pneumocystis carinii* pneumonia in homosexual men. Lancet II:1109-1111.

Jaffe, H. W., P. M. Feorino, W. W. Darrow, P. M. O'Malley, J. P. Getchell, D. T. Warfield, B. M. Jones, D. F. Echenberg, D. P. Francis, and J. W. Curran. 1985. Persistent infection with human T-lymphotropic virus type III/lymphadenopathy-associated virus in apparently healthy homosexual men. Ann. Intern. Med. 102:627-628.

Jarrett, W., O. Jarrett, L. Mackey, H. Laird, C. Hood, and D. Hay. 1975. Vaccination against feline leukemia virus using a cell membrane antigen system. Int. J. Cancer 16:134-139.

Jasmin, C., J. C. Chermann, C. Herve, A. Teze, P. Souchay, C. Boy-Soustau, N. Raybaud, F. Sinoussi, and M. Raynaud. 1974. *In vivo* inhibition of murine leukemia and sarcoma viruses by heteropolyanion 5-tungsto-2-antimoniate. J. Natl. Cancer Inst. 53:469-474.

Jenkins, F. J., and Y. C. Chen. 1981. Effect of ribavirin on Rous sarcoma virus transformation. Antimicrob. Agents Chemother. 19:364-368.

Johnson, R. T. 1985. Nononcogenic retrovirus infections as models for chronic and relapsing human disease: Introduction. Rev. Infect. Dis. 7:66-67.

Jones, E., J. Beniger, and C. Westoff. 1980. Pill and IUD discontinuation in the United States, 1970-1975: The influence of the media. Fam. Plann. Perspect. 12:293-300.

Kan, N. C., G. Franchini, F. Wong-Staal, G. C. Dubois, W. G. Robey, J. A. Lautenberger, and T. S. Papis. 1986. Identification of HTLV-III/LAV *sor* gene product and detection of antibodies in human sera. Science 231:1553-1555.

Kanki, P. J., J. Alroy, and M. Essex. 1985. Isolation of a T-lymphotropic retrovirus related to HTLV-III/LAV from wild-caught African green monkeys. Science 230:951-954.

Kanki, P. J., F. Barin, S. M'Boup, J. S. Allan, J. L. Romet-Lemonne, R. Marlink, M. F. McLane, T.-H. Lee, B. Arbeille, F. Denis, and M. Essex. 1986. New human T-cell retrovirus related to simian T-lymphotropic virus type III (STLV-III$_{AGM}$). Science 232:238-243.

Kennedy-Stoskopf, S., and O. Narayan. 1986. Neutralizing antibodies to visna lentivirus: Mechanism of action and possible role in virus persistence. J. Virol. 59:37-44.

Klapper, J. 1960. The Effects of Mass Communication. Glencoe, Ill.: The Free Press.

Klatzmann, D., and L. Montagnier. 1986. Approaches to AIDS therapy. Nature 319:10-11.

Klatzmann, D., E. Champagne, S. Chamaret, J. Gruest, D. Guetard, T. Hercend, J. C. Gluckman, and L. Montagnier. 1984. T-lymphocyte T4 molecule behaves as the receptor for human retrovirus LAV. Nature 312:767-768.

Knight, V., H. W. McClung, S. Z. Wilson, B. K. Waters, J. M. Quarles, R. W. Cameron,

S. E. Greggs, J. M. Zerwas, and R. B. Couch. 1981. Ribavirin small-particle aerosol treatment of influenza. Lancet II:945-949.

Krause, R. 1986. The NIH research effort on AIDS: To what extent has it been achieved by reprogramming funds originally allotted for other purposes? Background paper. Washington, D.C.: Committee on a National Strategy for AIDS.

Krown, S. E., F. X. Real, S. Cunningham-Rundles, P. L. Myskowski, B. Koziner, S. Fein, A. Mittelman, H. F. Oettgen, and B. Safai. 1983. Preliminary observations on the effect of recombinant leukocyte A interferon in homosexual men with Kaposi's sarcoma. N. Engl. J. Med. 308:1071-1076.

Kunreuther, H. 1978. Disaster Insurance Protection: Public Policy Lessons. New York: Wiley.

Lane, H. C., H. Masur, L. C. Edgar, G. Whalen, A. H. Rook, and A. S. Fauci. 1983. Abnormalities of B-cell activation and immunoregulation in patients with the acquired immunodeficiency syndrome. N. Engl. J. Med. 309:453-458.

Lane, H. C., J. M. Depper, W. S. Greene, G. Whalen, T. A. Waldmann, and A. S. Fauci. 1985. Qualitative analysis of immune function in patients with the acquired immunodeficiency syndrome: Evidence for a selective defect in soluble antigen recognition. N. Engl. J. Med. 313:79-84.

Lang, G., and L. Kurt. 1983. The Battle for Public Opinion. New York: Columbia University Press.

Lee, T. H., J. E. Coligan, J. S. Allan, M. F. McLane, J. E. Groopman, and M. Essex. 1985. A new HTLV-III/LAV protein encoded by a gene found in cytopathic retroviruses. Science 236:1546-1549.

Letvin, N. L., and R. D. Desrosiers. 1986. Animal models for AIDS and their use for vaccine and drug development. Background paper. Washington, D.C.: Committee on a National Strategy for AIDS.

Letvin, N. L., M. D. Daniel, P. K. Sehgal, R. C. Desrosiers, R. D. Hunt, L. M. Waldron, J. J. MacKey, D. K. Schmidt, L. V. Chalifoux, and N. W. King. 1985. Induction of AIDS-like disease in macaque monkeys with T-cell tropic retrovirus STLV-III. Science 230:71-73.

Levine, A. M., P. S. Gill, J. Cohen, J. G. Hawkins, S. C. Formenti, S. Aguilar, P. R. Meyer, M. Krailo, J. Parker, and S. Rasheed. 1985. Suramin antiviral therapy in the acquired immunodeficiency syndrome. Clinical, immunologic, and virologic results. Ann. Intern. Med. 105:32-37.

Leventhal, H., and P. Cleary. 1980. Review of the research: Theory of behavioral risk modification. Psychol. Bull. 88:370-405.

Lewis, M. G., L. E. Mathes, and R. G. Olsen. 1981. Protection against feline leukemia by vaccination with a subunit vaccine. Infect. Immun. 34:808-812.

Lichtenstein, E. 1982. The smoking problem. J. Consult. Clin. Psychol. 50:804-819.

Lifson, J. D., M. B. Feinberg, G. R. Reyes, L. Rabin, B. Banapour, S. Chakrabarti, B. Moss, F. Wong-Staal, K. S. Steimer, and E. Engleman. In press. Inductions of CD4 dependent cell fusion by the HTLV-III/LAV envelope glycoprotein. Nature.

Lifson, J. D., G. R. Reyes, B. S. Stein, and E. G. Engleman. 1986. AIDS retrovirus-induced cytopathology: Giant cell formation and involvement of CD4 antigen. Science 232:1123-1127.

Lutz, H., N. Pederson, J. Higgins, V. Hubscher, A. Troy, and G. H. Therten. 1980. Humoral immune reactivity to feline leukemia virus and associated antigens in cats naturally infected with feline leukemia virus. Cancer Res. 40:3642-3646.

Matthews, T. J., A. J. Langlois, W. G. Rovey, N. T. Chang, R. C. Gallo, P. J. Fischinger, and D. P. Bolognesi. In press. Restricted neutralization of divergent HTLV-III/LAV isolates by antibodies to the major envelope glycoprotein. Proc. Natl. Acad. Sci. USA.

McClosky, H., and A. Brell. 1983. Dimensions of Tolerance. New York: Russell Sage Foundation.

McCormick, J. B., S. W. Mitchell, J. P. Getchell, and D. R. Hicks. 1984. Ribavirin suppresses replication of lymphadenopathy-associated virus in culture of human lymphocytes. Lancet II:1367-1369.

McCormick, J. B., I. J. King, P. A. Webb, C. L. Schribner, R. B. Craven, K. M. Johnson, L. H. Elliott, and R. Belmont-Williams. 1986. Lassa fever: Effective therapy with ribavirin. N. Engl. J. Med. 314:20-26.

McGuire, T. C., D. S. Adams, G. C. Johnson, P. Klevjer-Anderson, D. D. Barbe, and J. R. Gorham. 1986. Acute arthritis in caprine arthritis encephalitis virus challenge exposure of vaccinated or persistently infected goats. Am. J. Vet. Res. 47:537-540.

Meusing, M. A., D. H. Smith, C. D. Cabradilla, C. V. Benton, L. A. Lasky, and D. J. Capon. 1985. Nucleic acid structure and expression of the human AIDS/lymphadenopathy retrovirus. Nature 313:450-457.

Miller, J. M., M. J. Van der Masten, and M. J. F. Schmen. 1985. Vaccination of cattle with binary ethylenimine treated bovine leukemia virus. Am. J. Vet. Res. 44:64-67.

Mitsuya, H., and S. Broder. 1986. Inhibition of the *in vitro* infectivity and cytopathic effect of HTLV-III/LAV by 2',3'-dideoxynucleosides. Proc. Natl. Acad. Sci. USA 83:1911-1915.

Mitsuya, H., M. Popovic, R. Yarchoan, S. Matsushita, R. C. Gallo, and S. Broder. 1984. Suramin protection of T cells *in vitro* against infectivity and cytopathic effect of HTLV-III. Science 266:172-174.

Mitsuya, H., K. J. Weinhold, P. A. Furman, M. H. St. Clair, S. N. Lehrman, R. C. Gallo, D. Bolognesi, D. W. Barry, and S. Broder. 1985. 3'-Azido-3'-deoxythymidine (BW A509U): Antiviral agent that inhibits the infectivity and cytopathic effect of human T-lymphotropic virus type III/lymphadenopathy-associated virus *in vitro*. Proc. Natl. Acad. Sci. USA 82:7096-7100.

Montelaro, R. C., B. Parekh, A. Orrego, and C. J. Issel. 1984. Antigenic infectious anemia virus, a retrovirus. J. Biol. Chem. 259:10539-10544.

Murray, H. W., R. A. Gellene, D. M. Libby, C. D. Rothermel, and B. Y. Rubin. 1985a. Activation of tissue macrophages from AIDS patients: *In vitro* response of alveolar macrophages to lymphokines and interferon-gamma. J. Immunol. 153:2374-2378.

Murray, H. W., J. K. Hillman, B. Y. Rubin, C. D. Kelley, J. L. Jacobs, L. W. Tyler, D. M. Donelly, S. M. Carriero, J. H. Godbold, and R. B. Roberts. 1985b. Patients at risk for AIDS-related opportunistic infections: Clinical manifestations and impaired gamma interferon production. N. Engl. J. Med. 313:1504-1509.

Narayan, O. 1986. Models of AIDS in the light of other natural lentivirus infections in domestic animals. Background paper. Washington, D.C.: Committee on a National Strategy for AIDS.

Narayan, O., D. E. Griffin, and J. E. Clements. 1978. Virus mutation during "slow infection": Temporal development and characterization of mutants of visna virus recovered from sheep. J. Gen. Virol. 41:343-352.

Narayan, O., D. Sheffer, D. E. Griffin, J. Clements, and J. Hess. 1984. Antibodies to caprine arthritis-encephalitis lentivirus in persistently infected goats can be overcome by immunization with inactivated *Mycobacterium tuberculosis*. J. Virol. 49:349-355.

Navarro, V. 1977. Political power, the state and their implications in medicine. Rev. Rad. Polit. Econ. 9:61-80.

Nelkin, D. 1973. Methadone Maintenance: A Technological Fix. New York: George Braziller.

Nelkin, D., and M. Brown. 1984. Workers at Risk. Chicago: University of Chicago Press.

Nelkin, D., and S. Hilgartner. 1986. Disputed dimensions of risk. Milbank Mem. Fund Q. Sept/Oct.

Olsen, R. G., E. A. Hoover, J. P. Schaller, L. E. Martes, and L. H. Wolff. 1977. Abrogation of resistance to feline oncornavirus disease by immunization with killed feline leukemia virus. Cancer Res. 37:2082-2096.

Olsen, R. G., M. Lewis, L. E. Marthes, and W. Hause. 1980. Feline leukemia vaccine: Efficacy testing in a large multicat household. Feline Pract. 10:13-16.

Osterhaus, A., K. Weijer, F. Uytdehaag, O. Jarrett, B. Sundquist, and B. Morein. 1985. Induction of protective immune response in cats by vaccination with feline leukemia virus iscom. J. Immunol. 135:591-596.

Pahwa, S., R. Pahwa, C. Saxinger, R. C. Gallo, and R. A. Good. 1985. Influence of HTLV-III/LAV on functions of human lymphocytes: Evidence for immunosuppressive effects and polyclonal B cell activation by banded viral preparations. Proc. Natl. Acad. Sci. USA 82:8198-8202.

Patrascu, I. V., S. Coman, I. Sandu, P. Stiube, I. Munteanu, T. Coman, M. Ionescu, D. Popescu, and D. Mihailescu. 1980. Specific protection against bovine leukemia virus infection conferred on cattle by the Romanian inactivated vaccine BL-VACC-RO. Virologie 31:95-102.

Pillemer, E. A., D. A. Kooistra, O. N. Witte, and I. L. Weissman. 1986. Monoclonal antibody to the amino-terminal L sequence of murine leukemia virus glycosylated *gag* polyproteins demonstrates their usual orientation in the cell membrane. J. Virol. 57:413-421.

Popovic, M., M. G. Sarngadharan, E. Read, and R. C. Gallo. 1984. Detection, isolation, and continuous production of cytopathic retroviruses (HTLV-III) from patients with AIDS and pre-AIDS. Science 224:497-500.

Quinnan, G. V., H. Masur, A. H. Rook, G. Armstrong, W. R. Frederick, J. Epstein, J. F. Manischewitz, A. M. Macher, L. Jackson, J. Ames, H. A. Smith, M. Parker, G. R. Pearson, J. Parrillo, C. Mitchell, and S. E. Strauss. 1984. Herpes virus infections in the acquired immune deficiency syndrome. JAMA 252:72-77.

Rabson, A. B., D. F. Daugherty, S. Ven Katesan, K. E. Boulukos, S. I. Benn, T. M. Folks, P. Feorino, and M. A. Martin. 1985. Transcription of novel open reading frames of AIDS retrovirus during infection of lymphocytes. Science 229:1388-1390.

Ratner, L., W. Haseltine, R. Patarca, K. J. Livak, B. Starcich, S. F. Josephs, E. R. Doran, J. Antoni Rafalski, E. A. Whitehorn, K. Baumeister, L. Ivanoff, S. R. Petteway, M. L. Pearson, J. A. Lautenberg, T. K. Papas, J. Ghrayeb, N. T. Chang, R. C. Gallo, and F. Wong-Staal. 1985. Complete nucleotide sequence of the AIDS virus, HTLV-III. Nature 313:277-284.

Resnick, L., F. diMarzo-Veronese, J. Schupbach, W. W. Tourtellotte, D. D. Ho, F. Muller, P. Shapshak, M. Vogt, J. E. Groopman, P. D. Markham, and R. C. Gallo. 1985. Intra-blood-brain-barrier synthesis of HTLV-III specific IgG in patients with neurologic symptoms associated with AIDS or AIDS-related complex. N. Engl. J. Med. 313:1498-1504.

Robert-Guroff, M., M. Brown, and R. C. Gallo. 1985. HTLV-III-neutralizing antibodies in patients with AIDS and AIDS-related complex. Nature 316:72-74.

Roberts, R. B., D. Scavuzzo, J. Laurence, O. Laskin, Y. Kim, and H. W. Murray. 1986. Effects of short term oral ribavirin in high risk patients for AIDS. P. 68 in Abstracts of the Second International Conference on AIDS, Paris, June 23-25, 1986.

Robinson, E. J. 1963. Analyzing the impact of science reporting. Journalist Quart. 40:306-314.

Rogers, E. 1983. Diffusion of Innovation. New York: The Free Press.

Roloff, M., and G. R. Miller. 1980. Persuasion: New Directions in Theory and Research. Beverly Hills: Sage Publications.

Roman, P., and H. Trice. 1972. Spirits and Demons at Work. Ithaca: New York State Industrial and Labor Relations Press.

Rook, A. H., H. Masur, H. C. Lane, F. Frederick, T. Kasahara, A. M. Macher, J. Y. Djeu, J. F. Manischewitz, L. Jackson, A. S. Fauci, and G. V. Quinnan, Jr. 1983. Interleukin-2 enhances the depressed natural killer and cytomegalovirus-specific cytotoxic activities of lymphocytes from patients with the acquired immune deficiency syndrome. J. Clin. Invest. 72:398-403.

Rosen, C. A., J. G. Sodroski, W. C. Goh, A. I. Dayton, J. Lippe, and W. A. Haseltine. 1986. Post-transcriptional regulation accounts for the trans-activation of the human T-lymphocyte virus type III. Nature 319:555-559.

Rossman, M., E. Arnold, J. W. Erikson, E. A. Frankenberger, J. P. Griffith, H. J. Hecht, J. E. Johnson, G. Kamer, M. Luo, A. G. Moser, R. R. Ruekert, B. Sherry, and G. Vriend. 1985. The structure of a human common cold virus and functional relationship to other picornaviruses. Nature 317:145-153.

Rouvroy, D., J. Bogaerts, J. B. Habyarimana, O. Nzaramba, and P. Van de Perre. 1985. Short-term results with suramin for AIDS-related conditions. Lancet I:878-879.

Rozenbaum, W., D. Dormont, B. Spire, E. Vilmer, M. Gentilini, C. Griscelli, L. Montagnier, F. Barre-Sinoussi, and J. C. Chermann. 1985. Antimoniotungstate (HPA 23) treatment of three patients with AIDS and one with prodrome. Lancet I:450-451.

Salahuddin, S. Z., P. D. Markham, R. R. Redfield, M. Essex, J. E. Groopman, M. G. Sarngadharan, M. F. McLane, A. Sliski, and R. C. Gallo. 1984. HTLV-III in symptom-free seronegative persons. Lancet I:1418-1420.

Salahuddin, S. Z., P. D. Markham, M. Popovic, M. G. Sarngadharan, S. Orndorff, A. Fladagar, A. Patel, J. Gold, and R. C. Gallo. 1985. Isolation of infectious human T-cell leukemia/lymphotropic virus type III (HTLV-III) from patients with acquired immunodeficiency syndrome (AIDS) or AIDS-related complex (ARC) and from healthy carriers: A study of risk groups and tissue sources. Proc. Natl. Acad. Sci. USA 82:5530-5534.

Sanchez-Pescador, R., M. D. Power, P. J. Barr, K. S. Steiner, M. M. Stempien, S. L. Brown-Shimer, W. W. Gee, A. Renard, A. Randolph, J. A. Levy, D. Dina, and P. A. Luciw. 1985. Nucleotide sequence and expression of an AIDS-associated retrovirus (ARV-2). Science 227:484-492.

Sandstrom, E. G., J. C. Kaplan, R. E. Byington, and M. S. Hirsch. 1985. Inhibition of human T-cell lymphotropic virus type III *in vitro* by phosphonoformate. Lancet I:1480-1482.

Sarin, P. S., Y. Taguchi, D. Sun, A. Thornton, R. C. Gallo, and B. Oberg. 1985. Inhibition of HTLV-III/LAV replication by foscarnet. Biochem. Pharmacol. 34:4075-4079.

Seligmann, M., L. Chess, J. L. Fahey, A. S. Fauci, P. J. Lachmann, J. L'Age-Stehr, J. Ngu, A. J. Pinching, F. S. Rosen, T. J. Spira, and J. Wybran. 1984. AIDS—an immunologic reevaluation. N. Engl. J. Med. 311:1286-1292.

Shannon, W. M. 1977. Selective inhibition of RNA tumor virus replication *in vitro* and evaluation of candidate antiviral agents *in vivo*. Ann. N.Y. Acad. Sci. 284:472-507.

Shaw, G. M., M. E. Harper, B. H. Hahn, L. G. Epstein, D. C. Gajdusek, R. W. Price, B. A. Navia, C. K. Petito, C. J. O'Hara, E.-S. Cho, J. M. Oleske, F. Wong-Stall, and R. C. Gallo. 1985. HTLV-III infection in brains of children and adults with AIDS encephalopathy. Science 227:177-182.

Sidwell, R. W., and D. F. Smee. 1981. Bovine leukemia virus inhibition *in vitro* by ribavirin. Antiviral. Res. 1:47-53.

Sidwell, R. W., L. B. Allen, J. H. Huffman, J. T. Witkowski, and L. N. Simon. 1975. Effect of 1-β-D-ribofuranosyl-1,2,4-triazole-3-carboxamide (ribavirin) of friend leukemia virus infections in mice (38647). Proc. Soc. Exp. Biol. Med. 148:854-858.

Singer, E., and T. Rogers. 1986. Public opinion about AIDS. AIDS and Public Policy J. 1:1.

Slovic, P., B. Fischoff, and S. Lichtenstein. 1981. Perceived risk: Psychological factors and social implications. Proc. R. Soc. London A376:17-34.

Sodroski, J. G., C. Rosen, and W. A. Haseltine. 1984. *Trans*-activating transcriptional activation of the long terminal repeat of human T-lymphotropic virus in infected cells. Science 225:381-385.

Sodroski, J., W. C. Goh, C. Rosen, K. Campbell, and W. A. Haseltine. 1986a. Role of HTLV-III/LAV envelope in syncytium formation and cytopathicity. Nature 322:470-474.

Sodroski, J. G., W. C. Goh, C. Rosen, A. Dayton, E. Terwilliger, and W. Haseltine. 1986b. A second post-transcriptional *trans*-activator gene required for HTLV-III replication. Nature 32:412-417.

Sodroski, J. G., W. C. Goh, C. Rosen, A. Tartar, D. Portetella, A. Burny, and W. Haseltine. 1986c. Replicative and cytopathic potential of HTLV-III/LAV with *sor* gene deletions. Science 231:1549-1553.

Sonigo, P., M. Alizon, K. Staskus, D. Klatzman, S. Cole, D. Danos, E. Retzel, P. Tiollais, A. Haase, and S. Wain-Hobson. 1985. Nucleotide sequence of visna lentivirus: Relationship to the AIDS virus. Cell 42:369-382.

Stein, C. A., W. Saville, R. Yarchoan, S. Border, and E. P. Gelmann. 1986. Suramin and function of the adrenal cortex. Ann. Intern. Med. 104:286-287.

Stewart, G. J., J. P. P. Tyler, A. L. Cunningham, J. A. Barr, G. L. Driscoll, J. Gold, and B. J. Lamont. 1985. Transmission of human T-cell lymphotropic virus type III (HTLV-III) by artificial insemination by donor. Lancet II:581-584.

Stoto, M. A., D. Blumenthal, J. S. Durch, and P. H. Feldman. 1986. Federal funding for AIDS: Decision process and results. Background paper. Washington, D.C.: Committee on a National Strategy for AIDS.

Sundquist, B., and B. Oberg. 1979. Phosphonoformate inhibits reverse transcriptase. J. Gen. Virol. 45:273-281.

Temin, H. M. 1986. Mechanisms of cell killing cytopathic effects by retrovirus. Background paper. Washington, D.C.: Committee on a National Strategy for AIDS.

Thormar, H. M., M. R. Barshatzky, K. Arnesen, and P. B. Kozlowski. 1983. The emergence of antigenic variants is a rare event in long term visna virus infection *in vivo*. J. Gen. Virol. 64:1427-1432.

Toltzis, R., and A. S. Huang. 1986. Effect of ribavirin on macromolecular synthesis in vesicular stomatitis virus-infected cells. Antimicrob. Agents Chemother. 29:1010-1016.

Townsend, A. R. M., F. M. Gotch, and J. Davey. 1985. Cytotoxic cells recognize fragments of the influenza nucleoprotein. Cell 42:457-467.

Troyer, R., and G. Markle. 1983. Cigarettes. New Brunswick: Rutgers University Press.

Tuchman, G. 1978. Making News. New York: The Free Press.

Wain-Hobson, S., P. Sonigo, O. Danos, S. Cole, and M. Alizon. 1985. Nucleotide sequence of the AIDS virus, LAV. Cell 40:9-17.

Weiss, R., N. Teich, H. Varmus, and J. Coffin, eds. 1982. The Molecular Biology of Tumor Viruses, 2d ed.: RNA Tumor Viruses. Cold Spring Harbor, N.Y.: Cold Spring Harbor Laboratory.

Weiss, R. A., P. R. Clapham, R. Cheingsong-Popov, A. G. Dalgleish, C. A. Carne, I. V. Weller, and R. S. Tedder. 1985. Neutralization of human T-lymphotropic virus type III by sera of AIDS and AIDS-risk patients. Nature 316:69-72.

Weissman, I. 1986. Approaches to understanding the pathogenic mechanisms in AIDS. Background paper. Washington, D.C.: Committee on a National Strategy for AIDS.

Williams, R. C., H. Masur, and T. J. Spira. 1984. Lymphocyte-reactive antibodies in acquired immune deficiency syndrome. J. Clin. Immunol. 4:118-123.

Wilson, I. A., J. J. Skehel, and D. C. Wiley. 1981. Structure of the haemoagglutinin membrane glycoprotein of influenza virus at 3 Å resolution. Nature 289:366-373.

Wyngaarden, J. B. 1985. Federal Biomedical Policy. Address before the New York Science Policy Association at the National Academy of Sciences, Washington, D.C., November 15, 1985.

Yanagihara, R., D. M. Asher, L. G. Epstein, A. V. Wolff, C. J. Gibbs, Jr., and D. C. Gajdusek. 1986. Current status of attempts to transmit acquired immunodeficiency syndrome (AIDS) to new and old world monkeys. P. 19 in Abstracts of the Second International Conference on AIDS, Paris, June 23-25, 1986.

Yarchoan, R., R. W. Klecker, K. J. Weinhold, P. D. Markham, H. K. Lyerly, D. T. Durack, E. Gelmann, S. N. Lehrman, R. M. Blum, D. W. Barry, G. M. Shearer, M. Fischl, H. Mitsuya, R. C. Gallo, J. M. Collins, D. P. Bolognesi, C. E. Myers, and S. Broder. 1986. Administration of 3'azido-3'-deoxythymidine, an inhibitor of HTLV-III replication, to patients with AIDS or AIDS-related complex. Lancet I:575-580.

Yohn, D. S., R. G. Olsen, J. P. Schaller, E. A. Hoover, L. E. Mathes, L. Heding, and G. W. Davis. 1976. Experimental oncornavirus vaccines in the cat. Cancer Res. 36:646-651.

Zagury, D., J. Bernard, R. Leonard, R. Cheynier, M. Feldman, P. S. Sarin, and R. C. Gallo. 1986. Immune induction of T cell death in long term culture of HTLV-III infected T cells: A cytopathogenic model for AIDS T-cell depletion. Science 231:850-853.

7

International Aspects of AIDS and HIV Infection

PROJECTIONS OF THE DISEASE OUTSIDE THE UNITED STATES

The 159 countries of the world, more than half of which have reported AIDS cases, appear to fall into three categories in regard to AIDS and HIV infection. The first category is made up of developed or relatively developed countries in which the distribution of AIDS and HIV infection resembles the demographic situation in the United States, although the number of reported cases is far fewer than in the United States. The groups most affected in these countries thus far are homosexual men and IV drug users, and heterosexual spread is beginning to be recognized. Such countries include Australia, Canada, Brazil, and the nations of Europe. In general, these countries have health care and public health systems with substantial resources. Many have put into place programs, similar to those in the United States, for controlling the spread of the epidemic through certain routes of transmission (e.g., parenteral). Also, many countries, such as the United Kingdom, have initiated national public education programs on AIDS.

The second category comprises developing countries where AIDS and HIV infection seem to occur among sexually active men and women in approximately equal proportions and in their offspring, and therefore where heterosexual spread is presumed to be the predominant mode of transmission. Such countries include, but may not be limited to, those of central Africa and certain countries in the Caribbean, including Haiti.

261

These countries have health care and public health systems with inadequate resources (many can spend only a few dollars per capita annually on all health care). Generally, they have not begun programs to screen blood donations or to provide education to reduce HIV transmission.

The third category includes those countries where AIDS or HIV infection is presently reported to be absent or at least rare. Given the modes of transmission of HIV, it is unlikely that these countries are or will remain free of infection or disease. Only some of these countries have health care and public health systems with resources adequate for mounting any programs to cope with AIDS or to reduce transmission.

Because diagnosis may not be reliable and reporting is generally inconsistent in many countries, the true number of AIDS cases worldwide cannot be accurately estimated. The number of persons infected with HIV is also difficult to estimate, because few studies of the prevalence of seropositivity have been done and because the ratio of symptomatic to infected persons in developing countries is not known. At the Second International Conference on AIDS held in Paris in June 1986, Halfdan Mahler, Director General of the World Health Organization (WHO), ventured an estimate of as many as 10 million persons infected with HIV worldwide, with a substantial proportion of these in central Africa (Mahler and Assaad, 1986). Within that region, however, the attention being devoted to studies and disease reporting varies greatly. Therefore, countries reporting the highest disease or infection levels do not necessarily have the highest levels or act as the foci of disease spread or origin.

Approximate projections for the number of pediatric AIDS cases can be made. In some areas in Africa, about 10 percent of pregnant women are seropositive for HIV, and approximately one-third of infants born to seropositive mothers become infected with HIV within one year after birth. Thus, at least 2 to 4 percent of newborns in these areas may be perinatally infected with HIV. These proportions, if valid for other areas in central Africa, would suggest that if seropositive pregnant women deliver, possibly tens to hundreds of thousands of infants in Africa will die of AIDS in the next decade. The adoption of birth control measures in Africa has not been great—for instance, Kenya has the world's highest fertility rate; hence the prospects for education and prevention in this matter seem bleak.

If the same proportion of HIV-infected individuals in developing countries can be expected to progress to AIDS as in the United States (at least 25 to 50 percent in 5 to 10 years), then there will probably be millions of deaths from AIDS in central Africa in the next decade unless a treatment is found and rapidly made available. Given the poor prospects for a vaccine in the next five years and probably longer, the fact that the resources for education to reduce risks are almost nonexistent, and the fact that no successful models of education to prevent sexually transmitted diseases are available, it must be presumed that the situation will significantly worsen in developing countries, as it will in the developed ones. Because AIDS strikes individuals in their most productive adult years, the economic as well as health burdens resulting from HIV infection will be enormous.

INTERNATIONAL ORGANIZATIONS

In response to the international threat of HIV infection, the World Health Organization has proposed an initiative on AIDS (World Health Organization, 1986a). Its main features are to develop activities in the following ways:

• Ensure the exchange of information on HIV, its epidemiology, laboratory, and clinical aspects, and prevention and control activities.
• Prepare and distribute guidelines, manuals, and educational materials.
• Assess commercially available HIV antibody test kits, develop a simple, inexpensive test for field application, and establish WHO reference reagents.
• Cooperate with member states in the development of national programs for the containment of HIV infection.
• Advise member states on the provision of safe blood and blood products.
• Promote research on the development of therapeutic agents and vaccines, simian retroviruses, and epidemiologic and behavioral aspects of HIV infection.
• Coordinate collaborative clinical trials of antiviral and other drugs that have been demonstrated in human early-phase trials to show efficacy in the treatment of AIDS or AIDS-related complex.

The WHO initiative will also seek additional funds from extrabudgetary sources for the support of national and collective programs of surveillance and epidemiology, laboratory services, clinical support, and prevention and control.

In addition to the WHO global program, regional organizations such as the African Regional Bureau of WHO and the Pan American Health Organization, which serves as the WHO regional office for the Americas, are undertaking programs initiated among member countries of their regions.

The European Economic Community, in addition to the research and prevention efforts in various individual countries of Western Europe, has established an advisory group of scientists drawn from its 12 member countries. This group promotes and funds activities aimed at ensuring "concerted action" among the various member states.

RATIONALE FOR U.S. INTERNATIONAL INVOLVEMENT

A variety of factors suggest that the United States should be actively involved internationally in efforts to control AIDS and HIV infection.

Foreign Policy Considerations

Over the last few decades, through a variety of mechanisms, the United States has actively promoted the technological development of less developed countries for economic, altruistic, and political reasons. HIV infection and AIDS are rapidly increasing in prevalence in a number of countries that have traditionally been assisted by U.S. development programs. The disease afflicts individuals in these countries at an age when they are entering or are in their most productive years. If it becomes more widespread, this disease, added to the other problems that beset these countries, may negate the benefits of all the technical assistance otherwise provided.

The strongest argument for U.S. involvement in international efforts is that such support would be a logical extension of our existing interests and efforts. Indeed, the effectiveness of other U.S. technical development assistance efforts may be jeopardized if HIV infection and AIDS are allowed to spread unchecked.

If the United States and other developed countries fail to vigorously support and, where appropriate, to become involved in efforts to control AIDS and HIV infection at all levels internationally, millions more than those now infected in poorer countries may die of this infection over the next decade or so, because the resources of developing countries to control this and other health problems are grossly inadequate. However, the United States should offer its assistance and expertise in appropriate ways. HIV infection is sexually transmitted and is therefore in some ways a sensitive political and diplomatic subject. But it is also transmitted in other ways, such as through the blood supply and through sharing of needles and syringes. Technical assistance in other sensitive areas has been successfully handled in the past. Also, the increasing willingness of the governments of affected countries to acknowledge the AIDS and HIV problem, as evidenced by reports from a number of developing countries at the Second International Conference on AIDS, bodes well for constructive U.S. involvement.

Health Improvement Assistance

Technical assistance programs have often included major contributions to efforts in improving health through programs in immunization and nutrition. Despite extremely constrained resources for health in developing countries, there has been some progress—for instance, immunization levels have increased. The addition of AIDS and other HIV-related conditions to the lengthy existing agenda of health problems in developing countries imposes a burden that may reverse the hard-won gains. Anecdotal reports from some areas and hospitals suggest that AIDS is already imposing a heavy demand on the health care systems in some developing countries. If so, resources will be unavailable for other health care demands.

The occurrence of pediatric AIDS will pose special problems in developing countries to immunization programs—one of the major and most successful interventions for health improvement—which currently receive major support from the United States. Data from central African countries suggest that many infants are acquiring HIV infection perinatally (Mann, 1986). When administered to infants infected with HIV, vaccines, particularly live replicating ones, may precipitate rapid progression to AIDS. In addition, it is theoretically possible that live vaccines might cause severe disease in HIV-infected individuals because of their compromised immunologic state. This has been reported with smallpox vaccine (live vaccinia virus) in a military recruit. However, Halsey et al. (1986) found no evidence of severe disease resulting from other live vaccines (measles, rubella, or BCG [for tuberculosis]) in Haiti in a small study. This situation needs further study to determine the extent of the theoretical risk.

These issues raise a question of how universal immunization programs should be pursued in areas where there are infants likely to have been infected perinatally. Selective or universal screening for HIV might be necessary to avoid precipitating disease in infected infants. If HIV screening is not part of immunization programs, and if many apparently healthy but HIV-infected infants do develop AIDS rapidly after immunization, perceptions that the immunization program itself was the cause of the infants' illnesses might become prevalent, diminishing the willingness of parents to permit immunization of their children. This situation would obviously decrease the control achieved over childhood infectious diseases and condemn many children to death and disability from them. Suspension of immunization efforts for fear of harming HIV-infected infants would have the same result. To these concerns must be added the concern for ensuring that immunization programs are carried out in such a way that they do not spread HIV infection through the use of unsterile needles and syringes.

Information about the HIV infection situation in many countries is incomplete, as is knowledge of the factors that influence disease progression. Decisions about how to pursue immunization programs without contributing to problems related to HIV need to be made in light of local conditions and existing knowledge. The advisable precautions should be regularly reviewed. Immunization programs must continue to be actively pursued and expanded. However, increases in the prevalence of HIV infection in certain countries will make undertaking such programs logistically and technically more difficult, which will almost certainly make them more expensive.

Not all of the tools needed to limit the spread of HIV are available. For example, a cheap, rapid, simple, highly specific, sensitive, and reliable test for HIV infection would be a tremendous aid to studies and health programs in all parts of the world.

International Spread of Diseases

In a world where millions of people travel readily from country to country and continent to continent, infectious diseases know no national boundaries. The spread of penicillin-resistant gonococci from Southeast Asia to the United States and elsewhere is a recent example of the global spread of sexually transmitted diseases. The mobile nature of today's society has also undoubtedly contributed to the spread of HIV. No country can be held responsible for the spread of an infectious disease, and all governments must contribute to decreasing the spread for the common good.

The United States has traditionally recognized a responsibility to promote better health worldwide. For example, at a time when smallpox posed only a small risk to U.S. residents, the United States contributed to control efforts abroad through bilateral arrangements and the WHO program, which eventually led to global eradication of the disease. Eradication of HIV infection is presently not a realistic goal without effective vaccines, and it may never be achievable if the virus has an animal reservoir. Nevertheless, educational programs and other community efforts must begin immediately to curb the spread of the virus.

Opportunities for Mutually Beneficial Research

There are additional reasons for U.S. international involvement. HIV poses a major problem for the United States, and there are many aspects of the infection and disease that need to be better understood before control will be achieved. Thus, while supporting local governments in present control efforts, the United States can and should contribute to the overall global research effort by supporting studies abroad. Not only is it desirable to understand the disease in all its settings, but new knowledge critical to prevention and treatment may be more readily obtained in situations outside the United States. The extent of perinatal and heterosexual transmission in central Africa offers opportunities for U.S. research resources to complement local expertise in mutually beneficial investigations. Only by thoroughly investigating the disease in all its settings will the factors become known that are unique to its occurrence in the United States and other countries, and the extent become understood to which findings can be extrapolated from one situation to another.

The understanding necessary to achieve control of HIV infection and related conditions will be most rapidly acquired if all of the resources of the international scientific community are brought to bear on the problem. Barriers to international exchange of information and resources should be identified and removed. For example, standardized reagents (e.g., virus stocks) have been identified as desirable (Katz, 1986). When these have been established, they should be made available to non-U.S. investigators. Reciprocity is a desirable feature of such arrangements, and U.S. efforts in this area should supplement and not compete with the efforts of WHO collaborating centers.

Agencies and Organizations with International Responsibilities or Operations

Certain agencies of the U.S. government have special international responsibilities or may be able to make contributions to the global effort to control the epidemic. The Agency for International Development sponsors technical assistance programs in a number of countries, including many health improvement programs in areas such as immunization. That agency, through its DIATECH program of diagnostic development, and the Food and Drug Administration, through its expertise in diagnostics and blood safety, could contribute to the development of sorely needed tools or to training.

Many commercial organizations in the United States also have considerable expertise in diagnostics, therapeutics, and vaccine development that could be put to the service of the international effort to control HIV infection and AIDS.

A further reason for U.S. involvement is that many federal agencies and other organizations require that their personnel visit or reside in other countries where HIV infection may be relatively prevalent. Policy considerations deriving from this situation relate either to the possibility that such service places an employee at risk of infection or to the need to ensure that individuals who are diagnosed with HIV-related conditions receive appropriate care.

As described in the next section, the major involuntary situations resulting in risk of infection would be accidents or illnesses requiring emergency medical treatment in local foreign facilities, where infection with HIV might occur as a result of the transfusion of blood from an infected donor or from the use of unsterile implements such as needles and syringes. Policies on these issues need to be developed in light of knowledge of local circumstances and the possibility that some individuals (e.g., hemophiliacs) may be more likely to require emergency treatments. In regard to employees abroad who are identified as infected with HIV, policies need to be formulated taking into account the individual's capacity to fulfill work-related responsibilities, the access to appropriate local care for HIV-related conditions, and local sensitivities to the presence of such persons, even though they may pose no health risk to others.

Agencies for which such issues are a particular concern are obviously the U.S. Department of State (including the Agency for International Development), the Peace Corps, and the U.S. Department of Defense. Private sector organizations with similar concerns would include any business or nonprofit groups (e.g., foundations, relief organizations, or churches) that have employees stationed abroad.

Importation

The U.S. government has recently proposed adding clinical AIDS to the list of "dangerous contagious diseases" for which aliens may be denied admission to the United States. This action acknowledges the risk that such people may pose to sexual contacts and the burden that they may put on the U.S. health care system. It overlooks, however, the risk posed by the larger number of seropositive aliens without AIDS and, more important, the vastly larger number of U.S. citizens already infected with the virus, who are the most likely source of infection for others in the United States. If much effort goes into excluding infected people from the United States, it will waste resources that could otherwise go to more effective control measures. It may also result in other countries establishing restrictions on travel from the United States.

INFECTION RISKS OUTSIDE THE UNITED STATES

Sexual Exposure

Sexual relations probably account for the largest amount of transmission of the virus both inside and outside of the United States. In a recent review, Mann (1986) concludes that the dominant mode of HIV transmission among adults in Africa is sexual, involving heterosexual, bidirectional transmission of the virus. If other factors—e.g., intercurrent sexually transmitted diseases or the disruption of cervical, vaginal, or penile epithelial integrity—enhance the efficiency of sexual transmission, it has not been proved. Also, the proportions of sexually active adult men and women already infected in the general population are unknown.

In addition, HIV infection has become a major problem among female prostitutes in many parts of the world, with prevalence rates as high as 80 percent in some areas. Business travelers, military personnel, and others who have sexual intercourse with prostitutes are at risk of infection.

Transmission of HIV between homosexual men is also well documented abroad, both in developed and certain developing countries. It must be presumed to be possible wherever behavior involving risk of infection is practiced. However, the risk of infection in different parts of the world will vary with the prevalence of HIV infection, knowledge of which is incomplete.

Knowledge of the frequency with which homosexual behaviors occur in different countries and cultures is also incomplete, and information may not be reliable because of problems of conducting sexual behavior research, especially cross-culturally.

In conclusion, people who live in or travel to countries where HIV infection is prevalent and who engage in sex with partners whose HIV infection status is not reliably known run a very real risk of infection. That risk is likely to increase sharply as international rates of infection rise, but it clearly can be avoided by abstaining from sexual relations with unknown individuals or lessened by following "safer sex" practices.

Exposure Through Blood Transfusion

Contamination of blood transfusions with HIV poses a decided risk of infection in many parts of the world, the exceptions being the countries (such as those of Western Europe) that have taken precautions with blood donations and have applied the serologic test to blood banking.

The risk varies with the prevalence of HIV infection among donors. In central Africa, 5 to 10 percent or greater prevalence of HIV infection among donors as measured by the serologic test has been reported (Mann, 1986). Thus, the risk to transfusion recipients is significant. In one study nearly 10 percent of AIDS patients reported at least one transfusion in the three years prior to onset of disease. Transfusions were twice as common among those infected as among those uninfected (Mann, 1986).

The WHO has issued guidelines on prevention of HIV transmission by transfused blood or blood products (World Health Organization, 1986d).

The recommendations urge self-exclusion from blood donation by persons at risk for HIV infection; testing of donated blood for HIV antibodies; improved antenatal care as a means of reducing the demand for blood; giving transfusions only when medically justified; using blood components rather than whole blood or plasma where appropriate; educating and selecting donors; and reviewing the manufacturing protocols of blood products to assess the acceptability of the product. Also, the WHO plans to provide reference materials for the evaluation and standardization of laboratory tests, establish uniform criteria for the treatment and testing of blood products, and revise its criteria to take new manufacturing and screening procedures into account. However, many of the countries that have not adopted procedures to prevent HIV transmission through blood transfusions lack the laboratory, financial, or trained personnel needed to institute such measures.

The risk of infection from blood transfusions in certain parts of the world is significant. But the application of currently available serologic tests will be possible only in some situations, since it is expensive for developing countries and requires highly trained personnel to apply and confirm. Simpler serologic tests, giving sensitive and specific results rapidly and reliably, are essential before widespread efforts to control HIV transmission via the blood supply in developing countries will be practicable.

IV Drug Use

Transmission of HIV by sharing of IV drug use equipment is well documented and undoubtedly can happen wherever this practice occurs. The risk of infection in any area will depend on the prevalence of HIV infection, which will in turn depend on when the virus was introduced into the IV drug-using population and the frequency with which needle and syringe sharing is practiced. In certain areas, such as sub-Saharan Africa, there is widespread agreement that nonmedical (illicit) IV drug use is extremely rare (Mann, 1986).

Use of Unsterile Needles and Implements

In Africa, injections administered for medical purposes may be a route of exposure. In one study of HIV infection, seropositive children one to two years of age whose mothers were seronegative had a mean of 44 reported lifetime injections (excluding vaccinations), as compared with 23 injections for children who were seronegative. In adults an association has been observed between the prevalence of seropositivity in hospital workers in Kinshasa, Zaire, and the number of injections received (Mann, 1986).

Among adults, interpretation of the data relating to infection is complicated by the possibility that injections were received as early treatment for HIV-related symptoms or for sexually transmitted diseases, which may be independent risk factors for exposure to HIV (Mann, 1986).

Evidence from needlesticks among health care workers suggests that viral transmission through skin penetration by contaminated needles is relatively inefficient.

There has been speculation that the use of unsterile implements in medical settings, ritual scarification, or female circumcision (genital mutilation) has the potential for HIV transmission. Mann et al. (1986a) have reported data suggesting an association, possibly indirect, between HIV infection and scarification, but the weight of evidence on the distribution of female circumcision and the findings from epidemiologic research on HIV in general suggest that they play at most a minor role in the spread of the epidemic (Hrdy, 1986; Mann, 1986).

Lack of Evidence for Transmission by Insect Vectors and Casual Contact

There is no evidence to support the hypothesis of HIV transmission by insect vectors or through casual contact in developing (or developed) countries. Notwithstanding a report that regions in DNA of various insects from central Africa are homologous with HIV proviral DNA (Becker et al., 1986), other sources of data suggest that vectorborne or casual contact transmission is unlikely. The age distribution of observed cases—peaking in infants and young adults but relatively absent among children between 1 and 14 years of age—is not consistent with either insect or casual transmission. Also, studies of nonspousal household contacts of AIDS patients and controls have revealed no differences in rates of HIV seropositivity. All observed infections among household contacts have been explicable on the basis of sexual or perinatal transmission (Mann et al., 1986b). Finally, the relative inefficiency of accidental needlestick transmission, the relatively small volume of blood carried by most common vectors such as mosquitoes, and the low blood titer of HIV all suggest that mechanical transmission by insects is unlikely (Zuckerman, 1986).

Conclusions

The risks of exposure to HIV by the various routes of transmission discussed above vary in different countries. In all settings, the dominant risk is probably sexual intercourse (heterosexual or homosexual), but the risk from contaminated blood transfusion in some areas is very real. American foreign travelers or residents abroad should be apprised of the risk they face.

INTERNATIONAL RESEARCH OPPORTUNITIES

The differences in epidemiologic patterns of HIV infection among countries offers a remarkable opportunity to define modes of spread and the effectiveness of alternative control strategies by concentrating resources where they could be most effectively used. Direct studies of the risk of heterosexual transmission would be useful but are hard to conduct in the United States because the number of heterosexual cases is small. Central Africa, where heterosexual transmission seems to predominate, may offer an opportunity for such studies.

Collaborative studies could define the relative ease of transmission from man to woman and from woman to man, the rate of transmission in varied sexual practices, and the effectiveness of different modifications of sexual behavior on the progression of the epidemic. The presence of large numbers of infected women of childbearing age offers both the opportunity and the need to study the factors affecting transmission from mother to child and the natural history of infection in children. The problem of mother-to-child transmission of HIV in Africa is potentially great, but to date relatively few pediatric cases of AIDS have been recognized there. Given the frequency of AIDS and HIV seropositivity in women of childbearing age, programs of identifying infected women and counseling them about the risk of transmission may, if effective, prevent rapid spread of the epidemic into the next generation. Studies of cohorts of infected and uninfected women who go on to have children may also help define cofactors that increase the probability of infection or illness in their offspring and lead to ways to intervene and lower those risks. Studies are also needed of seroconversion and risk factors in children born to seronegative mothers to identify the manner in which they became infected.

In Southeast Asian cities with a low prevalence of infection, techniques for prevention and control of the disease early in the course of a possible epidemic could be tested. Spread of infection from prostitutes into the general population could be studied in those countries in which cases were first seen in prostitutes.

There is great need for systematic surveillance of HIV infection in Africa and other developing countries. Knowledge of the present prevalence of the disease and of trends in its incidence would enable better allocation of local and international resources for control. It would also identify opportunities for research that might have international implications. As noted above, WHO has set up an AIDS program that will work with ministries of health in surveillance and control activities. The role of WHO as coordinator can complement bilateral agreements that several European and U.S. agencies have initiated with local governments or universities.

Investigation of the existence of cofactors (risk modifiers) for the acquisition and progression of infection and disease in both the United States and abroad is an example of opportunities for research in developing countries, but it also exemplifies an area in which particular care will be needed in extrapolating findings to the U.S. situation. It will be important to determine if any bacterial or parasitic disease endemic in Africa increases the probability of HIV infection and AIDS. Also, the differences in epidemiology of classical and aggressive Kaposi's sarcoma in Africa (as well as the differential susceptibility to Kaposi's sarcoma of male homosexuals compared with other AIDS patients in the United States) suggest the value of looking for an infectious agent or risk factor of aggressive Kaposi's sarcoma separate from HIV.

The heavy burden of parasitic and other infectious agents borne by many African populations generally and the distinctive infectious disease patterns seen in African AIDS patients suggest the importance of examining in far greater detail the interaction of HIV with a variety of infectious agents. It seems clear that the immunodeficiency characteristic of AIDS results in the presentation of AIDS patients with disseminated infections with agents common there, such as *Mycobacterium tuberculosis*. However, studies may show that chronic or repeated infections (for example, with malaria or enteric bacteria) increase the probability that latent infection with HIV may become manifest, or that infections that breach the skin or mucous membranes may predispose to HIV infection in the first place.

Recent identification of additional human retroviruses in western Africa (see Chapters 2 and 6), one of which appears similar to a virus identified in wild monkeys, suggests that extensive investigation of primate and human retroviruses is warranted in all areas of sub-Saharan Africa.

Support for establishing surveillance systems for HIV infection and programs for prevention of transmission and disease could result not only in definition and control of the AIDS problem but also in a model for surveillance and control of other infectious and noninfectious diseases in developing countries. Working through bilateral projects with individual countries or through multilateral arrangements, as with WHO, the United States could leverage its support of AIDS research and control to further public health practice internationally.

Any research conducted by U.S. investigators in other countries, particularly developing ones, is extremely sensitive, and this is especially true of research on sexually transmitted diseases. It is necessary that such research be done in truly collaborative fashion and in a manner that takes account of local cultural or social mores. Guidelines for such efforts should be developed to ensure that the long-term prospects for collaborative efforts are not damaged by cultural or political insensitivities.

THE U.S. CONTRIBUTION TO INTERNATIONAL EFFORTS

The United States has contributed greatly to the understanding of AIDS and HIV infection through its investment in domestic research. The mandates of various federal agencies recognize that the health of U.S. citizens can benefit from studies abroad. Hence, investigators supported by the Centers for Disease Control, the National Institutes of Health, and the Department of Defense have been involved in collaborative epidemiologic, serologic, and virologic studies of AIDS and HIV infection at various sites around the world, particularly in sub-Saharan Africa but also in Europe and Southeast Asia.

Until the fall of 1985 the Agency for International Development of the Department of State—the only federal agency with a direct mandate to be involved in international health activities—had no specific policy with regard to support of activities related to AIDS or HIV infection. (It should be noted that some countries affected by AIDS do not meet the general conditions for support from the Agency for International Development—e.g., Brazil, Tanzania.) In November 1985, however, its administrator, M. Peter McPherson, committed the agency to involvement in international efforts on the problem. This commitment resulted in an announcement in June 1986 of the provision to WHO of $2 million in FY 1986 (Agency for International Development, 1986). Of this amount, $1 million was to be a contribution to the central WHO effort to establish a global surveillance system, to provide epidemiologic and laboratory consultants to member countries, and to ensure the safety of the blood supply. The other $1 million would go directly to WHO's regional office for Africa in Brazzaville, Congo, to support WHO surveillance and educational activities in Africa with the assistance of the Centers for Disease Control. The plans of the regional office for Africa are to provide some basic support in most African countries and in four to six countries to establish pilot programs to establish diagnostic capabilities and reporting of AIDS and HIV infection and to assist these countries in establishing public health prevention and control activities for AIDS.

In addition to the monetary commitment to WHO, the Agency for

International Development's Bureau of Science and Technology Office of Health established in August 1986 a position to monitor and coordinate AIDS activities.

A federal interagency working group on the international aspects of AIDS and HIV infection also meets periodically. It is convened under the auspices of the U.S. Department of State.

It is the committee's understanding from its discussions with representatives of the Department of State and the Agency for International Development that the primary focus of these agencies' support to international activities will be through WHO. AIDS-related requests for technical assistance or support from foreign governments will be directed to that organization.

However, the committee believes that bilateral or multinational activities involving the United States outside the WHO program will be essential to enhancing the prospects for control of the disease. It agrees that to be most effective these must be coordinated with WHO's efforts. But a multiplicity of innovative activities may be needed to find the best ways to successfully tackle the problem, and a diversity of approaches would be useful in the search.

Bilateral or multinational efforts can usefully complement the WHO program for a number of reasons:

1. The WHO program is new and in the early phases of organization. It has a small staff and thus far has received less than 20 percent of the funds estimated to be required for the 1986-1987 biennium (World Health Organization, 1986b; J. Mann, World Health Organization, personal communication, 1986). Support for the program is still under consideration by a number of potential donors (*Lancet*, 1986; World Health Organization, 1986b,c). However, the need for action in some countries is urgent: all opportunities to supplement the WHO program, as it becomes established and expands, should be acted upon as soon as possible because of the seriousness of the epidemic.

2. The focus of the WHO program is prevention and control of AIDS and HIV infection. There will be opportunities for productive freestanding research projects or research projects that could usefully be coupled to prevention and control efforts but that do not fall within the scope of the WHO program. These could be pursued bilaterally, with funding from agencies such as the National Institutes of Health, the Centers for Disease Control, and the Department of Defense, as well as the Agency for International Development.

3. Many U.S. investigators or institutions with expertise in the study of AIDS or other infectious diseases have direct links with counterparts in

affected countries. These links provide the opportunity to respond rapidly to needs identified by the governments of such countries.

The committee further believes that efficient coordination and use of resources can be achieved by international exchange of information on national activities, perhaps with WHO as a central clearinghouse.

CONCLUSIONS AND RECOMMENDATIONS

AIDS and HIV infection pose a new global health problem that will affect most adversely the poorer developing countries, where health systems are least able to cope with the increased burden on resources. The impact of the epidemic could stall or reverse progress that has been achieved in health and economic areas—e.g., in child survival—in many developing countries.

The initial phases of data collection on the disease met with some reluctance in acknowledging the presence and magnitude of the problem. However, establishment of the WHO program and increasing recognition of the seriousness of the situation, as evidenced by reports from various countries at the Second International Conference on AIDS, have opened up opportunities for the United States to play a role worldwide in efforts to control HIV infection and AIDS. The United States should be a full participant in international efforts. U.S. involvement should be both through support of WHO programs and through bilateral arrangements in response to the needs and opportunities in individual countries. It should also be pursued in a fashion that is acceptable to host governments in these collaborating countries. The Agency for International Development is to be commended for moving rapidly to provide $2 million to the WHO to support efforts to control AIDS, but much more money will certainly be needed.

Increased contributions to international efforts in this area are needed through a variety of mechanisms—for instance, support of the World Health Organization, support of collaborative research (for example, through the National Institutes of Health, the U.S. Department of Defense, and the Centers for Disease Control), and support of bilateral technical assistance agreements.

Given the magnitude of the problem, particularly in central Africa and increasingly in Latin America, and the variety of reasons warranting U.S. participation in international efforts, the committee believes that the United States should make clear its commitment to global prevention and control of AIDS and HIV infection.

- By 1990, the total funding flowing to international efforts directed toward AIDS-related research and prevention should reach $50 million per year on a continuing basis. This amount is about 2.5 percent of the total expenditures that the committee recommends be spent annually in the United States for these purposes.

• Increased funding should be provided to the WHO program on the basis of demonstrated capacity to use such funds productively.

• Increased funds for research or technical assistance programs or projects abroad should be provided on the basis of review procedures involving individuals familiar with the conditions, such as the local availability and quality of laboratory resources and personnel, under which such projects are undertaken.

• The committee found that there was no tabulation or assessment of the extent and nature of work being undertaken on HIV-related conditions by U.S. investigators in other countries or of their collaborations with foreign researchers. It therefore recommends that an evaluation be initiated immediately to assess and coordinate the roles and responses of the various U.S. federal agencies, private voluntary groups, and foundations interested in international efforts on AIDS and HIV and to identify all work currently under way.

• Efforts to use funds and other resources of the United States, other industrialized countries, and the WHO would be aided by the establishment of national data bases or clearinghouses on AIDS and HIV-related work being undertaken in or involving collaboration with foreign countries. These groups should communicate regularly with WHO.

• Pending the more formal establishment of information centers, the office of the AIDS coordinator of the Public Health Service should serve as a clearinghouse for information on U.S. international activities on AIDS and HIV infection and should be provided with the resources to play a greater role in the United States' international efforts.

REFERENCES

Agency for International Development. 1986. U.S. Aid Assists World Health Organization to Control Global AIDS. News Release, June 13, 1986, Washington, D.C.

Becker, J.-L., O. Hazan, M.-T. Neugeyere, F. Rey, B. Spire, F. Barre-Sinoussi, A. Georges, L. Teulieres, and J. C. Chermann. 1986. Infection of insect cell lines by HIV, agent of AIDS, and evidence for HIV proviral DNA in insects from central Africa. C. R. Acad. Sci. (Paris) 303:33-36.

Halsey, N. A., R. Boulos, M. Robert-Guroff, J. Hughes, E. Holt, J. Rohde, and C. Boulos. 1986. Measles vaccination of infants born to LAV/HTLV-III positive mothers. P. 49 in Abstracts of the Second International Conference on AIDS, Paris, June 23-25, 1986.

Hrdy, D. 1986. Sexual preferences and other cultural practices contributing to the spread of AIDS in Africa. Background paper. Washington, D.C.: Committee on a National Strategy for AIDS.

Katz, S. O. 1986. Summary of a Workshop of AIDS Vaccine Development. Presented at the

Workshop on AIDS Vaccine Development, National Institutes of Health, Bethesda, Md., July 28-29, 1986.

Lancet. 1986. WHO's efforts to contain AIDS. Lancet I:1167.

Mahler, H., and F. Assaad. 1986. The World Health Organization's programme on AIDS. P. 5 in Abstracts of the Second International Conference on AIDS, Paris, June 23-25, 1986.

Mann, J. M. 1986. Epidemiology of LAV/HTLV-III in Africa. Paper presented at the Second International Conference on AIDS, Paris, June 23-25, 1986.

Mann, J. M., H. Francis, T. C. Quinn, P. K. Asila, N. Bosenge, N. Nzilambi, K. Bila, M. Tamfum, K. Ruti, P. Piot, J. McCormick, and J. W. Curran. 1986a. Surveillance for AIDS in a central African city: Kinshasa, Zaire. JAMA 255:3255-3259.

Mann, J. M., T. C. Quinn, H. Francis, N. Nzilambi, N. Bosenge, K. Bila, J. B. McCormick, K. Ruti, P. K. Asila, and J. W. Curran. 1986b. Prevalence of HTLV-III/LAV in household contacts of patients with confirmed AIDS and controls in Kinshasa, Zaire. JAMA 256:721-724.

World Health Organization. 1986a. WHO Activities for the Prevention and Control of Acquired Immunodeficiency Syndrome. Geneva: World Health Organization.

World Health Organization. 1986b. Global Strategy for the Prevention and Control of Acquired Immunodeficiency Syndrome: Projected Needs for 1986-1987. Geneva: World Health Organization.

World Health Organization. 1986c. Meeting of Participating Parties for the Prevention and Control of Acquired Immunodeficiency Syndrome. Geneva: World Health Organization.

World Health Organization. 1986d. WHO meeting and consultation on the safety of blood and blood products. WHO Weekly Epidemiol. Rec. 18:138-140.

Zuckerman, A. J. 1986. AIDS and insects. Br. Med. J. 292:1094-1095.

Appendixes

A

Clinical Manifestations of HIV Infection

OPPORTUNISTIC INFECTIONS

The deleterious effects inflicted on the immune system following HIV infection result in life-threatening opportunistic infections characterized by an aggressive clinical course, resistance to therapy, and a high rate of relapse. Opportunistic infections are the most common presenting clinical manifestations that ultimately lead to a diagnosis of AIDS (see Appendix E). The clinical recognition of these infections requires a high degree of suspicion, a familiarity with the many complexities of AIDS-related infections, and expert microbiological assistance.

Treatment of the varied AIDS-related opportunistic infections is as complex as their diagnosis. The duration of therapy is frequently long, and drug toxicities are seen much more often than when the same antibiotics are used in other patient populations.

Protozoal Infections

Pneumocystis carinii Pneumonia

Pneumocystis carinii pneumonia (PCP) is the most common AIDS-related opportunistic infection in U.S. patients, accounting for over 50 percent of all initial AIDS diagnoses. Patients with PCP typically complain of fever, cough (usually nonproductive or productive of clear to white sputum), shortness of breath and dyspnea on exertion, and chest tightness. Some or all of these symptoms are seen in approximately 80 percent of patients at the time of diagnosis. The time course between onset and medical evaluation is variable, ranging from several days in some cases to as long as two or more months in others (Kovacs et al., 1984).

At the time of PCP diagnosis, the chest X-ray is usually abnormal. More than 95 percent of cases show some increase in bronchovascular/interstitial markings. These infiltrates are typically diffuse. Pleural effusions are distinctly uncommon, and if seen suggest a secondary process. Similarly, mediastinal adenopathy is uncommonly associated with PCP alone (Catterall et al., 1985).

Identification of the organism is required before a diagnosis of PCP can be made. Tissue diagnosis can be made using several techniques. Initially, transbronchial biopsies were performed in most individuals, but broncho-alveolar lavage either with or without bronchoscopy is nearly as sensitive and is less invasive (Broaddus et al., 1985; Ognibene et al., 1984). In addition, induced sputum has been increasingly used to make a diagnosis. Sputum must be examined with particular care to find PCP organisms, but this procedure avoids more than 50 percent of invasive procedures (Bibgy et al., 1986). Serologic testing is not sufficient for the diagnosis, and empiric therapy should be avoided in most cases because of frequent drug toxicity.

The treatment of PCP consists of either trimethoprim-sulfamethoxazole or pentamidine isothianate (Hughes et al., 1978). However, toxicities are common with these drugs (Gordin et al., 1984), therapy must be longer than in other settings, and there is a high rate of relapse (Haverkos, 1984). Because conventional therapy is only partially effective with PCP, and because PCP is the most common direct cause of death in AIDS, there is currently a great deal of interest in identifying additional effective therapies. Trials are being conducted with dapsone (Hughes and Smith, 1984) and difluoromethoornithine (DFMO). Trials of prophylaxis using trimethoprim-sulfamethoxazole are also being conducted (Kaplan et al., 1986).

Toxoplasma gondii

Toxoplasmosis is one of the most common causes of central nervous system (CNS) disease in AIDS (Luft et al., 1984; Navia et al., 1986; Wong et al., 1984). It is also one of the most treatable AIDS-related opportunistic infections. Clinical features of CNS infection with *Toxoplasma gondii* include seizures, focal neurologic deficits, and encephalopathy. Because serologic testing for *Toxoplasma* is insensitive and nonspecific, diagnosis requires tissue confirmation. However, the morbidity of brain biopsy dictates that this is often not performed. Instead, many clinicians attempt empiric therapy in patients strongly suspected of having CNS toxoplasmosis.

A diagnosis of *T. gondii* infection of the CNS can be suspected when a patient with AIDS or in an AIDS risk group complains of seizures or focal neurologic deficits (Luft et al., 1984). Although encephalopathy can be seen with toxoplasmosis, it is more suggestive of HIV-related encephalopathy. The diagnosis of *Toxoplasma* CNS infection can be confirmed by computerized tomography (CT) scanning or magnetic resonance imaging (MRI) procedures. These typically show multiple lesions deep in the brain tissue with ring enhancement. These lesions are nearly diagnostic for toxoplasmosis in this population, and the only common alternative diagnosis considered is CNS lymphoma.

Therapy for toxoplasmosis is currently limited to a combination of pyramethamine and sulfadiazine with folinic acid. Response to therapy is generally prompt, with improvement on radiologic imaging seen within two weeks in most cases. However, relapses at some point after therapy are nearly universal. Also, drug toxicity is common and includes skin rashes, neutropenia, and thrombocytopenia. There is no standard second-line drug for the treatment of toxoplasmosis, but clindamycin is occasionally attempted.

After a two- to three-week course of sulfadiazine-pyramethamine, CT or MRI scanning can be repeated. If substantial regression of previously noted lesions has occurred, this is taken as presumptive evidence of the diagnosis. If, on the other hand, the disease is stable or worse, a brain biopsy can be performed to evaluate the possibility of other problems, including CNS lymphomas.

Cryptosporidium

Cryptosporidium is a unicellular coccidian parasite that produces a self-limited diarrhea in animals, travelers, and veterinarians. In AIDS patients, infection instead produces sustained, profuse diarrhea, often associated with malnutrition, malabsorption, and significant weight loss (Soave et al., 1984). Organisms are occasionally found in the lungs or gallbladder. Recognition of *Cryptosporidium* in stool requires special techniques.

No effective therapy for *Cryptosporidium* infection has been found in animal studies or human clinical trials to date. Drugs found ineffective include trimethoprim-sulfamethoxazole, iodoquinol, metronidazole, quinacrine, pentamidine, paramomycin, and tetracycline. Occasional clinical or parasitologic response to furazolidone have been encountered, but relapse occurs. Spiramycin, a macrolide antibiotic not commercially available in the United States with an antimicrobial spectrum similar to that of erythromycin, has been reported to be effective in uncontrolled trials (Collier et al., 1984), but this was not substantiated in one controlled trial. Further controlled studies of this agent are under way. DFMO has been used with differing results (Soave et al., 1985), though bone marrow toxicity, especially thrombocytopenia, has been commonly noted (Rolston et al., 1985).

Isospora belli

Isospora belli, another invasive coccidian parasite, produces a severe diarrhea clinically indistinguishable from that caused by *Cryptosporidium* in patients with AIDS (Whiteside et al., 1984). Oocysts are large but may evade detection in stool examination, even with special techniques. Trimethoprim-sulfamethoxazole or furazolidone were reported to be effective in a few cases, but relapse occurred after discontinuation (Westerman and Christensen, 1979).

Fungal Infections

Candida

Oral candidiasis (also known as thrush) is a very common infection in people with AIDS and at high risk for AIDS. The presence of thrush in high-risk patients without AIDS is strongly predictive of the subsequent development of a serious opportunistic infection (i.e., the development of AIDS) (Klein et al., 1984). However, only invasive esophageal candidiasis meets the Centers for Disease Control (CDC) surveillance definition of AIDS (see Appendix E).

There have been no treatment trials for either thrush or *Candida* esophagitis in AIDS, so treatment recommendations must be based on clinical experience and the results of treatment trials in other immunocompromised populations. Clotrimazole is commonly used to treat oral candidiasis in immunosuppressed non-AIDS patients and has been shown to be superior to placebo. Nystatin, the agent most commonly employed in patients who are not immunocompromised, has been only marginally effective in immunocompromised hosts.

Candida esophagitis may be asymptomatic, and most, but not all, patients will have thrush. Treatment options include nystatin and ketoconazole. Candidemia is rarely encountered, but treatment would be no different than that for other populations, using amphotericin B for disseminated disease.

Cryptococcus

The meninges are the sole site of cryptococcal infection in 75 percent of the cases seen in AIDS patients, though simultaneous or isolated infections of the blood, lungs, or other sites occur (Zuger et al., 1986). Cryptococcal antigen and/or culture are positive at the site of infection in over 90 percent of patients. In meningitis, cerebrospinal fluid (CSF) is otherwise normal in more than 50 percent of AIDS patients (Kovacs et al., 1984), a much higher percentage than with non-AIDS patients with cryptococcal meningitis.

There are no comparative trials of treatment for cryptococcal infections in patients with AIDS. However, in small series evaluated retrospectively, clinical failure and relapse are more frequent than in other immunosuppressed populations. In large, multicenter series evaluating treatment of cryptococcal meningitis in non-AIDS patients, amphotericin B in combination with 5-fluorocytosine achieved a better rate of cure and faster CSF sterilization than did amphotericin B alone given for a longer time.

Intravenous amphotericin B in combination with 5-fluorocytosine is the standard initial therapy for cryptococcal infection in patients with AIDS. Total doses administered vary widely, and dose does not appear to correlate with outcome. A convenient oral therapy for suppression after initial treatment and also for the treatment of isolated pulmonary *Cryptococcus* infection is much needed. Ketoconazole alone or in combination with other antifungal agents is efficacious in the laboratory and in animal studies. However, prospective trials are needed to establish the role of ketoconazole in the treatment of cryptococcal infection in patients with AIDS.

Bacterial Infections

Mycobacterium tuberculosis

Tuberculosis is seen with increasing frequency in groups at risk for AIDS, typically preceding the actual diagnosis of AIDS by several months (Louie et al., 1985). In Haitian patients infected with *Mycobacterium tuberculosis*, disseminated disease was found in 80 percent of patients with AIDS, whereas it was found in 20 percent of infected Haitians without AIDS (Pitchenik et al., 1984). Response to standard antituberculosis therapy is usually good.

Mycobacterium avium-intracellulare

Mycobacterium avium-intracellulare is a frequent isolate in blood, sputum, urine, and feces of AIDS patients and is found at multiple sites in about half of AIDS patients in whom postmortem evaluation is done (Zakowski et al., 1982). This infection is usually identified late in the course of AIDS, in association with fever, wasting, and fatigue, but often without the failure of specific organ systems despite their involvement. Many other AIDS-related infections and/or neoplasms are often present simultaneously.

In non-AIDS patients with *Mycobacterium avium-intracellulare*, dissemination is rare and treatment of pulmonary disease with multiple drugs or surgery is sometimes effective. Most strains of the bacterium are resistant to standard antituberculosis drugs. However, most isolates from AIDS patients have demonstrated *in vitro* sensitivity to two experimental agents: ansamycin, a rifamycin S derivative, and clofazimine, a dye derivative used to treat leprosy. Various combination therapies are also under evaluation, but further investigation of therapeutic agents is sorely needed.

Since *Mycobacterium tuberculosis* is a treatable disease in patients with AIDS and ARC, disseminated mycobacterial disease is probably best treated initially with triple drug therapy until cultures are available. If the patient has shown amelioration of systemic symptoms, some physicians would maintain that same regimen even if infection with *Mycobacterium avium-intracellulare* is documented. Others would treat with ansamycin with or without clofazimine, and still others would try four to six drugs chosen from INH, rifampin, ethambutol, an injectable aminoglycoside, ethionamide, and cycloserine. More specific recommendations cannot be made at this time. If the patient is premorbid or is asymptomatic, many would recommend no treatment to avoid drug toxicity. Pulmonary colonization alone does not necessitate treatment, but close observation for potential disseminated infection is warranted.

Salmonella Infections

Several recent reports have disclosed 14 cases of bacteremic *Salmonella* infections in AIDS and ARC patients. In the cases in New York and Washington, D.C., all were due to *Salmonella typhimurium*, an infrequent cause of *Salmonella* sepsis in other populations. Infections were severe, with sustained stool carriage and recurrent septicemia in some patients, despite therapy with antibiotics to which the organisms were sensitive *in vitro* (Glaser et al., 1985; Jacobs et al., 1985; Smith et al., 1985).

In California, five cases of *Salmonella dublin*, a *Salmonella* species closely linked to dairy cattle products such as raw milk, have been reported in AIDS patients. Recurrent bacteremia has been the rule with this infection as well.

Pyogenic Bacteria

Pyogenic infections are relatively uncommon in AIDS patients but do contribute to morbidity and mortality. Serious pneumococcal infections may be more common in AIDS patients than in the hospital population at large, and failure to respond to pneumococcal vaccine has been documented.

Viral Infections

Herpes Simplex Virus

A severe cutaneous herpes simplex virus (HSV) infection that persists for more than four weeks is considered diagnostic of AIDS. Such an infection may occur initially or be an ongoing problem throughout the course of an AIDS illness. Other identified types of herpes infections include severe orofacial herpes, encephalitis, myelitis, and pneumonia.

There are neither studies of the natural history nor comparative treatment trials of these viral infections in AIDS or ARC. Acyclovir used topically, intravenously, and orally reduces viral shedding and enhances the healing of cutaneous lesions in other immunocompromised populations (Epstein, 1983). Oral and intravenous acyclovir are also effective prophylaxes against recurrence in immunocompromised patients.

Herpes Zoster

Localized cutaneous zoster (shingles) is frequently encountered in patients with AIDS and ARC. However, there are no natural history studies of the relative severity of disease, the frequency of dissemination, or the incidence of postherpetic neuralgia. Disseminated disease and zoster encephalitis have been encountered.

Since most AIDS patients with herpes zoster are not sick enough to warrant hospitalization, treatment with intravenous acyclovir is best reserved for patients with cutaneous or visceral dissemination or systemic symptoms.

Cytomegalovirus

Serologic evidence of cytomegalovirus (CMV) infection is almost universal in homosexual men with AIDS and ARC. At bronchoscopy, more than one-third of patients have evidence of colonization by CMV, although histologic evidence of invasive disease is rare. In a small prospective study, the presence of CMV had no effect on the survival of

AIDS patients with *Pneumocystis carinii.* CMV can be associated with symptomatic retinitis, adrenalitis, colitis, and encephalitis.

To date no commercially available therapies are effective. A nucleoside analog, dihydroxymethyl propoxymethylguanine, has excellent *in vitro* activity against replication of CMV. The drug is currently undergoing clinical trials in AIDS patients, and preliminary results are encouraging (Bach et al., 1985; Felsenstein et al., 1985; Masur et al., 1986).

Other Infections in Members of Risk Groups

Given the large number of people in the United States infected with HIV, infections other than those considered diagnostic of AIDS are certain to occur. It can be very difficult to establish a direct relationship between these other medical problems and HIV-induced immune deficiency. This is especially so with certain infectious diseases that were well known to occur in members of AIDS risk groups prior to the introduction of HIV in those communities. In the case of IV drug users, these diseases are principally hepatitis B virus infection and endocarditis from a variety of organisms. So far, clinical or laboratory patterns of these infections and their response to conventional therapy do not seem to have changed.

Like IV drug users, homosexual and bisexual men have frequently been affected by infectious diseases. For example, they have a high incidence of sexually transmitted diseases (Rein, 1986), including gonorrhea, syphilis, genital herpes virus infections, genital warts, and bacterial and parasitic infections of the large bowel (Quinn, 1986). Although changes in life-styles of homosexual men in response to the AIDS epidemic have reduced the frequency of new diagnoses of sexually transmitted diseases in this group in recent years, they remain common.

Apart from sexually transmitted diseases such as persistent genital HSV infection, the relationship of other common infections to underlying cellular immune deficiency is unclear. In some instances, however, the features of such infections are suspected of having changed in people infected with HIV. Salmonellosis, for example, while not previously uncommon in homosexual men, is nonetheless being seen with increased incidence. In contrast to previous experience, it is increasingly resistant to drug therapy and typified by frequent relapses. Although evidence is still lacking, the fear remains that the delta agent may spread more readily in both homosexual men and IV drug users, given established chronic cases of hepatitis B and cellular immune deficiency.

Because infectious diseases are a common feature of at least two of the major AIDS risk groups independent of the AIDS epidemic, it may be extremely difficult to establish any direct connection between HIV infection and these other infections. Nevertheless, surveillance mechanisms should continue to record these other infections, particularly to find any evidence suggesting alterations in their clinical presentation or response to therapy.

MALIGNANCIES AND OTHER NEOPLASTIC DISEASES

Kaposi's Sarcoma

Before 1981, Kaposi's sarcoma was a distinctly uncommon cancer in the United States, and it had not previously been seen in healthy young adults. Its recognition in young homosexual men in mid-1981 was therefore an early and obvious alert that a new disease had arrived. Today, Kaposi's sarcoma remains a common and visible reminder of AIDS.

Throughout the AIDS epidemic, Kaposi's sarcoma has played an important role as an easily monitored clinical marker of the underlying immune deficiency. For this reason, plus the fact that Kaposi's sarcoma patients are frequently less severely immunocompromised than other AIDS groups, Kaposi's sarcoma has been the focus of many clinical therapy trials.

Kaposi's Sarcoma in Non-AIDS Populations

Prior to 1981, Kaposi's sarcoma, when seen, was limited to several groups, including elderly American men (especially those of Mediterranean descent), black Africans, and individuals with severe exogenous immunosuppression such as renal allograft recipients. While reports of Kaposi's sarcoma therapy in the elderly and African groups have little relevance to current cases in AIDS patients, Kaposi's sarcoma in renal transplant patients mimics the disease in AIDS patients. In both, Kaposi's sarcoma is often, though not always, an aggressive malignancy with extensive visceral spread; in both, opportunistic infections are common. Perhaps the most striking observation, however, is that in renal allograft patients Kaposi's sarcoma often regresses completely after the withdrawal of immunosuppressive drugs. This suggests that in AIDS-related Kaposi's sarcoma, drug-induced immune restoration might control the cancer. It also implies that Kaposi's sarcoma may, in the future, be useful as a clinical marker of the response to immunologic therapy.

Not all groups of AIDS patients are at equal risk of developing Kaposi's sarcoma. For reasons as yet unclear, Kaposi's sarcoma is much more frequent in homosexual men than in other AIDS patients (Cohn and Judson, 1984; Des Jarlais et al., 1984). Infection of homosexuals with cytomegalovirus (Drew et al., 1982) and the use of inhaled nitrites (Marmor et al., 1982) have been suggested as possible cofactors leading to the increased incidence of Kaposi's sarcoma in this population, but there are currently no data to support these contentions.

The clinical spectrum of Kaposi's sarcoma in AIDS is broad, possibly reflecting a variably severe underlying immune deficiency. In general, patients present with mucocutaneous lesions or lymphatic involvement. Although Kaposi's sarcoma lesions may begin in any site, initial lesions on the face or in the oral cavity are particularly common. While Kaposi's sarcoma frequently involves the plantar surface of the foot, the palms are rarely involved.

Kaposi's sarcoma lesions are easily recognized by alert patients or physicians. Typically, they are palpable but not exophytic, although protuberant, wartlike tumors are occasionally seen. Early lesions are usually red or violaceous and do not blanch on pressure. Rapidly enlarging tumors are often surrounded by a yellow-brown ecchymosis. Lesions are usually discrete, but with advanced disease plaques of coalesced lesions are common, especially over the medial aspect of the thigh. Lesions tend to be relatively circular, but lesions on the back or around the neckline can be linear and may appear to follow cutaneous lymphatics. Kaposi's sarcoma tumors in the early stages are painless, but pain may accompany more advanced disease, especially in the feet and lower extremities.

Visceral Kaposi's sarcoma is not uncommon but is often clinically silent. Pulmonary Kaposi's sarcoma, in contrast, is less common but more aggressive clinically (Nash and Fligiel, 1984). Patients with pulmonary Kaposi's sarcoma have an extremely poor prognosis, although some reports suggest longer survival in patients receiving systemic chemotherapy.

The diagnosis of Kaposi's sarcoma requires histologic confirmation even though the clinical suspicion may be extremely high. Biopsy can be performed at any site, but the skin is most convenient. Enlarged peripheral lymph nodes can also be biopsied and may in some cases be the only site of Kaposi's sarcoma. This is also true of gastrointestinal or endobronchial lesions, although endoscopic biopsies of gastrointestinal lesions may be too superficial for diagnostic purposes.

The choice of therapy for Kaposi's sarcoma in AIDS patients is difficult because of the variable natural history of the disease and the current lack of agents that can correct the immune defect underlying the disease (Mitsuyasu and Groopman, 1984). Conventional cytotoxic chemotherapy is often used, but this is controversial because it may further impair cellular immunity and thus increase infections (Mintzer et al., 1985). Clinical studies have demonstrated potential beneficial effects with alpha interferon against Kaposi's sarcoma (Volberding et al., 1984).

Non-Hodgkin's Lymphoma in AIDS

The first cases of high-grade (clinically aggressive) non-Hodgkin's lymphoma (NHL) in homosexual men were reported in 1982. Since then many such cases of lymphoma in patients at risk for AIDS have been reported (Ziegler et al., 1984). In June 1985 the CDC amended its surveillance definition of AIDS to include patients with high-grade B-cell NHL and documented HIV infection.

Non-Hodgkin's lymphoma has frequently been observed in association with abnormal cell-mediated immunity. Patients with primary immunodeficiency disorders, such as the Wiskott-Aldrich syndrome or ataxia-telangiectasia, have developed high-grade B-cell NHL in which immunoblastic lymphoma has been the most prevalent histologic pattern. A striking feature in these patients has been a marked generalized lymphadenopathy that was often present for several years before the diagnosis of lymphoma.

Circumstantial evidence supports a role for Epstein-Barr virus (EBV) in the etiology of these lymphomas. A majority of patients with these disorders have serologic evidence for either acute or reactivated EBV infection, and multiple copies of the EBV genome have been identified within the cells of many of these lymphomas.

Studies show that patients with AIDS-associated NHL respond significantly less well to aggressive combination chemotherapy than do immunocompetent patients suffering from the same high-grade lymphomas. Morbidity and mortality seem to be directly correlated with a previous history of an AIDS-related diagnosis. Patients who are asymptomatic at the time of diagnosis have the best treatment results. Those with a history of persistent generalized lymphadenopathy fare less well. Patients with a previous diagnosis of AIDS or with primary central nervous system lymphoma have the highest morbidity and mortality (Ioachim et al., 1985).

The prognosis for non-AIDS patients with primary central nervous system lymphoma is extremely poor. Despite the fact that such patients may respond to radiation therapy, most will die of recurrent disease within one year of diagnosis. No published series exists that evaluates treatment of patients with AIDS-associated primary central nervous system lymphoma, but these patients tend not to survive long. Moreover, treatment of primary central nervous system lymphoma even in immunocompetent patients has been largely unsuccessful.

Hodgkin's Disease in Homosexual Men

In contrast to other cancers in members of AIDS risk groups, a strong body of evidence links HIV infection to Hodgkin's disease in homosexual men (Schoeppel et al., 1985). Hodgkin's disease is being recognized more and more frequently in homosexual men. In this setting the disease is often advanced, with frequent extralymphatic sites of involvement, including the liver and bone marrow. Also, involvement of mesenteric nodes is common, in contrast to typical Hodgkin's disease.

Hodgkin's disease in homosexual men responds rapidly to conventional chemotherapeutic approaches, but hematologic toxicities are more severe than anticipated, with persistent and severe pancytopenia being particularly common. The high rate of secondary opportunistic infections in homosexual men with Hodgkin's disease receiving chemotherapy is also unusual.

Other Cancers in AIDS

While it may be very difficult to establish a direct relationship between cancers and AIDS, there is a growing suspicion that for some cancers a relationship exists. Besides Kaposi's sarcoma and B-cell lymphomas, which have been accepted as diagnostic of AIDS, members of AIDS high-risk groups have been seen to contract with apparently increased frequency squamous cell carcinomas of various sites, malignant melanoma, testicular cancers of all histologies, Hodgkin's disease, and primary hepatocellular carcinoma.

With the exception of Hodgkin's disease in homosexual men, there is as yet minimal direct evidence that these other cancers are caused by HIV-induced immune deficiency or that their mode of presentation or response to therapy is different from prior experience. Some of these cancers—in particular anal squamous cell carcinomas, malignant melanoma, and testicular malignancies—are known to have been relatively common in young men even before the beginning of the AIDS epidemic. Others, including hepatocellular carcinoma and squamous cell carcinomas, have only rarely been reported in members of AIDS risk groups. These may reflect a simultaneous occurrence of two separate diseases—HIV infection and a malignancy. Nevertheless, it is important to monitor populations at risk of AIDS for cancers, because even if they are not causally related, previous HIV infection may alter the clinical behavior or response to therapy of these spontaneously occurring malignancies.

NEUROLOGIC COMPLICATIONS

Clinical and Pathologic Features of Neurologic Diseases

Most of the attention to neurologic problems associated with AIDS initially focused on unusual infections of the central nervous system.

Toxoplasmosis, which was previously a rare opportunistic infection of the brain, is frequently seen in AIDS patients, where it appears as multiple abscesslike lesions. Cryptococcal meningitis is the second most common opportunistic infection of the central nervous system in AIDS and is most commonly seen in Africa. Disseminated herpesvirus infections of the nervous system (herpes simplex, varicella zoster, and cytomegalovirus) are seen less commonly. Progressive multifocal leukoencephalopathy, an otherwise rare demyelinating disease caused by papovavirus infection of oligodendrocytes, has occurred in patients with unprecedented frequency. A variety of other bacterial, viral, and fungal infections have also been reported (Snider et al., 1983).

Tumors of the central nervous system in patients with AIDS have largely been primary CNS lymphomas. Secondary lymphomas and metastatic Kaposi's sarcoma have occurred much more rarely. Metabolic encephalopathies associated with pulmonary, hepatic, and renal failure are found postmortem in approximately 10 percent of AIDS patients (Navia et al., 1986).

Although many of these infections and tumors have unusual presentation, five years of experience with AIDS have sharpened clinical evaluations and diagnoses and have allowed more timely and effective treatments, particularly for toxoplasmosis and cryptococcal meningitis.

Aseptic Meningitis

Healthy seropositive persons and ARC patients sometimes experience a self-limited aseptic meningitis. Though of minor clinical importance, this illness may have major significance in relation to disease pathogenesis. On several occasions, it has been noted at the time of seroconversion, and the virus has been isolated from cerebrospinal fluid (Cooper et al., 1985; Ho et al., 1985). Symptoms include fever, headache, meningeal signs, and in some cases cranial nerve palsies. Cerebrospinal fluid shows a mononuclear cell pleocytosis and protein elevation. This may represent HIV's initial invasion of the central nervous system. The frequency of its subclinical occurrence in HIV-infected persons is not known.

Subacute Encephalitis

Dementias that are sufficient to be detected by objective psychological tests and that are associated with subacute encephalitis appear to occur in over 50 percent of patients with AIDS. In a New York study, after excluding patients with metabolic encephalopathies and opportunistic infections, 46 of 70 AIDS patients had clinical evidence of dementia. This correlated with the severity of the subacute encephalitis found at autopsy in over 80 percent of the cases (Navia et al., 1986).

In the majority of cases, the cerebrospinal fluid shows an elevation of protein and mild pleocytosis with a striking reversal of the CD4 to CD8 ratio. Computerized tomography shows cortical atrophy and enlarged ventricles. Magnetic resonance imaging, which has been limited, may show remarkable white matter abnormalities. Multiple abnormal signals from white matter have been seen even in ambulatory, minimally affected patients. A diffuse abnormal signal in white matter may be present in patients with full-blown dementia.

Despite the severity of clinical disease and the dramatic findings on imaging studies, histopathologic changes are remarkably subtle. There is a diffuse pallor of white matter, perivascular infiltrations of lymphocytes and macrophages, and, in more advanced cases, multinucleated cells. These pathologic changes have been noted to be most striking in the white matter, basal ganglia, and temporal areas (Navia et al., 1986).

The dementia in children born with HIV infection frequently shows a more striking clinical course and pathology. During early development, they fail to thrive, develop microcephaly, and suffer from seizures, blindness, and abnormal movements. Their brains show decreased volume with gross atrophy, many microglial nodules and multinucleated cells in the white matter, and vascular calcifications (Epstein et al., 1985b; Sharer et al., 1986).

Myelopathy

Vacuolar myelopathy is found in approximately 20 percent of patients with AIDS. Clinically, this correlates with the development of progressive paraparesis accompanied by ataxia, spasticity, and incontinence. Pathologic vacuolar degeneration of myelin is found in the dorsal and lateral columns without inflammation (Petito et al., 1985).

Peripheral Neuropathies

Involvement of the peripheral nervous system takes three forms in AIDS. Many patients develop a severe painful sensory neuropathy with electrophysiologic characteristics indicative of axonal degeneration. The pathology of this neuropathy is undefined but may involve dorsal root ganglia. A second painful, less common multifocal neuropathy appears to be related to a vasculitis with multifocal nerve infractions. This has been found in patients with both AIDS and ARC.

Third, a group of patients, none with AIDS but seropositive and often with various signs of ARC, have developed acute or subacute demyelinating neuropathies resembling Guillain-Barré syndrome. These patients have been found to recover spontaneously or may respond to plasmapheresis. This has been postulated to represent an autoimmune phenomenon during a time of immunologic deregulation occurring prior to the onset of clinically apparent immunosuppression as manifested in clinical AIDS. In addition to the demyelination normally seen in the Guillain-Barré syndrome, this disease shows a strikingly greater degree of inflammation and vacuolar changes in cells than is the case with usual demyelinating neuropathies (Cornblath et al., in press).

HIV Infection of the Nervous System

HIV has been isolated from the nervous systems of AIDS and ARC patients with neurologic syndromes with remarkable consistency. Levy et al. (1985) recovered virus from the spinal fluid of 13 of 14 AIDS or ARC patients, including one without neurologic symptoms. Ho et al. (1985) recovered virus from at least one spinal fluid or tissue specimen from 24 of 33 AIDS patients. These specimens included spinal fluid isolates from 6 of 7 patients with chronic meningitis, the brains of 6 patients with dementias, the spinal cord of one patient with myelopathy, the spinal fluid from one patient who had an acute meningitis at the time of seroconversion, and a peripheral nerve of one patient with demyelinating neuropathy.

Further evidence for the direct replication of HIV in the brain comes from the demonstration of intrathecal antibody synthesis in patients. Comparisons of antibody levels in serum and in cerebrospinal fluid indicate antigenic stimulation within the nervous system (Resnick et al., 1985).

Initial *in situ* hybridization studies have also demonstrated that cells within the microglial nodules contain the RNA from HIV. Viral DNA sequences have also been found in brains by Southern blot analysis, where they occurred in greater quantities than in the spleen, lymph nodes, liver, or lung (Shaw et al., 1985).

These findings establish that the virus is present in the nervous system and that its presence correlates to some degree with neurologic disease. They fail to identify, however, whether the virus is in neural cells or in cells of hematogenous origin within the brain (Johnson and McArthur, 1986).

Cellular Localization of HIV

Electron microscope studies have demonstrated apparent virus particles within multinucleated cells, probably of macrophagic origin. In one case, particles resembling virus were also seen within astrocytes, but the failure to find budding particles leaves open the possibilities that these were phagocytosed (Epstein et al., 1985a).

A variety of studies have now been done with immunocytochemical staining for viral antigen, followed by double staining to identify cells with cell markers or *in situ* hybridization. In summary, all have shown low numbers of infected cells and a predominance of viral antigens and viral nucleic acids in macrophages within perivascular inflammatory responses (Gabuzda et al., in press; Koenig et al., 1986; Pumarola-Sune et al., in press; Wiley et al., in press). Several of these studies note that the presence of the virus in perivascular cells is more prominent in the white matter. Most of these studies have also found some infected parenchymal cells.

The most interesting and disparate findings are those of Wiley et al. (in press), who used immunocytochemistry together with *in situ* hybridization to find involvement in 9 of 12 cases of capillary vascular endothelial cells of the brain. This finding could be of major importance in terms of the virus's mode of entry, the potential pathogenesis of the diffuse white matter lesions, and the development of future therapeutic strategies.

Studies by Pert (1986) have attempted to map CD4 cell receptors in the brain of humans, monkeys, and rats. She has found the antigen to be predominantly in the outer layers of the cortex and in the hippocampus. The presence of these receptors is interesting, but their location fails to correlate with that of the histopathologic distribution of the viral antigens.

Unsolved Problems

The timing and frequency of nervous system infection by HIV is not known. The isolations of HIV with aseptic meningitis at the time of seroconversion raise the grim possibility that the virus may invade the nervous system very early in many patients. This is reminiscent of syphilis, where pathogenic organisms may invade the nervous system early but remain latent until disease develops up to 30 years later.

How much time elapses between involvement of the central nervous system and the development of the subacute encephalitis with dementia also remains unknown. Clearly, this has broad implications for the use of therapeutic immunomodulators, which could improve hematologic parameters and clear systemic infections but have little effect on an ongoing or latent infection within the central nervous system. It also has major implications for the use of drug therapies. If vascular endothelial cells are the primary site of infection, the systemic administration of drugs may be effective; if rare neurons or glial cells are involved, it may not.

The pathogenesis of the CNS lesions is also mysterious. Imaging studies suggest widespread severe white matter disease, but the histologic findings are subtle and the number of cells with evidence of HIV infection is very small. This does not appear to be analogous either to acute infections such as poliomyelitis, where selective infection of specific cells (the motor neurons) leads to paralysis, or to chronic infections such as progressive multifocal leukoencephalopathy, where oligodendrocytes harbor vast amounts of replicated papovavirus and are lysed, causing demyelinating disease. Instead, complex and indirect pathogenic mechanisms may be involved. For instance, recent studies of visna virus (Kennedy et al., 1986; Narayan et al., 1985) suggest that small amounts of visna virus in rare macrophages can cause the induction of a novel interferon, which in turn induces the expression of an Ia antigen on neural cells. This then evokes an inflammatory and demyelinating disease, despite a paucity of virus.

PEDIATRIC AIDS

Clinical Features and Diagnosis

The clinical manifestations of AIDS in children are significantly different from those in adults. In one series they included failure to thrive (65 percent), recurrent bacterial infections (43 percent), persistent candidiasis (70 percent), generalized lymphadenopathy (74 percent), recurrent (31 percent) or protracted (33 percent) diarrhea, hepatosplenomegaly, lymphadenopathy, parotitis (14 percent), interstitial pneumonitis (59 percent), chronic otitis media (48 percent), and encephalopathy. Kaposi's sarcoma (19 percent) and B-cell lymphoma occur but are less frequent than in adults (Parks and Scott, 1986).

In a minority of infants the same types of infections are seen that have been described in adults. Almost a third (32 percent) of AIDS cases in children have *Pneumocystis carinii* pneumonia. *Candida* esophagitis occurs in 22 percent of cases, and disseminated cytomegalovirus infection is found in 24 percent. On the other hand, disseminated cytomegalovirus was a well-known perinatally acquired infection before the emergence of HIV and, therefore, is not very specific evidence of AIDS. Even though Kaposi's sarcoma is found in some pediatric cases, the lesions are located in lymph nodes as opposed to the skin in adults. The lesions are usually found only at autopsy and thus are not of diagnostic help in caring for the patient.

In general, pediatric AIDS is characterized by the occurrence of unusually severe infections in a child without the presence of predisposing factors, such as congenital immunodeficiency or antineoplastic chemotherapy. Recurrent infection is by far the most frequent AIDS-related syndrome in the pediatric age group. In addition to oral and esophageal candidiasis resistant to the usual therapies and recurrent viral infections (including herpetic stomatitis, varicella/herpes zoster, condyloma, and molluscum contagiosum), children frequently suffer from bacterial infections. In this regard, infections in children are different from those in adults, in whom bacterial infections are much less frequent. Bacterial infections seen include recurrent pneumonia, bacterial sepsis (especially with *Streptococcus pneumoniae* and *Haemophilus influenzae*), and chronic draining otitis media.

Infants who are born infected tend to be small for gestational age and are usually symptomatic by six months of age. Recently, a specific phenotypic appearance of young infants with AIDS has been described, which suggests early *in utero* spread (Marion et al., 1986). Infants who are transfused with contaminated blood during the first year of life may be clinically well from one to four years before developing clinical symptoms.

Diagnostic Criteria

The conditions that have been listed above are similar to many that are usual in the general pediatric practice. What is unusual is that these problems are extremely severe and persistent in patients with AIDS. Lymphadenopathy with associated failure to thrive appears to be the most common finding.

Once the clinician's suspicion of the possible diagnosis of AIDS has been aroused, the appropriate laboratory tests should be ordered. The laboratory results will differ depending on whether they are performed early (before there are definitive clinical findings) or late (after one or more of the clinical findings previously described has occurred).

The earliest finding is that of a positive test for HIV antibodies, usually made using the ELISA test. This result must be confirmed with the Western blot test. Where the antibody test is positive, there is a very good chance that the virus will be isolated. A common finding is a polyclonal hypergammaglobulinemia, which results from increased stimulation of B cells and/or decreased suppression by T lymphocytes. Usually this involves IgG, but sometimes also IgA and IgM. Some patients may have hypogammaglobulinemia.

In the later stages of the disease, the laboratory findings are consistent with a deterioration of T-lymphocyte function along with one or more of the clinical syndromes already described and HIV positivity. Children tend to have levels of lymphocytes higher than those seen in adults or older patients, presumably because children normally have much higher levels of lymphocytes than do adults. Special testing may reveal that CD4 cells have been depleted relative to CD8 cells, producing an inverted

T-lymphocyte subset ratio. This finding, in combination with polyclonal increase in IgG levels, is sufficient for laboratory confirmation of a tentative or presumptive diagnosis of AIDS in an infant.

In addition to HIV, a variety of other viruses are often present, including hepatitis B virus, cytomegalovirus, Epstein-Barr virus, and herpes simplex. When there is severe disease, there may be a negative HIV antibody test.

It is important to exclude other congenital immunodeficiency syndromes, such as the Nezelof syndrome or combined immune deficiency syndrome. The combination of selected clinical findings and laboratory results provides the physician with a presumptive diagnosis of AIDS in infants. But it has become clear that it is impractical to try to make the diagnostic criteria for AIDS in children fit those of adults. It seems that grouping the clinical findings into different syndromes may be the most effective way to recognize clinical AIDS when Kaposi's sarcoma and opportunistic infections do not occur. Because most clinicians still try to use the adult diagnostic criteria to diagnose AIDS in small children, this disorder is underreported in the pediatric age group. Additional work is needed to further clarify the natural history of AIDS in children.

REFERENCES

Bach, M. C., S. P. Bagwell, N. P. Knapp, K. M. Davis, and P. S. Hedstron. 1985. 9-(1,3-Dihydroxy-2-propoxymethyl)guanine for cytomegalovirus infections in patients with the acquired immunodeficiency syndrome. Ann. Intern. Med. 103:381-382.

Bigby, T. D., D. Margolskee, J. L. Curtis, P. F. Michael, D. Sheppard, W. K. Hadley, and P. C. Hopewell. 1986. The usefulness of induced sputum in the diagnosis of *Pneumocystis carinii* pneumonia in patients with the acquired immunodeficiency syndrome. Am. Rev. Respir. Dis. 133:515-518.

Broaddus, C., M. D. Dake, M. S. Stulbarg, W. Blumenfeld, K. Hadley, J. A. Golden, and P. C. Hopewell. 1985. Bronchoalveolar lavage and transbronchial biopsy for the diagnosis of pulmonary infections in the acquired immunodeficiency syndrome. Ann. Intern. Med. 102:747-752.

Catterall, J. R., I. Potasman, and J. S. Remington. 1985. *Pneumocystis carinii* pneumonia in the patient with AIDS. Chest 88:758-762.

Cohn, D. C., and F. N. Judson. 1984. Absence of Kaposi's sarcoma in hemophiliacs with AIDS. N. Engl. J. Med. 101:401.

Collier, A. C., R. A. Miller, and J. D. Meyers. 1984. Cryptosporidiosis after marrow transplantation: Person-to-person transmission and treatment with spiramycin. Ann. Intern. Med. 101:205-206.

Cooper, D. A., J. Gold, P. Maclean, B. Donovan, R. Finlayson, T. G. Barnes, H. M. Michelmore, P. Brooke, and R. Penny. 1985. Acute AIDS retrovirus infection: Definition of a clinical illness associated with seroconversion. Lancet I:537-540.

Cornblath, D. R., J. C. McArthur, and J. W. Griffin. In press. Inflammatory demyelinating peripheral neuropathies associated with AIDS retrovirus infection. Ann. Neurol.

Des Jarlais, D. C., M. Marmor, P. Thomas, M. Chamberland, S. Zolla-Pazner, and D. J.

Sencer. 1984. Kaposi's sarcoma among four different AIDS risk groups. N. Engl. J. Med. 310:1119.

Drew, W. L., R. C. Miner, J. C. Ziegler, J. H. Gullett, D. I. Abrams, M. A. Conant, E.-S. Huang, J. R. Groundwater, P. Volberding, and L. Mintz. 1982. Cytomegalovirus and Kaposi's sarcoma in young homosexual men. Lancet II:125-127.

Epstein, E. 1983. Acyclovir for immunocompromised patients with herpes zoster. N. Engl. J. Med. 309:1254.

Epstein, L. G., L. R. Sharer, E.-S. Cho, M. Myerhofer, B. A. Navia, and R. W. Price. 1985a. HTLV-III/LAV-like retrovirus particles in the brains of patients with AIDS encephalopathy. AIDS Res. 1:447-454.

Epstein, L. G., L. R. Sharer, V. V. Joshi, M. M. Fojas, M. R. Koenigsberger, and J. M. Oleske. 1985b. Progressive encephalopathy in children with acquired immunodeficiency syndrome. Ann. Neurol. 17:488-496.

Felsenstein, D., D. J. D'Amico, M. S. Hirsch, D. M. Cederberg, P. de Miranda, and R. T. Schooley. 1985. Treatment of cytomegalovirus retinitis with 9-[2-hydroxy-1-(hydroxy-methyl)ethoxymethyl]guanine. Ann. Intern. Med. 103:377-380.

Gabuzda, D. H., D. D. Ho, S. M. de al Monte, M. S. Hirsch, T. R. Rota, and R. A. Sobel. In press. Immunohistochemical identification of HTLV-III antigen in brains of patients with AIDS. Ann. Neurol.

Glaser, J. B., L. Morton-Kute, S. R. Berger, J. Weber, F. P. Siegel, C. Lopez, W. Robbins, and S. H. Landesman. 1985. Recurrent Salmonella typhimurium bacteremia associated with the acquired immunodeficiency syndrome. Ann. Intern. Med. 102:189-193.

Gordin, F. M., G. L. Simon, C. B. Wofsy, and J. Mills. 1984. Adverse reactions to trimethoprim-sulfamethoxazole in patients with AIDS. Ann. Intern. Med. 100:495-499.

Haverkos, H. W. 1984. Assessment of therapy for Pneumocystis carinii pneumonia. Am. J. Med. 76:501-508.

Ho, D. D., T. R. Rota, R. T. Schooley, J. C. Kaplan, J. D. Allan, J. E. Groopman, L. Resnick, D. Felsenstein, C. A. Andrews, and M. C. Hirsch. 1985. Isolation of HTLV-III from cerebrospinal fluid and neural tissues of patients with neurologic syndromes related to the acquired immunodeficiency syndrome. N. Engl. J. Med. 313:1493-1497.

Hughes, W. T., and B. C. Smith. 1984. Efficacy of diaminodiphenylsulfone and other drugs in murine Pneumocystis carinii pneumonia. Antimicrob. Agents Chemother. 26:436.

Hughes, W. T., S. Feldman, S. C. Chaudhary, M. J. Ossi, F. Cox, and S. K. Sanyal. 1978. Comparison of pentamidine isothionate and trimethoprim-sulfamethoxazole in the treatment of Pneumocystis carinii pneumonia. J. Pediatr. 92:285-291.

Ioachim, H. C., M. C. Cooper, and G. C. Hellman. 1985. Lymphomas in men at high risk for acquired immune deficiency syndrome (AIDS). A study of 21 cases. Cancer 56:2831-2842.

Jacobs, J. L., M. W. M. Gold, H. W. Murray, R. B. Roberts, and D. Armstrong. 1985. Salmonella infections in patients with the acquired immunodeficiency syndrome. Ann. Intern. Med. 102:186-188.

Johnson, R. T., and J. C. McArthur. 1986. AIDS and the brain. Trends Neurosci. 9:91-94.

Kaplan, L. D., R. Wong, C. Wofsy, and P. A. Volberding. 1986. Trimethoprim-sulfamethoxazole (TMP-SMZ) prophylaxis of Pneumocystis carinii pneumonia (PCP) in AIDS. P. 53 in Abstracts of the Second International Conference on AIDS, Paris, June 23-25, 1986.

Kennedy, P. G. E., O. Narayan, Z. Ghotbi, J. Hopkins, H. E. Gendelman, and J. E. Clements. 1986. Persistent expression of Ia antigen and viral genome in visna-maedi virus-induced inflammatory cells. J. Exp. Med. 162:1970-1982.

Klein, R. S., C. A. Harris, C. B. Small, B. Moll, M. Lesser, and G. H. Friedland. 1984. Oral candidiasis in high risk patients as the initial manifestation of the acquired immunodeficiency syndrome. N. Engl. J. Med. 311:354-358.

Koenig, S., H. E. Gendelman, M. C. DelCanto, M. Yungbluth, G. H. Pezeskpour, T. Folks, M. Martin, H. C. Lance, and A. S. Fauci. 1986. Detection of AIDS retroviral RNA in nonlymphoid cells in the brain of an AIDS patient with encephalopathy. Clin. Res. 34:722A.

Kovacs, J. A., J. W. Hiemenz, A. M. Macher, D. Stover, H. W. Murray, J. Shelhamer, H. C. Lane, C. Urmacher, C. Honig, D. L. Longo, M. M. Parker, C. Natanson, J. E. Parrillo, A. S. Fauci, P. A. Pizzo, and H. Masur. 1984. *Pneumocystis carinii* pneumonia: A comparison between patients with acquired immunodeficiency syndrome and patients with other immunodeficiencies. Ann. Intern. Med. 100:663-671.

Levy, J. A., J. Shimabukuro, H. Hollander, J. Mills, and L. Kaminsky. 1985. Isolation of AIDS-associated retrovirus from cerebrospinal fluid and brains of patients with neurological symptoms. Lancet II:586-588.

Louie, E., L. B. Rice, and R. S. Holzman. 1985. *Mycobacterium tuberculosis* (Mtb) infection in patients with AIDS. P. 38 in Abstracts of the International Conference on AIDS, Atlanta, Ga., April 14-17, 1985.

Luft, B. J., R. G. Brooks, F. K. Conley, R. E. McCabe, and J. S. Remington. 1984. Toxoplasmic encephalitis in patients with acquired immune deficiency syndrome. JAMA 252:913-917.

Marion, R. W., A. A, Wiznia, G. Hutcheon, and A. Rubenstein. 1986. Human T-cell lymphotropic virus type III (HTLV-III/LAV) embryopathy. A new dysmorphic syndrome associated with intrauterine HTLV-III infection. Am. J. Dis. Child. 140:638-640.

Marmor, M., A. E. Friedman-Kien, L. Laubenstein, R. D. Byrum, D. C. William, S. D'Onofrio, and N. Dubin. 1982. Risk factors for Kaposi's sarcoma in homosexual men. Lancet I:1083-1087.

Masur, M., H. C. Lane, and A. Palestine. 1986. Effect of 9-(1,3-dihydroxy-2-propoxy-methyl) guanine on serious cytomegalovirus disease in eight immunosuppressed homosexual men. Ann. Intern. Med. 104:41-44.

Mintzer, D. M., F. X. Real, L. Jovino, and S. E. Krown. 1985. Treatment of Kaposi's sarcoma and thrombocytopenia with vincristine in patients with the acquired immunodeficiency syndrome. Ann. Intern. Med. 102:200-202.

Mitsuyasu, R. T., and J. E. Groopman. 1984. Biology and therapy of Kaposi's sarcoma. Semin. Oncol. 11:53-59.

Narayan, O., D. Sheffer, J. E. Clements, and G. Tennekoon. 1985. Restricted replication of lentiviruses: Visna viruses induce a unique interferon during interaction between lymphocytes and infected macrophages. J. Exp. Med. 162:1954-1969.

Nash, G., and S. Fligiel. 1984. Pathologic features of the lung in the acquired immune deficiency syndrome (AIDS): An autopsy study of seventeen homosexual males. Am. J. Clin. Pathol. 81:6-12.

Navia, B. A., E.-S. Cho, C. K. Petito, and R. W. Price. 1986. The AIDS dementia complex: II. Neuropathology. Ann. Neurol. 19:525-535.

Ognibene, F. P., J. Shelhamer, V. Gill, A. M. Macher, D. Loew, M. M. Parker, E. Gelmann, A. S. Fauci, J. E. Parrillo, and H. Masur. 1984. The diagnosis of *Pneumocystis carinii* pneumonia in patients with the acquired immunodeficiency syndrome using subsegmental bronchoalveolar lavage. Am. Rev. Respir. Dis. 129:929-932.

Parks, W. P., and G. B. Scott. 1986. An Overview of Pediatric AIDS: Approaches to Diagnosis and Outcome Assessment. Background paper. Washington, D.C.: Committee on a National Strategy for AIDS.

Pert, C. B. 1986. HTLV-III virus visualization of the OKT4 antigen in brain. Paper presented at the National Institute of Mental Health AIDS Conference. Bethesda, Md.

Petito, C. A., B. A. Navia, E.-S. Cho, B. D. Jordan, D. C. George, and R. W. Price. 1985. Vacuolar myelopathy pathologically resembling subacute combined degeneration in patients with the acquired immunodeficiency syndrome. N. Engl. J. Med. 312:874-879.

Pitchenik, A. E., C. Cole, B. W. Russel, M. A. Fischl, T. J. Spira, and D. E. Snider, Jr. 1984. Tuberculosis, atypical mycobacteriosis and the acquired immunodeficiency syndrome among Haitian and non-Haitian patients in south Florida. Ann. Intern. Med. 101: 641-645.

Pumarola-Sune, T., B. A. Navia, C. Cordon-Cardo, E.-S. Cho, and R. W. Price. In press. LAV/HTLV-III antigen in the brains of patients with the AIDS dementia complex.

Quinn, T. C. 1986. Clinical approach to intestinal infections in homosexual men. Med. Clin. North Am. 70:611-634.

Rein, M. F. 1986. Clinical approach to urethritis, mucocutaneous lesions, and inguinal lymphadenopathy in homosexual men in AIDS and other medical problems in the male homosexual. Med. Clin. North Am. 70:587-609.

Resnick, L., F. diMarzo-Veronese, J. Schupbach, W. W. Tourtellotte, D. D. Ho, F. Muller, P. Shapshak, M. Vogt, J. E. Groopman, P. D. Markham, and R. C. Gallo. 1985. Intra-blood-brain-barrier synthesis of HTLV-III specific IgG in patients with neurologic symptoms associated with AIDS or AIDS-related complex. N. Engl. J. Med. 313:1498-1504.

Rolston, K., V. Fainstein, P. Mansell, A. Sjoerdsma, and G. P. Bodey. 1985. Alpha-difluoromethylornithine (DFMO) in the treatment of cryptosporidiosis in AIDS patients: Preliminary evaluation. P. 77 in Abstracts of the International Conference on AIDS, Atlanta, Ga., April 14-17, 1985.

Schoeppel, S. C., R. T. Hoppe, R. F. Dorfman, S. J. Horning, A. C. Collier, T. G. Chew, and L. M. Weiss. 1985. Hodgkin's disease in homosexual men with generalized lymphadenopathy. Ann. Intern. Med. 102:68-70.

Sharer, L. R., L. G. Epstein, E.-S. Cho, V. V. Joshi, M. F. Myenhofer, L. F. Rankin, and C. K. Petito. 1986. Pathology of AIDS encephalopathy in children: Evidence for LAV/HTLV-III infection in brain. Human Pathol. 17:271-284.

Shaw, G. M., M. E. Harper, B. H. Hahn, L. G. Epstein, D. C. Gajdusek, R. W. Price, B. A. Navia, C. K. Petito, C. J. O'Hara, E.-S. Cho, J. M. Oleske, F. Wong-Staal, and R. C. Gallo. 1985. HTLV-III infection in brains of children and adults with AIDS encephalopathy. Science 227:177-182.

Smith, P. D., A. M. Macher, M. A. Bookman, R. V. Boccia, R. G. Steis, V. Gill, J. Manischewitz, and E. P. Gelmann. 1985. *Salmonella typhimurium* enteritis and bacteremia in the acquired immunodeficiency syndrome. Ann. Intern. Med. 102:207-209.

Snider, W. D., D. M. Simpson, G. Nielson, J. W. M. Gold, C. Metroka, and J. B. Posner. 1983. Neurologic complications of acquired immunodeficiency syndrome: Analysis of 50 patients. Ann. Neurol. 14:403-418.

Soave, R., R. L. Danner, C. L. Honig, P. Ma, C. C. Hart, T. Nash, and R. B. Roberts. 1984. Cryptosporidiosis in homosexual men. Ann. Intern. Med. 100:504-511.

Soave, R., A. Sjoerdsma, and M. J. Cawein. 1985. Treatment of cryptosporidiosis in AIDS patients with alpha-difluoromethylornithine. P. 77 in Abstracts of the International Conference on AIDS, Atlanta, Ga., April 14-17, 1985.

Volberding, P. A., R. Valero, J. Rothman, and G. Gee. 1984. Alpha interferon therapy of Kaposi's sarcoma in AIDS. Ann. N.Y. Acad. Sci. 437:439-446.

Westerman, E. L., and R. P. Christensen. 1979. Chronic *Isospora belli* infection treated with co-trimoxazole. Ann. Intern. Med. 91:413-414.

Whiteside, M. E., J. S. Barkin, R. G. May, S. D. Weiss, M. A. Fischl, and C. L. MacLeod. 1984. Enteric coccidiosis among patients with the acquired immunodeficiency syndrome. Am. J. Trop. Med. Hyg. 33:1065-1072.

Wiley, C. A., R. D. Schrier, J. A. Nelson, P. W. Lampert, and M. A. B. Oldstone. In press. Cellular localization of human immunodeficiency virus infection within the brains of acquired immunodeficiency syndrome (AIDS) patients. Proc. Natl. Acad. Sci. USA.

Wong, B., J. W. Gold, A. E. Brown, M. Lang, R. Fried, M. Grieco, D. Mildvan, J. Giron, M. L. Topper, C. W. Lerner, et al. 1984. Central nervous system toxoplasmosis in homosexual men and parenteral drug abusers. Ann. Intern. Med. 100:36-42.

Zakowski, P., S. Fligiel, G. W. Berlin, and L. Johnson, Jr. 1982. Disseminated *Mycobacterium avium-intracellulare* infection in homosexual men dying of acquired immunodeficiency syndrome. JAMA 248:2980-2982.

Ziegler, J. L., J. A. Beckstead, P. A. Volberding, D. I. Abrams, A. M. Levine, R. J. Lukes, P. S. Gill, R. L. Burkes, P. R. Meyer, C. E. Metroka, J. Mouradian, A. Moore, S. A. Riggs, J. J. Butler, F. C. Cabanillas, E. Hersh, G. R. Newell, L. J. Laubenstein, D. Knowles, C. Odajnyk, B. Raphael, B. Koziner, C. Urmacher, and B. D. Clarkson. 1984. Non-Hodgkin's lymphoma in 90 homosexual men. Relation to generalized lymphadenopathy and the acquired immunodeficiency syndrome. N. Engl. J. Med. 311:565-570.

Zuger, A., E. Louie, R. S. Holtzman, M. S. Simberkoff, and J. J. Rahal. 1986. Cryptococcal disease in patients with acquired immunodeficiency syndrome. Ann. Intern. Med. 104: 234-240.

B

Serologic and Virologic Testing

The standard tests used to define individuals who have been exposed to HIV detect antibodies to the virus in the serum. Antibodies to HIV can be detected by several techniques, including enzyme-linked immunosorbent assays (ELISA), immunofluorescent assays (IFA), and Western blot analysis. Each of these techniques, when performed by expert technicians, is very accurate at detecting antibody either to the whole virus or to viral subcomponents.

In contrast to some viral infections, HIV induces antibodies that do not, in most cases, appear to effectively neutralize the establishment or consequences of viral spread in an infected host. Therefore, most patients with positive tests for HIV antibodies are considered to be simultaneously and actively infected by HIV. The resulting concerns about the equation of seropositivity with extant infection, continuing transmissibility, risk of disease in an infected individual, and issues of social stigmatization have caused HIV serologic testing to be very controversial.

The tests currently in use attempt to measure specific antibodies to proteins or polyproteins produced as a result of infection with HIV. The virus's *gag* and *env* genes encode for the predominant viral antigen to which antibodies detected by today's tests are directed. The *gag* gene, which encodes the protein constituents of the viral core, initially produces a 55-kilodalton (kd) polyprotein that is present in large amount in virus-infected cells. This nonglycosylated protein is subsequently cleaved to form p17 (a phosphoprotein), p24, and gag peptides. Although p24 and p17 are detectable in both extracellular virus and disrupted virus-infected

304

cells, the 55-kd precursor protein is not present in significant amounts in virus harvests used to prepare antigen. Antibodies to HIV core protein p24 and its group antigen precursor are thought to appear earliest following infection and are readily detected in a number of ELISA tests.

The *env* gene encodes for a polyprotein of about 90 kd in its nonglycosylated form. Since it has numerous glycosylation sites, it migrates as a glycoprotein of about 160 kd in electrophoretic analyses and is found as such in infected cells. This glycoprotein gives rise to two principal proteins, gp120 and gp41. Both are present in infectious virus particles and infected cells. Antibodies to these proteins are thought to appear somewhat later than core antibodies and are present in most sera from HIV-infected individuals.

Additional immunoreactive viral gene products include those nonstructural proteins encoded by *sor*, a short open reading frame of unspecified function; *tat*, which is responsible for certain critical aspects of viral expression; and 3'-*orf*, another open reading frame that encodes for a 27-kd protein of unknown function. The proteins encoded by the *pol* gene of HIV, which catalyze essential enzymatic processes in viral replication, are strongly immunogenic and recognized by sera from the vast majority of infected persons. The distribution of antibodies against the proteins encoded for by these genes is becoming better understood as newer and potentially improved tests are being developed using recombinant DNA technologies to produce specific viral proteins. While all are potential substrates for improved serologic tests, so far no patterns of serologic reactivity have been found to correlate with disease stage or prognosis.

The configuration of the ELISA test most frequently employed in serologic analyses involves coating plastic microtiter wells or plastic beads with HIV antigen and adding test serum in various dilutions. An antigen-antibody reaction is detected by the use of so-called second-stage antibodies, which react with any human antibodies remaining bound to the viral antigens in the ELISA plate. The second-stage antibodies are modified to facilitate their detection by conjugation with enzymes such as horseradish peroxidase or alkaline phosphatase. If antibodies in the serum tested are bound to viral antigens, then the antihuman antibody will bind to the antiviral antibodies, if present, and the attached enzyme will be free to catalyze a chemical reaction after the addition of the appropriate substrate. The extent of the reaction is detected colorimetrically. A control serum is used. "Positives" are distinguished from "negatives" on the basis of the relative degree of absorbance of the test serum and control. Where the cutoff point is set affects the sensitivity and specificity of the serologic test.

While the ELISA test can identify the presumptive presence of antibodies against HIV in a serum sample, another test, the Western blot analysis, permits the documentation of antibodies to specific viral proteins and thus a more specific level of resolution of serologic reactivity. The Western blot analysis is basically an immunoelectrophoretic test in which viral proteins from purified disrupted virus are fractionated by size using polyacrylamide gel electrophoresis. The fractionated viral proteins are then transferred to nitrocellulose paper to permit subsequent immunologic detection. Control molecular-weight standards are included to identify migration of proteins of various sizes. Samples being tested for antibody are added to the strip, followed by appropriate stages of inoculation and washing. Enzyme-linked antihuman IgG globulin is added and incubated. Then an appropriate substrate is added and the enzyme catalyzes the colorimetric reaction, which detects bound antibody. Again, the extent of the reaction is measured by the intensity of the color produced.

There has been considerable variation in what different laboratories have interpreted as positive in Western blots. In the past the presence of antibody to the gag p24 alone was considered positive by the Centers for Disease Control (CDC) criteria. With accumulating experience of HIV Western blot determination, it became apparent that many patients who have only this antibody appear to represent false positives. Recently, a consensus has developed that serum specimens are considered specifically reactive with HIV if antibody to the following proteins is demonstrated in the presence or absence of other bands: (1) p24 and p41, (2) p24 and p55, (3) p41. If only p24 antibody is demonstrated, the reaction is considered equivocal and must be repeated on the same serum sample.

Other tests for antibody detection include the radioimmunoprecipitation and cytoplasmic or membrane immunofluorescence tests. Both tests work well but are less well suited for screening purposes and appear to be more appropriate for use in research laboratories. In good hands, immunofluorescent testing is as accurate as ELISA testing, but it is much harder to standardize and therefore is not used as often.

In the first generation of the ELISA tests made available, the intact virus was used to detect antibodies. In more recent versions, recombinant antigens are employed. Even with the first generation of test kits, accuracy has been very high. Sensitivity and specificity (see below) are in the 95 to 99 percent range.

PERFORMANCE CHARACTERISTICS OF THE TESTS

In evaluating the utility of a test, the terms "sensitivity," "specificity," "prevalence," "predictive value," "gold standard," and "cutoff point" are often used. The sensitivity of a test is the percentage of infected persons who will have a positive test. This often varies depending upon the stage or severity of the disease. With HIV infection, seropositivity appears to rise slowly after initial infection and then to remain relatively stable.

Estimates of the true sensitivity of the HIV test are hampered by the lack of a "gold standard"—an independent verification of the presence of infection. For example, if one could isolate virus in all cases, one would be able to determine the exact sensitivity of a serologic test. In the case of HIV, however, the virus isolation techniques are far from 100 percent sensitive. Many investigators calculate sensitivity using small numbers of samples that are not generally representative. Also, the use of sera from AIDS patients to determine the sensitivity of a test may be very misleading if the test is applied to low-risk populations to detect early infections. Given the better appreciation of reactivity with certain particularly immunogenic viral proteins, it has become increasingly important to determine the protein content of the different antigens used for the test and to relate this to what is being learned about changes in the antibody profile to various proteins over time.

Specificity is the percentage of uninfected persons who have a negative test. One would like to have 100 percent specificity, especially for an infection with the implications of HIV infection. The way the antigen is prepared may affect specificity, in that one may be measuring antibodies present in the test sera reacting with cellular products that contaminate viral preparations. This may be particularly troublesome in patients who use drugs or have chronic illnesses. Again, failure to use a large number of broadly representative sera may give falsely high estimates of specificity. For example, measurements of specificity in well populations may underestimate the problems encountered when the test is later used in alternate populations.

The cutoff point is the point above which one calls a test positive and below which one calls it negative. No test is 100 percent sensitive and 100 percent specific, so one is usually trading off either sensitivity or specificity. One sets the cutoff point to maximize one or the other, depending on whether it is important to detect all those who are infected and then sort out true positives from false positives or whether one is willing to miss a certain number of true positives in order to minimize the risk of false positives.

Chapter 4 describes general aspects of the uses of these tests, their applications in improving the safety of the blood supply, their emerging use as an indicator of infection in individuals, and the problems associated with these uses. Chapter 6 contains recommendations regarding desirable future efforts in this area.

BIBLIOGRAPHY

American Medical Association Council on Scientific Affairs. 1985. Status report on the acquired immunodeficiency syndrome: Human T-cell lymphotropic virus type III testing. JAMA 254:1342-1345.

National Institutes of Health. 1985. Workshop on experience with HTLV-III antibody testing: Update on screening, laboratory and epidemiologic conditions. Bethesda, Md., July 31.

National Institutes of Health. 1986. Program and abstracts: Impact of routine HTLV-III antibody testing on public health. Bethesda, Md., July 7-9.

Silberner, J. 1986. AIDS blood screens: Chapters 2 and 3. Science News 130:56-57.

C

Risk of HIV Transmission from Blood Transfusion

The risk (R) of receiving a blood transfusion containing HIV depends on a number of factors, including the prevalence (P) of HIV viremia in the donor population, the likelihood (L) of donation during the preantibody phase of viremia, the sensitivity (S) of the ELISA screening test to detect HIV antibody when antibody is in fact present, and the number (n) of units of blood (or blood products) received.

The risk (D) that a donated unit of blood contains HIV can be expressed as:

$$D = PL + P(1 - L)(1 - S). \tag{1}$$

The first part of the expression to the right of the equals sign, PL, represents the portion of risk due to blood donation during the preantibody phase of infection. The remainder of the equation, $P(1 - L)$ $(1 - S)$, represents the portion of risk due to donors with antibody whose blood escapes detection by the screening test.

The pertinent concern from the vantage point of a blood recipient is the following: Given the number of units transfused, what is the risk (R) that one or more units contain HIV? This is approached by first asking the computationally simpler, related question: What is the likelihood that *none* of the transfused units contains HIV?

If n units are transfused, the likelihood (C) that none contains virus can be expressed as:

$$C = (1 - D)^n. \tag{2}$$

TABLE C-1 Definitions of Variables Entering Estimates of Risk of HIV Transmission from Blood Transfusion

Symbol	Definition
P	Probability of HIV viremia in a donor
t_1	Mean time between development of HIV viremia and antibody formation
t_2	Mean time between development of HIV viremia and development of clinical indications of disease (i.e., duration of possible unknowing transmission)
£	Relative likelihood of blood donation soon after HIV exposure compared with later donation
L	Likelihood of donation during the preantibody phase of viremia
D	Risk that a donated unit of blood contains HIV
C	Likelihood that no unit of blood contains HIV
n	Number of units of blood transfused into a blood recipient
R	Risk of exposure to HIV from n units of transfused blood

Then the risk, R, of exposure to HIV in an individual receiving transfused blood is:

$$R = 1 - C. \qquad (3)$$

Each of the elements entering Equation 1 is uncertain, though some data are available to provide a basis for estimates. Tables C-1 and C-2 summarize the definitions, baseline assumptions, and optimistic and pessimistic ranges in assumptions for each variable.

Following are comments on the variables entering the equations:

P: The nationwide experience with blood donor screening suggests that the frequency of HIV in the United States donor population may be between 1 and 10 per 10,000 (Schorr et al., 1985). Lower figures may

TABLE C-2 Assumptions in the Estimation of Risk of HIV Transmission from Blood Transfusion

Symbol	Assumptions and Calculations				
	Baseline	Optimistic	Very Optimistic	Pessimistic	Very Pessimistic
P	0.0004	0.0002	0.0001	0.001	0.001
t_1 (weeks)	4	4	4	4	4
t_2 (weeks)	260	410	520	260	130
£	1.0	0.75	0.50	1.0	1.0
S	0.99	0.995	0.995	0.985	0.98

prevail in low-prevalence areas and also may be realized through increased efforts to discourage donors who have engaged in high-risk behaviors and by eliminating those who previously tested positive for HIV antibodies. In areas with a higher prevalence of HIV infection, the frequency of HIV among donors can be expected to be higher. Also, as more heterosexuals become infected (e.g., the female partners of men who are bisexual or intravenous drug users), the frequency of HIV infection may increase among donors who have no known history of risk behaviors.

L: The likelihood of donation by an infected person during the preantibody phase depends on the average duration of time (t_1) in which the patient may be viremic prior to formation of detectable antibody, the average length of time (t_2) during which a blood donor may be unknowingly infectious (i.e., the interval between viremia and development of clinical indications of disease), and the relative likelihood (£) of donating blood soon after exposure. Specifically:

$$L = £t_1/t_2. \tag{4}$$

Evidence from a small number of patients suggests that the mean interval between exposure and antibody formation is approximately eight weeks (*Lancet,* 1984; Tucker et al., 1985). Though hard data are lacking, it is reasonable to assume that viremia is extremely unlikely during the first third of this interval, moderately likely during the second third, and almost surely present during the final third. The net result would be an effective average period of viremia prior to antibody formation of approximately four weeks (t_1). The duration of time that a donor may unknowingly be an HIV carrier is speculative. The baseline estimate for this mean interval time (t_2) between development of viremia and development of clinical disease is 5 years (Jaffe et al., 1985), with a range from 2.5 to 10 years. The likelihood of donating blood soon after exposure may be lower than the likelihood of donating later because, for example, an isolated homosexual encounter may be forgotten or discounted in memory over time. A countervailing tendency may be for some to donate soon after an exposure to reassure themselves about their freedom from disease. The baseline relative likelihood (£) of early versus later donation is 1.0 (equal likelihood). The optimistic range extends down to 0.5; the calculations based on pessimistic assumptions retain the baseline value of 1.0 for the relative likelihood (£).

S: Practically no diagnostic test is perfect. The sensitivity of the ELISA screening test refers to its ability to detect antibody when antibody is present. (The test's specificity, or its ability to exclude antibody when none is present, is another measure of performance, though one not relevant to this analysis.) Measurements of test sensitivity require an

TABLE C-3   Risk of Exposure to HIV from Blood Transfusion
(expressed as 1 per nearest thousandth)

Number of Units Transfused	Baseline	Optimistic	Very Optimistic	Pessimistic	Very Pessimistic
1	1/99,000	1/407,000	1/1,133,000	1/33,000	1/20,000
2	1/50,000	1/204,000	1/566,000	1/17,000	1/10,000
2.9[a]	1/34,000	1/140,000	1/391,000	1/11,000	1/7,000
3	1/33,000	1/136,000	1/378,000	1/11,000	1/7,000
4	1/25,000	1/102,000	1/283,000	1/8,000	1/5,000
5	1/20,000	1/81,000	1/227,000	1/7,000	1/4,000
6	1/17,000	1/68,000	1/189,000	1/6,000	1/3,000
7	1/14,000	1/58,000	1/162,000	1/5,000	1/3,000
8	1/12,000	1/51,000	1/142,000	1/4,000	1/2,000
9	1/11,000	1/45,000	1/126,000	1/4,000	1/2,000
10	1/10,000	1/41,000	1/113,000	1/3,000	1/2,000
15	1/7,000	1/27,000	1/76,000	1/2,000	<1/1,000
20	1/5,000	1/20,000	1/57,000	1/2,000	<1/1,000
30	1/3,000	1/14,000	1/38,000	<1/1,000	<1/1,000

[a]The approximate average number of units transfused, based on the total number of units of blood used annually in the United States (10 million) divided by the average number of patients receiving blood in a year (3.5 million).

independent truth standard that could demonstrate unequivocally the presence of antibody. No such absolute standard exists; hence, estimates of sensitivity cannot be regarded as firmly established. Various manufacturers have provided estimates of ELISA test sensitivities ranging from 0.95 to 0.996 (Reesink et al., 1986; Weiss et al., 1986). The baseline sensitivity for this analysis is 0.99, with a range from 0.98 to 0.995.

n: The number of units of blood received in transfusion depends, of course, on individual clinical circumstances. The average number of units received by a patient may be approximated by dividing the total number of units of blood used annually in the United States (10 million) by the number of patients receiving blood during a year (3.5 million). This figure of approximately 2.9 units per patient is probably a slight underestimation because a single patient receiving blood on separate hospital admissions would be counted as two separate patients in the year's tabulations.

Table C-3 summarizes the results of the risk of exposure to HIV for recipients of varying numbers of units of transfused blood. The results are shown using baseline assumptions and using the range of optimistic and pessimistic assumptions taken from Table C-2.

The risk to a hypothetical blood recipient from an average number of units transfused is, under baseline assumptions, approximately 1 in 34,000.

Progressively more optimistic assumptions yield estimates of approximately 1 in 140,000 and 1 in 391,000. Progressively more pessimistic assumptions produce estimates of approximately 1 in 11,000 and 1 in 7,000.

The risk rises as the number of units transfused increases. For example, under baseline assumptions the risk from a single unit of blood is approximately 1 in 99,000; from 5 units the risk is 1 in 20,000; and from 10 units the risk is 1 in 10,000. The recipient of 4 units under optimistic assumptions has about the same risk (1 in 102,000) as does the recipient of 1 unit under baseline assumptions (1 in 99,000). The recipient of 1 unit under pessimistic assumptions has about the same risk (1 in 33,000) as does the recipient of 3 units under baseline assumptions (1 in 33,000).

The introduction of antibody testing has reduced the risk of HIV transmission to blood recipients by a substantial margin. In other words, instead of nearly 4,000 recipients of viremic units, the baseline calculations project the transfusion of only about 100 (3,500,000/34,000) HIV-infected units each year. Most of the current risk from HIV in blood transfusion relates to the possibility of blood donation during the preantibody phase of HIV infection. This emphasizes the importance of self-selection by potential donors to eliminate those who have engaged in high-risk behaviors.

The wide range in the estimated risk under different sets of assumptions highlights the uncertainty in these projections. As experience and additional data become available, more accurate estimates of risk may be possible.

REFERENCES

Jaffe, H. W., W. W. Darrow, D. F. Echenberg, P. M. O'Malley, J. P. Getchell, V. S. Kalyanaraman, R. H. Byers, D. P. Drennan, E. H. Braff, J. W. Curran, and D. P. Francis. 1985. The acquired immunodeficiency syndrome in a cohort of homosexual men. A six-year follow-up study. Ann. Intern. Med. 103:210-214.

Lancet. 1984. Needlestick transmission of HTLV-III from a patient infected in Africa. Lancet II:1376-1377.

Reesink, H. W., J. G. Huisman, M. Gonsalves, et al. 1986. Evaluation of six enzyme immunoassays for antibody against human immunodeficiency virus. Lancet II:483-486.

Schorr, J. B., A. Berkowitz, P. D. Cumming, A. Katz, and S. G. Sandler. 1985. Prevalence of HTLV-III antibody in American blood donors. N. Engl. J. Med. 313:384-385.

Tucker, J., C. A. Ludham, A. Craig, et al. 1985. HTLV-III infection associated with glandular fever like illness in a hemophiliac. Lancet II:585.

Weiss, S. H., J. J. Goedert, M. G. Sarngadharan, et al. 1985. Screening test for HTLV-III (AIDS-agent) antibodies: Specificity, sensitivity, and applications. JAMA 253:221-225.

D

U.S. Public and Private Sector Resources for Fighting AIDS

Following is a list of public and private sector resources in the United States that could be brought to bear on problems related to AIDS and HIV infection. (The list is simply alphabetical; no hierarchical arrangement is intended.)

PUBLIC SECTOR

Federal

NATIONAL SCIENCE FOUNDATION

U.S. DEPARTMENT OF DEFENSE
    U.S. Army Medical Research and Development Command
      Walter Reed Army Institute of Research
        U.S. Army Medical Research Institute for Infectious Diseases

U.S. DEPARTMENT OF EDUCATION

U.S. DEPARTMENT OF HEALTH AND HUMAN SERVICES
    Health Care Financing Administration
    Public Health Service/Office of the Assistant Secretary for Health
      Alcohol, Drug Abuse, and Mental Health Administration
      Centers for Disease Control
      Food and Drug Administration
      Health Resources and Services Administration

314

National Center for Health Services Research and Health Care
Technology Assessment
National Institutes of Health
National Cancer Institute
National Heart, Lung, and Blood Institute
National Institute of Allergy and Infectious Diseases

U.S. DEPARTMENT OF STATE
Agency for International Development

State, City, and Local Authorities

Public health agencies (including research laboratories and education
boards)
State legislatures (through policymaking and funding of research and
prevention efforts)

PRIVATE SECTOR

Commercial Entities

Mass media
Electronic (e.g., radio, television)
Print (e.g., newspapers, magazines, advertising)
Pharmaceutical companies, both major and new biotechnology-based
(research and development on drugs and vaccines)
Various commercial concerns (through employee education or volunteer
services)

Noncommercial Organizations

Community action/volunteer groups (education/support)
National organizations
Philanthropic foundations
(funding of biomedical or health services research)
Universities and other nonfederal researchers

E

The Centers for Disease Control's Surveillance Definition of AIDS

For the purposes of national reporting of some of the severe late manifestations of infection with human immunodeficiency virus (HIV) in the United States, the Centers for Disease Control (CDC) defines a case of acquired immunodeficiency syndrome (AIDS) as an illness characterized by (1) one or more of the opportunistic diseases listed below (diagnosed by methods considered reliable) that are at least moderately indicative of underlying cellular immunodeficiency, and (2) the absence of all known underlying causes of cellular immunodeficiency (other than HIV infection) and the absence of all other causes of reduced resistance reported to be associated with at least one of those opportunistic diseases.

Despite having the above, patients are excluded as AIDS cases if they have a negative result(s) on testing for serum antibody to HIV, do not have a positive culture for HIV, and have both a normal or high number of CD4 T cells and a normal or high ratio of CD4 to CD8 T cells. A single negative test for HIV may be applied here if it is an antibody test by ELISA, immunofluorescent, or Western blot methods, because such tests are very sensitive. Viral cultures are less sensitive but more specific, and so may be relied on if positive but not if negative. If multiple antibody tests have inconsistent results, the result applied to the case definition

SOURCE: Based on ''The Case Definition of AIDS Used by CDC for National Reporting (CDC-reportable AIDS),'' Document No. 0312S, August 1, 1985, Centers for Disease Control, Atlanta, Ga.

should be that of the majority. A positive culture, however, would overrule negative antibody tests. In the absence of test results, patients satisfying all other criteria in this definition are included as cases.

This general case definition can be made more explicit by specifying the particular diseases considered at least moderately indicative of cellular immunodeficiency that are used as indicators of AIDS. In the following list of diseases, the required diagnostic methods with positive results are shown in parentheses. "Microscopy" may include cytology.

Protozoal and Helminthic Infections

1. Cryptosporidiosis, intestinal, causing diarrhea for over one month (on histology or stool microscopy).
2. *Pneumocystis carinii* pneumonia (on histology or microscopy of a "touch" preparation, bronchial washings, or sputum).
3. Strongyloidosis causing pneumonia, central nervous system infection, or infection disseminated beyond the gastrointestinal tract (on histology).
4. Toxoplasmosis causing infection in internal organs other than the liver, spleen, or lymph nodes (on histology or microscopy of a "touch" preparation).

Fungal Infections

1. Candidiasis causing esophagitis (on histology, microscopy of a "wet" preparation from the esophagus, or endoscopic or autopsy findings of white plaques on an erythematous mucosal base, but not by culture alone).
2. Cryptococcosis causing central nervous system or other infection disseminated beyond lungs and lymph nodes (on culture, antigen detection, histology, or India ink preparation of cerebrospinal fluid).

Bacterial Infections

1. *Mycobacterium avium* or *intracellulare* (*Mycobacterium avium* complex) or *Mycobacterium kansasii* causing infection disseminated beyond lungs and lymph nodes (on culture).

Viral Infections

1. Cytomegalovirus causing infection in internal organs other than the liver, spleen, or lymph nodes (on histology or cytology but not by culture or serum antibody titer).
2. Herpes simplex virus causing chronic mucocutaneous infection with ulcers persisting more than one month or pulmonary, gastrointestinal

tract (beyond mouth, throat, or rectum), or disseminated infection, but not encephalitis alone (on culture, histology, or cytology).

3. Progressive multifocal leukoencephalopathy, presumed to be caused by papovavirus (on histology).

Cancer

1. Kaposi's sarcoma (on histology).
2. Lymphoma limited to the brain (on histology).

Other Opportunistic Infections with Positive Test for HIV

In the absence of the above opportunistic diseases, any of the following diseases is considered indicative of AIDS if the patient had a positive test for HIV:

1. Disseminated histoplasmosis (on culture, histology, or cytology).
2. Bronchial or pulmonary candidiasis (on microscopy or visualization grossly of characteristic white plaques on the bronchial mucosa, but not by culture alone).
3. Isosporiasis causing chronic diarrhea of over one month (on histology or stool microscopy).

Chronic Lymphoid Interstitial Pneumonitis

In the absence of the above opportunistic diseases, a histologically confirmed diagnosis of chronic (persisting over two months) lymphoid interstitial pneumonitis in a child (under 13 years of age) is indicative of AIDS unless test(s) for HIV are negative. The histologic examination of lung tissue must show diffuse interstitial and peribronchiolar infiltration by lymphocytes, plasma cells with Russell bodies, plasmacytoid lymphocytes, and immunoblasts. Histologic and culture evaluation must not identify a pathogenic organism as the cause of this pneumonia.

Non-Hodgkin's Lymphoma with Positive Test for HIV

If the patient had a positive test for HIV, then the following histologic types of lymphoma are indicative of AIDS, regardless of anatomic site:

1. Small *non*cleaved lymphoma (Burkitt's tumor or Burkitt-like lymphoma), but not small cleaved lymphoma.
2. Immunoblastic sarcoma (or immunoblastic lymphoma) of B-cell or unknown immunologic phenotype (not of T-cell type). Other terms that may be equivalent include diffuse undifferentiated non-Hodgkin's lymphoma, large-cell lymphoma (cleaved or noncleaved), diffuse histiocytic lymphoma, reticulum cell sarcoma, and high-grade lymphoma.

Lymphomas should not be accepted as indicative of AIDS if they are described in any one of the following ways: low grade, of T-cell type (immunologic phenotype), small cleaved lymphoma, lymphocytic lymphoma (regardless of whether well or poorly differentiated), lymphoblastic lymphoma, plasmacytoid lymphocytic lymphoma, lymphocytic leukemia (acute or chronic), or Hodgkin's disease (or Hodgkin's lymphoma).

F

CDC Classification System for HIV Infections*

INTRODUCTION

Persons infected with the etiologic retrovirus of acquired immunodeficiency syndrome (AIDS) (1-4)* may present with a variety of manifestations ranging from asymptomatic infection to severe immunodeficiency and life-threatening secondary infectious diseases or cancers. The rapid growth of knowledge about human T-lymphotropic virus type III/ lymphadenopathy-associated virus (HTLV-III/LAV) has resulted in an increasing need for a system of classifying patients within this spectrum of clinical and laboratory findings attributable to HTLV-III/LAV infection (5-7).

Various means are now used to describe and assess patients with manifestations of HTLV-III/LAV infection and to describe their signs, symptoms, and laboratory findings. The surveillance definition of AIDS has proven to be extremely valuable and quite reliable for some epidemiologic studies and clinical assessment of patients with the more severe manifestations of disease. However, more inclusive definitions and classifications of HTLV-III/LAV infection are needed for optimum patient care, health planning, and public health control strategies, as well as for epidemiologic studies and special surveys. A broadly applicable, easily understood classification system should also facilitate and clarify communication about this disease.

In an attempt to formulate the most appropriate classification system, CDC has sought the advice of a panel of expert consultants[†] to assist in defining the manifestations of HTLV-III/ LAV infection.

GOALS AND OBJECTIVES OF THE CLASSIFICATION SYSTEM

The classification system presented in this report is primarily applicable to public health purposes, including disease reporting and surveillance, epidemiologic studies, prevention and control activities, and public health policy and planning.

Immediate applications of such a system include the classification of infected persons for reporting of cases to state and local public health agencies, and use in various disease coding and recording systems, such as the forthcoming 10th revision of the International Classification of Diseases.

---

*The AIDS virus has been variously termed human T-lymphotropic virus type III (HTLV-III), lymphadenopathy-associated virus (LAV), AIDS-associated retrovirus (ARV), or human immunodeficiency virus (HIV). The designation human immunodeficiency virus (HIV) has recently been proposed by a subcommittee of the International Committee for the Taxonomy of Viruses as the appropriate name for the retrovirus that has been implicated as the causative agent of AIDS (4).

[†]The following persons served on the review panel: DS Burke, MD, RR Redfield, MD, Walter Reed Army Institute of Research, Washington, DC; J Chin, MD, State Epidemiologist, California Department of Health Services; LZ Cooper, MD, St Luke's-Roosevelt Hospital Center, New York City; JP Davis, MD, State Epidemiologist, Wisconsin Division of Health; MA Fischl, MD, University of Miami School of Medicine, Miami, Florida; G Friedland, MD, Albert Einstein College of Medicine, New York City; MA Johnson, MD, DI Abrams, MD, San Francisco General Hospital; D Mildvan, MD, Beth Israel Medical Center, New York City; CU Tuazon, MD, George Washington University School of Medicine, Washington, DC; RW Price, MD, Memorial Sloan-Kettering Cancer Center, New York City; C Konigsberg, MD, Broward County Public Health Unit, Fort Lauderdale, Florida; MS Gottlieb, MD, University of California—Los Angeles Medical Center; representatives of the National Institute of Allergy and Infectious Diseases, National Cancer Institute, National Institutes of Health; Center for Infectious Diseases, CDC.

SOURCE: Reprinted from *Morbidity and Mortality Weekly Report* 35 (May 23, 1986):334-339.

DEFINITION OF HTLV-III/LAV INFECTION

The most specific diagnosis of HTLV-III/LAV infection is by direct identification of the virus in host tissues by virus isolation; however, the techniques for isolating HTLV-III/LAV currently lack sensitivity for detecting infection and are not readily available. For public health purposes, patients with repeatedly reactive screening tests for HTLV-III/LAV antibody (e.g., enzyme-linked immunosorbent assay) in whom antibody is also identified by the use of supplemental tests (e.g., Western blot, immunofluorescence assay) should be considered both infected and infective (8-10).

Although HTLV-III/LAV infection is identified by isolation of the virus or, indirectly, by the presence of antibody to the virus, a presumptive clinical diagnosis of HTLV-III/LAV infection has been made in some situations in the absence of positive virologic or serologic test results. There is a very strong correlation between the clinical manifestations of AIDS as defined by CDC and the presence of HTLV-III/LAV antibody (11-14). Most persons whose clinical illness fulfills the CDC surveillance definition for AIDS will have been infected with the virus (12-14).

CLASSIFICATION SYSTEM

This system classifies the manifestations of HTLV-III/LAV infection into four mutually exclusive groups, designated by Roman numerals I through IV (Table 5). *The classification system applies only to patients diagnosed as having HTLV-III/LAV infection (see previous section, DEFINITION OF HTLV-III/LAV INFECTION).* Classification in a particular group is not explicitly intended to have prognostic significance, nor to designate severity of illness. However, classification in the four principal groups, I-IV, is hierarchical in that persons classified in a particular group should not be reclassified in a preceding group if clinical findings resolve, since clinical improvement may not accurately reflect changes in the severity of the underlying disease.

Group I includes patients with transient signs and symptoms that appear at the time of, or shortly after, initial infection with HTLV-III/LAV as identified by laboratory studies. All patients in Group I will be reclassified in another group following resolution of this acute syndrome.

TABLE 5. Summary of classification system for human T-lymphotropic virus type III/ lymphadenopathy-associated virus

---

Group I. Acute infection

Group II. Asymptomatic infection*

Group III. Persistent generalized lymphadenopathy*

Group IV. Other disease
    Subgroup A. Constitutional disease
    Subgroup B. Neurologic disease
    Subgroup C. Secondary infectious diseases
        Category C-1.   Specified secondary infectious diseases listed in the CDC surveillance definition for AIDS[†]
        Category C-2.   Other specified secondary infectious diseases
    Subgroup D. Secondary cancers[†]
    Subgroup E. Other conditions

---

*Patients in Groups II and III may be subclassified on the basis of a laboratory evaluation.

[†]Includes those patients whose clinical presentation fulfills the definition of AIDS used by CDC for national reporting.

Group II includes patients who have no signs or symptoms of HTLV-III/LAV infection. Patients in this category may be subclassified based on whether hematologic and/or immunologic laboratory studies have been done and whether results are abnormal in a manner consistent with the effects of HTLV-III/LAV infection.

Group III includes patients with persistent generalized lymphadenopathy, but without findings that would lead to classification in Group IV. Patients in this category may be subclassified based on the results of laboratory studies in the same manner as patients in Group II.

Group IV includes patients with clinical symptoms and signs of HTLV-III/LAV infection other than or in addition to lymphadenopathy. Patients in this group are assigned to *one or more* subgroups based on clinical findings. These subgroups are: A. constitutional disease; B. neurologic disease; C. secondary infectious diseases; D. secondary cancers; and E. other conditions resulting from HTLV-III/LAV infection. There is no *a priori* hierarchy of severity among subgroups A through E, and these subgroups are not mutually exclusive.

Definitions of the groups and subgroups are as follows:

Group I. Acute HTLV-III/LAV Infection. Defined as a mononucleosis-like syndrome, with or without aseptic meningitis, associated with seroconversion for HTLV-III/LAV antibody (*15-16*). Antibody seroconversion is required as evidence of initial infection; current viral isolation procedures are not adequately sensitive to be relied on for demonstrating the onset of infection.

Group II. Asymptomatic HTLV-III/LAV Infection. Defined as the absence of signs or symptoms of HTLV-III/LAV infection. To be classified in Group II, patients must have had no previous signs or symptoms that would have led to classification in Groups III or IV. Patients whose clinical findings caused them to be classified in Groups III or IV should not be reclassified in Group II if those clinical findings resolve.

Patients in this group may be subclassified on the basis of a laboratory evaluation. Laboratory studies commonly indicated for patients with HTLV-III/LAV infection include, but are not limited to, a complete blood count (including differential white blood cell count) and a platelet count. Immunologic tests, especially T-lymphocyte helper and suppressor cell counts, are also an important part of the overall evaluation. Patients whose test results are within normal limits, as well as those for whom a laboratory evaluation has not yet been completed, should be differentiated from patients whose test results are consistent with defects associated with HTLV-III/LAV infection (e.g., lymphopenia, thrombocytopenia, decreased number of helper [T_4] T-lymphocytes).

Group III. Persistent Generalized Lymphadenopathy (PGL). Defined as palpable lymphadenopathy (lymph node enlargement of 1 cm or greater) at two or more extra-inguinal sites persisting for more than 3 months in the absence of a concurrent illness or condition other than HTLV-III/LAV infection to explain the findings. Patients in this group may also be subclassified on the basis of a laboratory evaluation, as is done for asymptomatic patients in Group II (see above). Patients with PGL whose clinical findings caused them to be classified in Group IV should not be reclassified in Group III if those other clinical findings resolve.

Group IV. Other HTLV-III/LAV Disease. The clinical manifestations of patients in this group may be designated by assignment to one or more subgroups (A-E) listed below. Within Group IV, subgroup classification is independent of the presence or absence of lymphadenopathy. Each subgroup may include patients who are minimally symptomatic, as well as patients who are severely ill. Increased specificity for manifestations of HTLV-III/LAV infection, if needed for clinical purposes or research purposes or for disability determinations, may be achieved by creating additional divisions within each subgroup.

Subgroup A. Constitutional disease. Defined as one or more of the following: fever persisting more than 1 month, involuntary weight loss of greater than 10% of baseline, or diarrhea persisting more than 1 month; and the absence of a concurrent illness or condition other than HTLV-III/LAV infection to explain the findings.

Subgroup B. Neurologic disease. Defined as one or more of the following: dementia, myelopathy, or peripheral neuropathy; and the absence of a concurrent illness or condition other than HTLV-III/LAV infection to explain the findings.

Subgroup C. Secondary infectious diseases. Defined as the diagnosis of an infectious disease associated with HTLV-III/LAV infection and/or at least moderately indicative of a defect in cell-mediated immunity. Patients in this subgroup are divided further into two categories:

Category C-1. Includes patients with symptomatic or invasive disease due to one of 12 specified secondary infectious diseases listed in the surveillance definition of AIDS[§]: *Pneumocystis carinii* pneumonia, chronic cryptosporidiosis, toxoplasmosis, extraintestinal strongyloidiasis, isosporiasis, candidiasis (esophageal, bronchial, or pulmonary), cryptococcosis, histoplasmosis, mycobacterial infection with *Mycobacterium avium* complex or *M. kansasii*, cytomegalovirus infection, chronic mucocutaneous or disseminated herpes simplex virus infection, and progressive multifocal leukoencephalopathy.

Category C-2. Includes patients with symptomatic or invasive disease due to one of six other specified secondary infectious diseases: oral hairy leukoplakia, multidermatomal herpes zoster, recurrent *Salmonella* bacteremia, nocardiosis, tuberculosis, or oral candidiasis (thrush).

Subgroup D. Secondary cancers. Defined as the diagnosis of one or more kinds of cancer known to be associated with HTLV-III/LAV infection as listed in the surveillance definition of AIDS and at least moderately indicative of a defect in cell-mediated immunity[¶]: Kaposi's sarcoma, non-Hodgkin's lymphoma (small, noncleaved lymphoma or immunoblastic sarcoma), or primary lymphoma of the brain.

Subgroup E. Other conditions in HTLV-III/LAV infection. Defined as the presence of other clinical findings or diseases, not classifiable above, that may be attributed to HTLV-III/LAV infection and/or may be indicative of a defect in cell-mediated immunity. Included are patients with chronic lymphoid interstitial pneumonitis. Also included are those patients whose signs or symptoms could be attributed either to HTLV-III/LAV infection or to another coexisting disease not classified elsewhere, and patients with other clinical illnesses, the course or management of which may be complicated or altered by HTLV-III/LAV infection. Examples include: patients with constitutional symptoms not meeting the criteria for subgroup IV-A; patients with infectious diseases not listed in subgroup IV-C; and patients with neoplasms not listed in subgroup IV-D.

Reported by Center for Infectious Diseases, CDC.

Editorial Note: The classification system is meant to provide a means of grouping patients infected with HTLV-III/LAV according to the clinical expression of disease. It will require periodic revision as warranted by new information about HTLV-III/LAV infection. The defini-

---

[§]This subgroup includes patients with one or more of the specified infectious diseases listed whose clinical presentation fulfills the definition of AIDS as used by CDC for national reporting.

[¶]This subgroup includes those patients with one or more of the specified cancers listed whose clinical presentation fulfills the definition of AIDS as used by CDC for national reporting.

tion of particular syndromes will evolve with increasing knowledge of the significance of certain clinical findings and laboratory tests. New diagnostic techniques, such as the detection of specific HTLV-III/LAV antigens or antibodies, may add specificity to the assessment of patients infected with HTLV-III/LAV.

The classification system defines a limited number of specified clinical presentations. Patients whose signs and symptoms do not meet the criteria for other groups and subgroups, but whose findings are attributable to HTLV-III/LAV infection, should be classified in subgroup IV-E. As the classification system is revised and updated, certain subsets of patients in subgroup IV-E may be identified as having related groups of clinical findings that should be separately classified as distinct syndromes. This could be accomplished either by creating additional subgroups within Group IV or by broadening the definitions of the existing subgroups.

Persons currently using other classification systems (*6-7*) or nomenclatures (e.g., AIDS-related complex, lymphadenopathy syndrome) can find equivalences with those systems and terminologies and the classification presented in this report. Because this classification system has only four principal groups based on chronology, presence or absence of signs and symptoms, and the type of clinical findings present, comparisons with other classifications based either on clinical findings or on laboratory assessment are easily accomplished.

This classification system does not imply any change in the definition of AIDS used by CDC since 1981 for national reporting. Patients whose clinical presentations fulfill the surveillance definition of AIDS are classified in Group IV. However, not every case in Group IV will meet the surveillance definition.

Persons wishing to comment on this material are encouraged to send comments in writing to the AIDS Program, Center for Infectious Diseases, CDC.

References
1. Gallo RC, Salahuddin SZ, Popovic M, et al. Frequent detection and isolation of cytopathic retroviruses (HTLV-III) from patients with AIDS and at risk for AIDS. Science 1984;224:500-3.
2. Barré-Sinoussi F, Chermann JC, Rey F, et al. Isolation of a T-lymphotropic retrovirus from a patient at risk for acquired immune deficiency syndrome (AIDS). Science 1983;220:868-71.
3. Levy JA, Hoffman AD, Kramer SM, Landis JA, Shimabukuro JM, Oshiro LS. Isolation of lymphocytopathic retroviruses from San Francisco patients with AIDS. Science 1984;225:840-2.
4. Coffin J, Haase A, Levy JA, et al. Human immunodeficiency viruses [Letter]. Science 1986;232:697.
5. CDC. Revision of the case definition of acquired immunodeficiency syndrome for national reporting—United States. MMWR 1985;34:373-5.
6. Haverkos HW, Gottlieb MS, Killen JY, Edelman R. Classification of HTLV-III/LAV-related diseases [Letter]. J Infect Dis 1985;152:1095.
7. Redfield RR, Wright DC, Tramont EC. The Walter Reed staging classification for HTLV-III/LAV infection. N Engl J Med 1986;314:131-2.
8. CDC. Antibodies to a retrovirus etiologically associated with acquired immunodeficiency syndrome (AIDS) in populations with increased incidences of the syndrome. MMWR 1984;33:377-9.
9. CDC. Update: Public Health Service Workshop on Human T-Lymphotropic Virus Type III Antibody Testing—United States. MMWR 1985;34:477-8.
10. CDC. Additional recommendations to reduce sexual and drug abuse-related transmission of human T-lymphotropic virus type III/lymphadenopathy-associated virus. MMWR 1986;35:152-5.
11. Selik RM, Haverkos HW, Curran JW. Acquired immune deficiency syndrome (AIDS) trends in the United States, 1978-1982. Am J Med 1984;76:493-500.
12. Sarngadharan MG, Popovic M, Bruch L, Schüpbach J, Gallo RC. Antibodies reactive with human T-lymphotropic retroviruses (HTLV-III) in the serum of patients with AIDS. Science 1984;224:506-8.
13. Safai B, Sarngadharan MG, Groopman JE, et al. Seroepidemiological studies of human T-lymphotropic retrovirus type III in acquired immunodeficiency syndrome. Lancet 1984;I:1438-40.
14. Laurence J, Brun-Vezinet F, Schutzer SE, et al. Lymphadenopathy associated viral antibody in AIDS. Immune correlations and definition of a carrier state. N Engl J Med 1984;311:1269-73.

15. Ho DD, Sarngadharan MG, Resnick L, Dimarzo-Veronese F, Rota TR, Hirsch MS. Primary human T-lymphotropic virus type III infection. Ann Intern Med 1985;103:880-3.
16. Cooper DA, Gold J, Maclean P, et al. Acute AIDS retrovirus infection. Definition of a clinical illness associated with seroconversion. Lancet 1985;I:537-40.

G

PHS Plan for Prevention and Control of AIDS and the AIDS Virus

Foreword

In 1985, the Public Health Service's Executive Task Force on AIDS published a comprehensive plan that included a set of objectives to control and prevent the spread of acquired immune deficiency syndrome by the year 2000 (1). In the year since the plan was developed, considerable progress has been made. Our knowledge base has expanded many fold during 5 cumulative years of experience with AIDS and the AIDS virus. New information permits tentative long-range demographic projections, a better understanding of pathogenesis, a refined approach to research and development of vaccines and therapeutic agents, a refocus of prevention and control efforts, and the incorporation of patient care issues.

The Public Health Service (PHS) convened a meeting at the Coolfont Conference Center in Berkeley Springs, WV, June 4-6, 1986. Eighty-five experts in various aspects of AIDS, including clinicians, epidemiologists, public health policy makers, and basic research scientists were invited to review and modify the plan according to current information, needs, and demographic projections through 1991. The following plan is the result of that meeting; it represents a renewed commitment by the Public Health Service to prevent and control AIDS infection and its sequelae.

Donald Ian Macdonald, MD
Acting Assistant Secretary for Health

Purpose

This document provides a framework for the steps that must be taken in five broad areas—pathogenesis and clinical manifestations, therapeutics, vaccines, public health control measures, and patient care and health care needs—to achieve prevention and control of AIDS. The current plan is based on estimated changes in the demographics of AIDS through 1991. It calls for concerted action by Federal agencies, State and local health departments, professional organizations, and volunteer groups.

Goals

The following goals were first published in the 1985 plan and remain valid for guiding the continuing national effort.

• By 1987, reduce the transmission of the HTLV-III/LAV infection.
• By 1990, reduce the increase in the incidence of AIDS.
• By 2000, eliminate transmission of HTLV-III/LAV infection with a decline in the incidence of AIDS thereafter.

Background

Five years have elapsed since the initial report of *Pneumocystis carinii* pneumonia from Los Angeles marked the recognition of what has become known as AIDS. By 1984, a human retrovirus, HTLV-III/LAV (human T-cell lymphotropic virus type III/lymphadenopathy-associated virus) had been determined to be the etiologic agent of AIDS. (The International Committee on the Taxonomy of Viruses proposed the name "human immunodeficiency virus" for these viruses (2).) By early 1985, serologic tests for antibody to the virus were licensed and widely available.

In retrospect, when AIDS was initially reported in June 1981, some 5 years already had elapsed since the introduction of HTLV-III/LAV into the United States, and 3 years had elapsed since the first clinical cases had occurred. AIDS cases have been reported from all 50 States, the District of Columbia, and 4 Territories. Cases have been reported from more than 100 foreign countries.

The rapid development and implementation of sensitive and specific assays for HTLV-III/LAV antibodies have permitted screening of donated blood and plasma, and the research use of these

SOURCE: *Public Health Reports* 101(July-August 1986):341-348.

'During 1991 alone, more than 145,000 cases of AIDS will require medical care and more than 54,000 AIDS patients are predicted to die, bringing the cumulative number of deaths due to AIDS to more than 179,000.'

and other assays has elucidated the modes of transmission, the natural history of infection, and a better understanding of the clinical manifestations of HTLV-III/LAV infections.

The predominant defect in AIDS is a profound and, so far, irreversible immune dysfunction that results when HTLV-III/LAV preferentially infects the helper-inducer subset of T-lymphocytes. Although the virus can also infect other cells of the immune system, as well as cells of the central nervous system, it is the infection of these T-lymphocytes that ultimately leads to a breakdown in the ability of an infected individual to mount an immune response. In the past 5 years, more effective therapies for some of the opportunistic infections that accompany AIDS have been found, but no cure for AIDS is yet available.

Studies of the molecular biology of HTLV-III/LAV have revealed that a copy of the viral genetic material becomes an integral and permanent component of the DNA of an infected individual. As a result, such an individual is likely to be a carrier of the virus for the rest of his or her life and, for purposes of public health control, is assumed to be capable of transmitting the virus to others.

The HTLV-III/LAV genome has been completely sequenced and the functions of several of its genes are known. Considerable differences in some genes have been found among various isolates. In addition, related viruses have been identified in man and nonhuman primates. These related viruses cause a range of different diseases. Studies in animals indicate the feasibility of vaccination against retroviruses, and one veterinary vaccine is available for the prevention of feline leukemia virus. Although some promising approaches are under way, as yet no effective vaccine for AIDS exists.

HTLV-III/LAV is transmitted by sexual, parenteral, and perinatal contact with the virus. Although this infection has been most often recognized in homosexual men and intravenous (IV) drug abusers, it is clear that this virus does not discriminate by sex, age, race, ethnic group, or sexual orientation. Behaviors which are high risk for the acquisition of HTLV-III/LAV infection include sexual contact or sharing of drug injection equipment with an infected person. Studies now clearly demonstrate that AIDS is not spread by casual contact, such as sneezing, coughing, or sharing meals with an AIDS patient.

There were 21,517 cases of AIDS reported in the United States as of June 1986. Blacks and Hispanics represent 39 percent of total cases. Women who report no history of IV drug abuse represent half of the 1,400 cases in women. Approximately 304 cases of AIDS occurred in infants and children under age 13. Between 2 and 3 percent of the cases have occurred in transfusion recipients or hemophiliacs.

Projections

The following projections, including those in the table, are based on the Centers for Disease Control (CDC) surveillance data and epidemiologic studies of populations at high risk to infection with the virus.

• Twenty to 30 percent of the estimated 1 to 1.5 million Americans infected with HTLV-III/LAV as of June 1986 are projected to develop AIDS by the end of 1991. The latency period between infection and overt AIDS averages 4 or more years in adults; therefore, most persons who will develop AIDS between 1986 and 1991 will be those who are already infected with HTLV-III/LAV.

• Based on an empirical model that uses reported cases of AIDS, by the end of 1991, the cumulative cases of AIDS in the U.S. meeting the CDC surveillance definition will total more than 270,000. During 1991 alone, more than 145,000 cases of AIDS will require medical care and more than 54,000 AIDS patients are predicted to die, bringing the cumulative number of deaths due to AIDS to more than 179,000.

• The empirical model may underestimate by at least 20 percent the serious morbidity and mortality attributable to AIDS, because of underreporting or underascertainment of cases.

Projected cases of AIDS,[1] United States

Category	1986	1991	1991 range
Cases diagnosed			
Cumulative cases at start of year	19,000	196,000	155,000 to 219,000
Diagnosed during year..................................	16,000	74,000	46,000 to 92,000
Cumulative cases at end of year	35,000	270,000	201,000 to 311,000
Alive at start of year.....................................	10,000	71,000	50,000 to 83,000
Alive at any time during year	26,000	145,000	96,000 to 174,000
Deaths			
Cumulative deaths at start of year.........................	9,000	125,000	105,000 to 137,000
Deaths during year......................................	9,000	54,000	36,000 to 64,000
Cumulative deaths at end of year	18,000	179,000	141,000 to 201,000
Infections			
Persons with HTLV-III/LAV infection.......................	1 million- 1.5 million (estimate)	. . .	

[1]These numbers refer only to those cases that meet the CDC definition for AIDS (see Morbidity and Mortality Weekly Report 34:373-375, June 28, 1985) and do not include other manifestations of infection, such as AIDS-related complex and lymphadenopathy syndrome.

• In 1985, 9,000 cases of AIDS were diagnosed in the United States and reported to the Centers for Disease Control. The empirical model predicts that cases will continue to increase through 1991, that there will be nearly 16,000 cases reported in 1986, and that more than 74,000 cases are projected for 1991. The estimates for 1991 range from 46,000 to 90,000.

• More than 70 percent of the cases will be diagnosed among homosexual or bisexual men, and 25 percent of the cases will occur among IV drug abusers with some overlap to continue between the groups. Because the periods between infection and disease are long and variable, cases will continue to be reported among transfusion recipients and persons with hemophilia.

• Additional cases in heterosexual men and women are projected; the 1,100 (7 percent of the total) for 1986 will increase to nearly 7,000 (more than 9 percent) by 1991. This group includes patients who reported heterosexual contact with an infected person or someone in a risk group. It also includes patients in groups in which epidemiologic studies suggest heterosexual transmission as the major risk factor. By 1991, more than 3,000 cases will have been diagnosed in infants and children.

• Through 1985, fewer than 60 percent of cases were diagnosed in persons outside New York City and San Francisco, but by 1991 more than 80 percent of cases are predicted to be reported from other localities.

• Homosexual-bisexual men and men and women who use drugs of abuse intravenously will continue to be the populations at highest risk for HTLV-III/LAV infection during the next 5 years. Using estimates published by Kinsey (3), more than 2.5 million (4 percent) of U.S. men between 16 and 55 years of age are exclusively homosexual throughout their lives; an estimated 5-10 million more will have some homosexual contact. An estimated 750,000 Americans inject heroin or other drugs intravenously at least once a week; a similar number inject drugs less often.

• The prevalence of HTLV-III/LAV seropositivity among homosexual men and IV drug users parallels the frequency of AIDS in various cities. In 1984-85, 20 to 50 percent of homosexual men who participated in research studies had evidence of HTLV-III/LAV infection. Similarly, seroprevalence estimates among IV drug abusers ranged from 10 percent to more than 50 percent in various U.S. cities. By extrapolating all available data, we estimate that there are approximately 1 to 1.5 million infected persons in those two groups at present. Thus estimates of a 20 to 30 percent progression to AIDS by 1991 in this group are consistent with the total number of AIDS cases predicted by the empirical model.

• Uninfected homosexual men have continued to acquire HTLV-III/LAV infections during the past year, but at a lower rate than would be predicted from the increases in previous years and from the increase in the number of potentially infectious persons. This observation is consistent with changes reported in sexual behavior and declines in other sexually transmitted infections in homosexual men. Nonetheless, due to the large present and future populations at risk, hundreds of thousands of additional homosexual men, IV drug abusers, and others may become infected during the next 5 years.

• Because of heat and chemical treatment of clotting factor concentrates, donor deferral, and serologic screening of donated blood and plasma, only a very small number of additional infections are likely to occur through blood and plasma transfusions.

• Current information is insufficient to predict the future incidence of HTLV-III/LAV infection in heterosexual populations, but increases in heterosexual transmission are likely. Those at highest risk will be heterosexual sexual partners of infected persons and those who have sexual contact with past or present IV drug abusers, bisexual men, prostitutes, or others at increased risk for HTLV-III/LAV infection. As is true for homosexual men, sexual contact with multiple partners will increase one's risk for HTLV-III/LAV infection.

• Additional increases in HTLV-III/LAV infection in infants are expected as more women in child-bearing years become infected.

The following five sections summarize the deliberations and recommendations made by the work groups at the Coolfont meeting.

Pathogenesis and Clinical Manifestations

Infection with HTLV-III/LAV results in a broad range of clinical manifestations including an acute retroviral syndrome, asymptomatic disease, chronic lymphadenopathy, and serious diseases including Kaposi's sarcoma and other malignant neoplasms, fatal opportunistic infections, and neurological and psychiatric disorders.

The factors that determine the expression and progression of disease in an individual are largely unknown. Techniques are available to diagnose and treat many of these opportunistic diseases, although they often recur. However, once Kaposi's sarcoma or certain opportunistic infections occur, an ultimately fatal outcome for the patient has been the rule.

• Clinical and epidemiologic studies need to be conducted to

— Clarify the natural history of infection, including the role which may be played by exogenous or endogenous factors in determining which clinical manifestations occur, and

— Continue to expand the spectrum of clinical manifestations.

• Basic scientific studies on the virology and immunopathogenesis of HTLV-III/LAV need to be expanded, especially to

— Assess target cell susceptibility;
— Identify viral and host cell determinants of transmissibility and pathogenicity including portals of viral entry, mechanisms of cytopathic effects, and dysfunction;
— Further elucidate mechanisms of viral latency and activation;
— Identify and assess direct and indirect immunopathogenic mechanisms;
— Further delineate the pathogenesis of neurologic and psychiatric abnormalities; and
— Ascertain more fully the functions of viral gene products and determine the meaning and mechanisms of genetic heterogeneity.

More suitable animal models for HTLV-III/LAV infection need to be developed to allow more comprehensive understanding of pathogenesis and rapid evaluation of treatment and prophylaxis. Dedicated efforts must be made to maximize efficiency of use of limited animal resources.

Improved methodologies are needed to detect infected and infectious individuals and to identify and quantitate virus, viral antigen, and viral antibody.

Therapeutics

No drug with proven clinical efficacy for AIDS is currently known. Both antiviral agents and immunomodulators are being developed, and several drugs are under clinical investigation at present. The ability of an agent to reverse the disease process or halt its progression may vary depending upon the stage of infection. Research is now in progress to develop new methods to inhibit viral replication and correct the immune deficiencies. A safe and effective antiviral agent is not likely to be in general use for the next several years. Experimental products are also under study for treatment of opportunistic infections and neoplasms associated with HTLV-III/LAV infection.

The following points should be considered in

order to develop drugs for the treatment of AIDS in the most expeditious manner:

• Further expansion of the multiinstitutional, multidisciplinary approach to identify and develop agents for the treatment and prevention of HTLV–III/LAV infection and associated diseases, including central nervous system disease, is necessary. Part of this effort must be the establishment of a large capacity screening program to measure the antiviral and immunomodulator activity and toxic effects of newly identified natural and synthetic compounds.

• A system for classifying HTLV–III/LAV associated disease manifestations which is useful in the design, implementation, and analyses of therapeutic trials must be developed. Standard clinical criteria for the measurement of efficacy and toxicity must be formulated to facilitate the performance of well organized multicenter clinical trials.

• The most efficient design of clinical trials of candidate antiviral agents will require the use of placebo controls. Once an agent has been shown to be safe and efficacious in a clinical trial, this agent can generally be substituted for the placebo control in subsequent clinical trials and can be used as the standard against which other agents are compared.

• New therapeutic approaches must be developed to control or eliminate latent virus and to specifically direct antiviral compounds to the appropriate target tissues. Combination strategies to control viral replication and restore the immune system must be developed and evaluated.

• Since antiviral drugs currently under development are likely to repress rather than eliminate the AIDS virus infection, long-term therapy is expected and with it the emergence of drug-resistant strains.

• New and existing strategies in the diagnosis, treatment, and prophylaxis of the opportunistic infections and neoplasms associated with AIDS all need to be developed, tested, and improved.

Vaccines

A number of vaccine candidates for human beings are currently under development, and limited clinical testing for some could begin within 2 years. Field trials to demonstrate efficacy may require additional years. Vaccines are not anticipated to be useful in individuals who are already infected. A vaccine for general use is not anticipated before the next decade, and its use would

'In the absence of a vaccine and therapy, prevention and control of HTLV-III/LAV infection depends largely upon effective approaches to decrease sexual transmission, transmission among IV drug users, and perinatal transmission from infected mothers.'

not affect the number of persons infected by that time.

The following steps need to be taken:

• Vaccines employing recombinant DNA derived antigens, virus subunits, killed viruses, synthetic peptides, live recombinant or attenuated viruses, and antiidiotypes will need to be evaluated as potential candidates for human trials.

• Vaccination methods will need to be devised to induce immunity to antigenically distinct strains of HTLV-III/LAV.

• Reliable *in vitro* and *in vivo* systems need to be developed for the evaluation of vaccine immunogenicity safety and efficacy before commencing human trials.

• A program for clinical and field evaluation of vaccine(s) needs to be established, including resolution of difficult aspects of design such as identification of target populations and the definition of parameters of vaccine efficacy.

• Protocols need to be developed for the *in vitro* and *in vivo* evaluation of anti-HTLV-III/LAV immunoglobulin to explore its value in passive immunization.

Public Health Control Measures

In the absence of a vaccine and therapy, prevention and control of HTLV-III/LAV infection depends largely upon effective approaches to decrease sexual transmission, transmission among IV drug users, and perinatal transmission from infected mothers. A strategy to control and prevent AIDS should involve voluntary counseling and testing for persons at increased risk of HTLV-III/LAV infection and imparting to infected patients those Public Health Service recommendations concerning personal behaviors that must be observed if spread of the virus is to be halted. Throughout this section, serological testing is intended to be voluntary, conducted with confidentiality, and accompanied by appropriate pretest and post-test counseling.

Public health activities directed toward the control and prevention of AIDS have required significant funding and staffing at national, State, and local levels. The projected increases in AIDS and HTLV-III/LAV infection over the next 5 years will pose substantial continuing demands for resources for these efforts.

The recommendations of the conference participants concerning public health measures focused on five areas.

1. Information base.
• Information is needed to better determine the size of the population at greatest risk in the United States, particularly the numbers of homosexual men, bisexual men, IV drug abusers, and heterosexuals who have multiple partners.
• Better information is needed on the number of persons infected with HTLV-III/LAV. Extensive and repeated seroepidemiologic surveys are needed to determine the incidence and prevalence of infection by age, race, ethnicity, sex, geographic area, and sexual preference. States should be encouraged to obtain and report data on incidence and prevalence to CDC for publication.
• The Public Health Service should encourage and assist in the evaluation and comparison of all interventions for prevention and control of AIDS and HTLV-III/LAV infection.
• PHS should continue to support key epidemiologic studies.
• The United States should continue to play a role in understanding and assisting efforts to control the disease worldwide, particularly in areas with seemingly different epidemiologic patterns.

2. Information and education. National information and education campaigns on AIDS and HTLV-III/LAV infection should be targeted to individuals and groups whose behavior places them at high risk for AIDS, other sexually active adults, adolescents, preadolescents, and health care providers. A major target of mass information-education programs is the currently uninfected population, to assure that those persons know how to protect themselves. An additional purpose is to persuade infected persons to take appropriate steps to safeguard their own health and to avoid infecting others.
• PHS should explore the advantages of using paid radio, TV, and printed media advertising as well as public service announcements to inform the public on AIDS and HTLV-III/LAV infection.
• PHS, State and local health departments, State and local boards of education, colleges, universities, and other organizations should support and encourage comprehensive health education that includes information about AIDS and HTLV-III/LAV infection.
• With the assistance of appropriate organizations, programs should be implemented to provide culturally sensitive, meaningful information and education to blacks and Hispanics, including homosexuals, IV drug abusers, blood donors, women both at risk themselves and also at risk for transmitting infection perinatally, and to other segments of the public.
• Health care providers need current information and training on the diagnosis, psychosocial counseling, and management of HTLV-III/LAV infected persons.

3. Prevention of IV drug abuse transmission. IV drug abusers serve as the major reservoir for transmission of infection to heterosexual adults and their infants, as well as among themselves. As a group, they are not well organized, often poorly educated, and tend to have less interaction with the health care delivery system than other groups who participate in high-risk behaviors. Efforts to change drug abuse behavior must proceed with the understanding that addictive behavior is not often changed without specific drug treatment.

• A systematically increased capacity for treating IV drug abusers is needed. Until adequate capacity is available, persons in need of treatment should be prioritized. Decisions may vary by locality, but highest priority should be given to those presently on waiting lists for treatment.
• All treatment and prevention approaches should include information and counseling on sexual and perinatal transmission of HTLV-III/LAV, availability of family planning services, and availability of voluntary serological testing for HTLV-III/LAV.
• Until treatment capacity is adequate for persons who continue to abuse IV drugs, studies are needed to evaluate the efficacy and feasibility of promoting safer use of drug paraphernalia (for example, increased availability of sterile needles or

"works") and education regarding use of sterile needles and sharing of needles.

4. Prevention of sexual transmission. Sexual contact will remain the primary mode of HTLV-III/LAV infection for the foreseeable future, with greater increase in the proportion of heterosexual transmission over the next 5 years.

A central goal of local disease control programs should be to reach the greatest number of HTLV-III/LAV infected persons with testing and counseling (provision of pretest and post-test information, including psychological support) about their infections and methods to reduce the likelihood of transmission to others, in order to change high-risk sexual behaviors. At present, only a small proportion of the already infected population has been reached.

Several methods may help achieve this goal, although they may have differing efficacies in various settings and populations. These include encouragement of voluntary serological screening, self referral of sexual and drug abuse contacts, notification and counseling of contacts by health authorities, and targeted educational programs.

• Serological testing of persons whose behavior places them at risk should be encouraged and made widely available. In all communities, appropriate medical care encompasses offering counseling and testing to all persons at risk, including persons with a sexually transmitted disease, IV drug abusers, and persons seen in private practice who engage in high-risk behaviors. (Anonymous testing should be available as an option.)
• Self-referral of an infected person's sexual and needle-sharing contacts should be encouraged. In some areas or populations, additional contact notification activities may be offered to infected persons by the health agency.
• Research is needed on the efficacy of counseling or knowledge of personal serological status or both in modifying sexual and needle-sharing behavior to reduce or eliminate the risk of transmission.
• For persons who know that they are infected with HTLV-III/LAV yet continue to practice high-risk sexual or needle-sharing activities, temporary involuntary isolation should be considered an option only in rare instances and after due process. Enforced isolation is not a practical way to minimize spread of the infection, since infected persons probably remain infectious for life. Education, counseling, and social services—including

'PHS estimates that the direct health care costs of persons with AIDS will be between $8 and $16 billion in 1991. The $8 billion figure is based on the projection of 71,000 AIDS patients alive in 1991 and 74,000 new cases by then.'

drug treatment—are the main interventions for dealing with this problem and are appropriately applied to recalcitrant infected persons and their potential consenting partners. Uninfected persons must avoid behavior which would permit infection from persons who know or do not know they are infected.

5. Prevention of transmissibility by blood and blood products. The risk of transmission of HTLV-III/LAV by transfusion of blood and blood products is extremely low, due to deferral of high-risk donors, serological screening of donated blood and plasma, and the heat and chemical treatment of clotting factor concentrates. Nonetheless, some additional measures are appropriate to further reduce this low risk.

• Increase the effectiveness of deferral by all persons at increased risk of HTLV-III/LAV infection by:

—Collecting demographic and other data from donors found to have confirmed HTLV-III antibody. This will require some type of case reporting and subsequent interviews, but it is essential to the continued evolution of the high-risk donor deferral strategy;
—Improving communications to potential donors about self-deferral, taking into consideration their language skills and literacy;
—Exploring the usefulness of providing means at the time of donation for blood donors, who do not self-exclude but who have remaining doubts about their suitability, to designate that their donated unit not be used for transfusion;
—Implementing the use of a signed donor consent form in all blood banks that clearly indicates the absence of specific risk factors for transmission of infections;
• Continue to require that blood and plasma establishments maintain deferral lists of donors who have repeatedly reactive ELISA tests.

• Continue to encourage development and use of more sensitive serologic tests for HTLV-III/LAV infection.

• Recommend that current recommendations for HTLV-III antibody testing for donors of organs, tissues, cells, and semen be made mandatory.

• Encourage increased activities to eliminate unnecessary transfusions.

Patient Care and Health Care Needs

Over the period 1986 to 1991, AIDS and associated conditions will place an increasing burden on the health care delivery system through an increased number of patients and increased aggregate costs of care. The burden will be shared by a larger number of communities, including some which will have a less complete capacity for response. There will be increasing fragmentation and less health care control of services provided if more nonmedical, less traditional, and some unethical providers become involved.

PHS estimates that the direct health care costs of persons with AIDS will be between $8 and $16 billion in 1991. (The $8 billion figure is based on the projection of 71,000 AIDS patients alive in 1991 and 74,000 new cases by then. An additional 29,000 cases was added to account for the 20 percent underreporting or underascertainment of cases. The cost for treating a patient with AIDS used in the calculation was $46,000. For the higher range, the $8 billion figure was doubled.) These sums represents 1.2 to 2.4 percent of the expected total U.S. personal health care expenditures in 1991 of about $650 billion. Because people with AIDS are concentrated in certain urban centers, however, these costs will be disproportionately borne.

These estimates may be conservative by 10 to 50 percent because of the increased need for care for the large population of patients with the other conditions associated with HTLV-III/LAV infection and the significant nonmedical care costs necessary for management of these illnesses. Development of community-based health and social services support systems can reduce costs and enhance care during this 5-year period.

To improve care for AIDS patients, all sectors of the health care delivery system should work together to

• Develop a coordinated Federal, State, and local response to manage the health services and health financing crisis posed by the escalating AIDS epidemic. This response must reflect the pluralistic character of the American health care system and must involve the coordinated participation of the public, private, and voluntary sectors, as well as ambulatory, in-hospital, and long-term care providers;

• Explore the feasibility and need for convening a national, blue-ribbon commission representing the necessary constituencies to canvass needs and resources available and to make recommendations regarding how each sector of our society can help to fill financing and resource needs;

• Emphasize the needs of institutional and community-based providers for training, continuing education, and psychosocial support;

• Upon request, assist State and local governments and community-based organizations to assess, develop, and implement comprehensive service delivery systems of care for AIDS patients in a cost-effective manner;

• Develop organized consortia of service delivery systems responsive to the care of AIDS patients; such consortia should include all the necessary components of care (that is, ambulatory, hospital, mental health, and dental health services, counseling, home health care, and hospice care.)

• Explore efforts to set up regionalized consortia of services for AIDS patients;

• Utilize studies of the special health services needs and barriers to prevention of HTLV-III/LAV infection in blacks and Hispanics, and best methods of information dissemination to foster inclusion of culturally sensitive service delivery for children with AIDS, IV drugs abusers, hemophiliacs, and minorities in all appropriate metropolitan areas;

• Initiate demonstrations of the appropriate care needed at different stages of the illness, costs of services, and most cost effective provisions of needed services, including Model Medical Waiver programs; and

• Support health services research on AIDS that emphasizes cost of services for different risk groups, stages of illness, and treatment modalities and assesses potential improvement of methods and increased cost-effectiveness of care.

References ....

1. Public Health Service plan for the prevention and control of acquired immune deficiency syndrome (AIDS). Public Health Rep 100: 453-455, September-October 1985.
2. Coffin, J., et al.: Human immunodeficiency viruses. [Letter]. Science 232: 697, May 9, 1986.
3. Kinsey, A. C., Pomeroy, W. B., and Martin, C. E.: Sexual behavior in the human male. W. B. Saunders, Philadelphia, 1948.

H

List of Background Papers

The following background papers (listed alphabetically by author) were prepared for the Committee on a National Strategy for AIDS. Copies of the papers are available from the Institute of Medicine, 2101 Constitution Avenue, NW, Washington, DC 20418.

AIDS and Biomedical Research: A Comparative Analysis
  Evridiki Chatziandreou and John D. Graham, Ph.D.
Beyond the Political Model of Reporting: Non-Specific Symptoms in Media Communications About AIDS
  William A. Check, Ph.D.
Genetic Variation in AIDS Viruses
  John M. Coffin, Ph.D.
AIDS Among Intravenous Drug Users: Current Research in Epidemiology, Natural History, and Prevention Strategies
  Don C. Des Jarlais, Ph.D.
Animal Models for AIDS and Their Use for Vaccine and Drug Development
  Ronald C. Desrosiers, Ph.D., and Norman L. Letvin, M.D.
The Human T-Cell Lymphotropic Virus Type-III (HTLV-III) and Drug Abusers
  Harold M. Ginzburg, M.D., J.D., M.P.H., and Stanley H. Weiss, M.D.
The AIDS Epidemic: A Projection of Its Impact on Hospitals, 1986-1991
  Jesse Green, Ph.D., Madeleine Singer, M.P.H., and Neil Wintfeld, Ph.D.

Cultural Practices Contributing to the Transmission of AIDS in Africa
Daniel B. Hrdy, M.D., Ph.D.

Drug Use After Drug Abuse Treatment: Followup of 1979-1980 TOPS Admission Cohorts
Robert L. Hubbard, Ph.D., Mary Ellen Marsden, Ph.D., Elizabeth Cavanaugh, and J. Valley Rachal

The NIH Research Effort on AIDS: To What Extent Has It Been Achieved by Reprogramming Funds Originally Allotted for Other Purposes?
Richard M. Krause, M.D.

Ethical Dilemmas About Intensive Care in Patients with AIDS
Bernard Lo, M.D., Thomas A. Raffin, M.D., Neal H. Cohen, M.D., Robert M. Wachter, M.D., John M. Luce, M.D., and Philip C. Hopewell, M.D.

Neurological Manifestations of Human Immunodeficiency Virus Infections
Justin C. McArthur, M.B., B.S.

Models of AIDS in the Light of Other Natural Lentivirus Infections in Domestic Animals
Opendra Narayan, D.V.M., Ph.D.

Social Science Research Relating to AIDS: Existing Knowledge and Research Needs
Dorothy Nelkin, Ph.D.

An Overview of Pediatric AIDS: Approaches to Diagnosis and Outcome Assessment
Wade P. Parks, M.D., Ph.D., and Gwendolyn B. Scott, M.D.

Issues of Ethics, Cost, and the Utilization of Scarce Medical Resources in the Terminal Care of AIDS Patients
Thomas A. Raffin, M.D., and Bernard Lo, M.D.

Intensive Care for Patients with the Acquired Immunodeficiency Syndrome
Thomas A. Raffin, M.D., Bernard Lo, M.D., Robert M. Wachter, M.D., John M. Luce, M.D., and Neal H. Cohen, M.D.

Federal Funding for AIDS: Decision Process and Results
Michael Stoto, Ph.D., David Blumenthal, M.D., M.P.P., Jane S. Durch, M.A., and Penny H. Feldman, Ph.D.

Mechanisms of Cell Killing Cytopathic Effects by Retroviruses
Howard M. Temin, Ph.D.

Public Perceptions, Plural and Individual Behaviors in Response to AIDS Epidemic: Present Knowledge
Charles Turner, Ph.D.

Approaches to Understanding the Pathogenic Mechanisms in AIDS
Irving Weissman, M.D.

I

List of Presentations at Public Meetings

Following is a list of the presentations (arranged alphabetically by author) made at the two public meetings held by the Committee on a National Strategy for AIDS.

SAN FRANCISCO, CALIFORNIA, APRIL 8, 1986

Insurance; Screening Issues; AIDS in Prisons
  Chris Bowman, Concerned Republicans for Individual Rights
Federal Incentives for Vaccine Development, Education: Gaps in Federal Response
  Harry Britt, Supervisor, San Francisco
Insurance: Discrimination
  Larry Bush, Aide, and Art Agnos, California State Legislature
Need for State Health Department Involvement in Policy Formation
  Kristine M. Gebbie, Oregon State Health Division
A Public Health Policy Approach to Care and Treatment of AIDS Patients
  Hadley Hall, Visiting Nurses Association
The Role of the Community-Based Physician in the AIDS Crisis
  Richard Hamilton, San Francisco
Insurance Costs
  Carl Heimann, Schmidt & Schmidt Insurance Association
Public Education
  Luis Maura, AIDS Project Los Angeles

AIDS in the Workplace
  Nancy Merrit, Bank of America
Insurance Coverage
  Jim Spahr, Concerned Insurance Professionals for Human Rights
Screening Issues
  W. L. Warner, Bay Area Physicians for Human Rights
Intermediate and Long-Term Care Needs: Education
  David Werdegar, San Francisco Department of Public Health

NEW YORK CITY, MAY 15, 1986

Jim Campbell, private citizen
GMHC Activities
  Robert Cecchi, Gay Men's Health Crisis, Inc.
Public Education
  Reuben Dworski, Community Service Programs, AIDS Institute, New York State Department of Health
Developing Community-Based Outpatient Services for IV Drug Abuse AIDS Patients
  Charles Eaton, ADAPT, St. Luke's-Roosevelt Hospital Center
AIDS: Concerns of a Substance Abuse Agency
  L. Allen Grooms, Jr., The Washington Area Council on Drug Abuse, Inc.
AIDS Among IV Drug Abusers; Education of Female Sexual Partners
  Joyce Jackson, New Jersey State Department of Health
The New York City Response to AIDS: Strategies for Prevention and Provision of Health Care
  Stephan Joseph, New York City Department of Health
AIDS-Related Discrimination
  Mitchell Karp, Commission on Human Rights, City of New York
Need for Increased Federal Funding for Biomedical Research
  Mathilde Krim, American Foundation for AIDS Research
Long-Term Care Needs
  Harold Leeds, Village Nursing Home AIDS Project
Research Needs; Education; Access to Health Care; Social Issues
  Alvin Novick, American Association of Physicians for Human Rights
Volunteer Services for Minority Patients with AIDS
  Suki Parks, Minority Task Force on AIDS, The Council of Churches of the City of New York
Settlement of AIDS Disputes
  Robert E. Stein, Environmental Mediation International
Impact of AIDS on the Well Child
  Brenda Stoller, Nurses Network on AIDS

Dual Diagnosis: AIDS and Chemical Dependency
  Ron Vachon, National Association of Lesbian and Gay Alcoholism Professionals

Myths About Men: The Faulty Foundation of Public Health Policies to Counter AIDS
  Darrell Yates-Rist, Gay and Lesbian Alliance Against Defamation

J

Acknowledgments

The following list includes members of the Epidemiology Working Group, people who prepared background papers for or sent preprints to the Committee on a National Strategy for AIDS, and invited speakers at meetings. The committee extends its appreciation to all and apologizes for any inadvertent omissions.

EDMUND ABRAMOVITZ, New Jersey Hospital Association
GEORGE ALLEN, George Allen Associates, New York City
STEPHEN ANDERMAN, New York State Department of Health
PETER ARNO, University of California, San Francisco
JOAN ARON, The Johns Hopkins University School of Hygiene and
    Public Health, Baltimore, Md.
WILLIAM H. BANCROFT, Walter Reed Army Medical Center,
    Washington, D.C.
RONALD C. BAYER, The Hastings Center, Hastings-on-Hudson, N.Y.
MARY F. BELMONT, St. Luke's-Roosevelt Hospital, New York City
WILLIAM A. BLATNER, National Institutes of Health, Bethesda, Md.
DAVID BLUMENTHAL, John F. Kennedy School of Government,
    Cambridge, Mass.
KENT BOTTLES, University of California, San Francisco
SUSAN D. BROWN, Greater New York Hospital Association
DONALD BURKE, Walter Reed Army Medical Center, Washington,
    D.C.
ELIZABETH CAVANAUGH, Research Triangle Institute, Research
    Triangle Park, N.C.

339

EVRIDIKI CHATZIANDREOU, Harvard School of Public Health, Boston, Mass.
WILLIAM A. CHECK, Medical and Scientific Communications, Atlanta, Ga.
THOMAS J. COATES, University of California, San Francisco
JOHN M. COFFIN, Tufts University School of Medicine, Boston, Mass.
NEAL H. COHEN, University of California, San Francisco
JAMES CURRAN, Centers for Disease Control, Atlanta, Ga.
WENDY DAVIS, Health Resources and Services Administration, Washington, D.C.
WILLIAM DeJONG, Education Development Center, Inc., Newton, Mass.
DON C. DES JARLAIS, New York State Division of Substance Abuse Services, New York City
RONALD C. DESROSIERS, New England Regional Primate Research Center, Southboro, Mass.
MARGUERITE DONOGHUE, National Institutes of Health, Bethesda, Md.
WALTER DOWDLE, Public Health Service, Washington, D.C.
JANE S. DURCH, John F. Kennedy School of Government, Cambridge, Mass.
MAX ESSEX, Harvard School of Public Health, Boston, Mass.
ANTHONY FAUCI, National Institutes of Health, Bethesda, Md.
DOUGLAS FELDMAN, New York University, New York City
PENNY H. FELDMAN, John F. Kennedy School of Government, Cambridge, Mass.
PETER J. FISCHINGER, National Institutes of Health, Bethesda, Md.
DONALD P. FRANCIS, Department of Health Services, State of California, Berkeley
JEFFREY FRERICHS, Cabrini Medical Center, New York City
L. PATRICK GAGE, Hoffmann-La Roche, Inc., Nutley, N.J.
ROBERT GALLO, National Institutes of Health, Bethesda, Md.
MURRAY B. GARDNER, University of California, Davis
HAROLD M. GINZBURG, Public Health Service, Rockville, Md.
JOHN D. GRAHAM, Harvard School of Public Health, Boston, Mass.
PETER HARTSTOCK, Public Health Service, Rockville, Md.
WILLIAM A. HASELTINE, Harvard School of Public Health, Boston, Mass.
HARRY W. HAVERKOS, National Institutes of Health, Bethesda, Md.
KING HOLMES, University of Washington, Seattle
PHILIP C. HOPEWELL, San Francisco General Hospital Medical Center
DANIEL B. HRDY, University of California at Davis Medical Center, Sacramento

ROBERT L. HUBBARD, Research Triangle Institute, Research Triangle Park, N.C.

WILLIAM JARRETT, University of Glasgow, Scotland

ALBERT R. JONSEN, University of California, San Francisco

RICHARD A. KASLOW, National Institutes of Health, Bethesda, Md.

LEWIS KELLER, Association of California Life Insurance Companies, Sacramento

DANNIE KING, Burroughs Wellcome Company, Research Triangle Park, N.C.

RHONDA KOTELCHUCK, New York City Health and Hospital Corporation

IVAN KRAMER, University of Maryland, Baltimore

RICHARD M. KRAUSE, Emory University School of Medicine, Atlanta, Ga.

CLIFF LANE, National Institutes of Health, Bethesda, Md.

LAURENCE A. LASKY, Genentech, Inc., South San Francisco

PHILIP R. LEE, University of California, San Francisco

NORMAN L. LETVIN, New England Regional Primate Research Center, Southboro, Mass.

CAROL LEVINE, The Hastings Center, Hastings-on-Hudson, N.Y.

JAY LEVY, University of California, San Francisco

BERNARD LO, University of California, San Francisco

JOHN M. LUCE, San Francisco General Hospital Medical Center

PAUL LUCIW, Chiron Corporation, Emeryville, Calif.

MARY ELLEN MARSDEN, Research Triangle Institute, Research Triangle Park, N.C.

DAVID W. MARTIN, Genentech, Inc., South San Francisco

JEANNE PARKER MARTIN, Hospice of San Francisco

JUSTIN C. McARTHUR, The Johns Hopkins Hospital, Baltimore, Md.

PAUL R. McCURDY, National American Red Cross, Washington, D.C.

KENNETH McINTOSH, The Children's Hospital, Boston, Mass.

HARRY MEYERS, Food and Drug Administration, Rockville, Md.

MEADE MORGAN, Centers for Disease Control, Atlanta, Ga.

MAUREEN MYERS, National Institutes of Health, Bethesda, Md.

OPENDRA NARAYAN, The Johns Hopkins Hospital, Baltimore, Md.

NEIL NATHANSON, University of Pennsylvania, Philadelphia

ROBERT NEWMAN, Beth Israel Medical Center, New York City

JACK OBIJESKI, Genentech, Inc., South San Francisco

WADE P. PARKS, University of Miami School of Medicine, Fla.

B. FRANK POLK, The Johns Hopkins University School of Hygiene and Public Health, Baltimore, Md.

ISOBEL K. POLLACK, Health Insurance Plan of Greater New York

THOMAS QUINN, The Johns Hopkins Hospital, Baltimore, Md.

J. VALLEY RACHAL, Research Triangle Institute, Research Triangle Park, N.C.

THOMAS A. RAFFIN, Stanford University Medical Center

GEORGE B. RATHMANN, Amgen, Thousand Oaks, Calif.

ROBERT REDFIELD, Walter Reed Army Medical Center, Washington, D.C.

IRA REISS, University of Minnesota, Minneapolis

DOROTHY P. RICE, University of California, San Francisco

MERLE A. SANDE, University of California, San Francisco

HELEN SCHEITINGER, Shanti AIDS Resident Program, San Francisco

ANDY SCHNEIDER, Subcommitteee on Health and the Environment, U.S. House of Representatives, Washington, D.C.

NEIL R. SCHRAM, Kaiser Permanente, Harbor City, Calif.

ANNE A. SCITOVSKY, Palo Alto Medical Research Foundation

GWENDOLYN B. SCOTT, University of Miami School of Medicine

MADELEINE SINGER, New York University Medical Center, New York City

JANE SISK, Office of Technology Assessment, U.S. Congress, Washington, D.C.

DAVID W. SMITH, St. Clare's Hospital and Health Center, New York City

MICHAEL STOTO, John F. Kennedy School of Government, Cambridge, Mass.

DANIEL SUSOTT, New York City Health and Hospital Corporation, New York City

CHARLES TURNER, National Research Council, National Academy of Sciences, Washington, D.C.

PABLO VALENZUELA, Chiron Corporation, Emeryville, Calif.

HAROLD E. VARMUS, University of California, San Francisco

JOHN VASCONCELLOS, California State Assembly, San Jose

BRUCE C. VLADECK, United Hospital Fund of New York, New York City

ROBERT M. WACHTER, San Francisco General Hospital Medical Center

ROGER WEAVING, St. Vincent's Hospital and Medical Center of New York

STANLEY H. WEISS, National Institutes of Health, Bethesda, Md.

WARREN WINKELSTEIN, University of California, Berkeley

NEIL WINTFELD, New York University Medical Center, New York City

CONSTANCE WOFSY, University of California, San Francisco

SUSAN WOLF, The Hastings Center, Hastings-on-Hudson, N.Y.

TIM WOLFRED, San Francisco AIDS Foundation

K

Biographical Notes on Committee Members

DAVID BALTIMORE is director of the Whitehead Institute for Biomedical Research and professor of biology at the Massachusetts Institute of Technology. From 1974 until 1982, when he was named director of the institute, he was with the Center for Cancer Research of the Massachusetts Institute of Technology. He has taught in the Department of Biology at the Massachusetts Institute of Technology since being appointed to the faculty in 1968. In 1975 he received the Nobel Prize, along with Howard Temin and Renato Dulbecco, for the discovery of reverse transcriptase and for related work on retroviruses. That same year he was an organizer of the Asilomar Conference in California, which focused attention on the development of genetic engineering, and he was later a member of the National Institutes of Health Recombinant DNA Advisory Committee. Dr. Baltimore received his B.A. degree in chemistry from Swarthmore College and his Ph.D. in biology from Rockefeller University.

JOHN J. BURNS is an adjunct member of the Roche Institute of Molecular Biology and adjunct professor of the Rockefeller University. From 1967 to 1984 he was vice president of research and development at Hoffmann-La Roche, Inc., Nutley, New Jersey. Prior to that time, he was director of research at Wellcome Research Laboratory, Tuckahoe, New York, and deputy chief of the Laboratory of Chemical Pharmacology, National Heart Institute. Dr. Burns is a member of the National Academy of Sciences and of the Institute of Medicine and has served as president of the International Union of Pharmacology, president of the American Society for Pharmacology and Experimental Therapeutics, chairman of the Committee on Problems of Drug Safety of the National Research Council, senior consultant to the Pharmacology-Toxicology Program, National Institute of General Medical Sciences, and member of the National Advisory Food and Drug Committee of the Department of Health, Education, and Welfare. His research interests have been the metabolic fate of drugs, drug interactions, the metabolism of vitamin C, and the pharmacology of recombinant DNA products. Dr. Burns received a B.S. degree from Queens College and a Ph.D. in chemistry from Columbia University.

JAMES CHIN is chief of the Infectious Disease Branch of the California State Department of Health Services and clinical professor of epidemiology at the School of Public Health, University of California, Berkeley. He has served on several national committees related to infectious disease control, including the Committee on Infectious Diseases of the American Public Health Association, the National Advisory Committee on Immunization Practices, and the Armed Forces Epidemiology Board. He received a B.S. degree from the University of Michigan, an M.D. from the State University of New York, Downstate, and an M.P.H. from the School of Public Health, University of California, Berkeley.

WILLIAM J. CURRAN is Frances Glessner Lee Professor of Legal Medicine in the faculties of both medicine and public health at Harvard University. Before that he was a lecturer in legal medicine at Harvard Law School and a professor at Boston University in both the law and medical schools. He is widely known for his regular column, "Law-Medicine Notes," in the *New England Journal of Medicine* and also practices law in Boston as counsel and specialist in health care and hospital law with the firm of Warner and Stackpole. He is an adviser on health legislation for the World Health Organization and has engaged in research and investigation for the WHO in many countries. In public offices he served as chairman from 1978 to 1982 of the Massachusetts Commission on Medicolegal Investigation and was a member in the 1970s of the Secretary's Commission on Medical Malpractice, U.S. Department of Health, Education, and Welfare. He received his undergraduate and J.D. degrees from Boston College, his LL.M. from Harvard Law School, and an S.M. in hygiene from the Harvard School of Public Health.

LEON EISENBERG is Maude and Lillian Presley Professor and chairman of the Department of Social Medicine and Health Policy and professor of psychiatry at the Harvard Medical School in Boston, Massachusetts. Prior to his move to Boston in 1967, he was professor of child psychiatry at the Johns Hopkins University School of Medicine. His research interests center on the role of social factors as determinants of health and illness. He is a member of the Institute of Medicine, has served on the Advisory Committee to the Director of the National Institutes of Health, and is a consultant to the Division of Mental Health of the World Health Organization. He received his A.B. and M.D. degrees from the University of Pennsylvania.

BERNARD N. FIELDS is professor and chairman of the Department of Microbiology and Molecular Genetics at Harvard Medical School, a position he has held since 1982. His research has focused on the molecular basis of viral pathogenesis. He has served on a number of scientific advisory boards, was chairman of the Experimental Virology Study Section of the National Institutes of Health, and is an editor of the *Journal of Virology*. He is a member of the National Academy of Sciences. He received his M.D. degree from New York University Medical School and his B.A. from Brandeis University.

HARVEY V. FINEBERG is dean of the Harvard School of Public Health. A graduate of Harvard Medical School and the John F. Kennedy School of Government, he was formerly director of the Graduate Program in Health Policy and Management at the Harvard School of Public Health and professor of health policy and management. On July 1, 1984, he assumed the deanship of the school. As a member of the Public Health Council of Massachusetts from 1976 to 1979, he participated in decision making on matters of hospital investment and health policy. In 1982 he was appointed to a three-year term as chairman of the Health Care Technology Study Section of the National Center for Health Services Research. He has also served as a consultant to the World Health Organization, and recently he chaired the Massachusetts Task Force on Liver Transplantation. Dean Fineberg's research has addressed several areas of health policy, including the processes of policy development and implementation, assessment of medical technology, and dissemination of medical innovations. Some of his research involves the application of decision analysis and cost-effectiveness evaluation to medical practices. Dean Fineberg helped found and has served as president of the Society of Medical Decision Making and is a member of the Institute of Medicine. He is the coauthor of two books, *Clinical Decision Analysis* and *The Epidemic That Never Was*, an analysis of the controversial federal immunization program against swine flu in 1976.

DAVID W. FRASER is president of Swarthmore College and adjunct professor of medicine at the University of Pennsylvania. For nine years he was an epidemiologist with the Centers for Disease Control, where his work focused on emerging diseases, such as Legionnaire's disease, toxic shock syndrome, and Lassa fever. He has also served as a medical epidemiologic consultant to the Office of Management and Budget. He received his M.D. degree from Harvard Medical School and his B.A. degree from Haverford College.

J. THOMAS GRAYSTON is professor of epidemiology and pathobiology in the School of Public Health and Community Medicine, University of Washington, Seattle. His research, which has been on a variety of infectious diseases both in the United States and the Far East, has for many years concentrated on chlamydial infections. From 1971 until 1983 he served as vice president for health sciences at the University of Washington. He is a member of the Institute of Medicine and has served on a number of advisory boards, committees, and consultative groups related to infectious disease research and to health professions education. Dr. Grayston received his M.D. degree and residency and fellowship training at the University of Chicago.

JEROME E. GROOPMAN is associate professor of medicine at Harvard Medical School and chief of the Division of Hematology/Oncology at the New England Deaconess Hospital. He has been an active clinical and laboratory researcher in AIDS since the recognition of the disease in 1980. His major contributions include epidemiologic studies of heterosexual transmission of the virus, transfusion-associated AIDS, and infection of different body fluids. He has developed an assay for neutralizing antibodies to HIV that may prove useful in formulating a prototype subunit vaccine. He has published extensively on testing of new drugs for AIDS and ARC and has conducted the first randomized prospective study of recombinant alpha-2A interferon in Kaposi's sarcoma and AIDS. He is also on the editorial board of *Blood*.

JEFFREY E. HARRIS is professor in the Department of Economics at the Massachusetts Institute of Technology and a practicing internist at the Massachusetts General Hospital. He has served on the Diesel Impacts Study Committee of the National Research Council and on the Committee on Strategies to Reduce the Incidence of Low Birthweight of the Institute of Medicine. He has been a contributor, consulting editor, and senior reviewer to several Surgeon General's reports on smoking and health. He has written widely on medical economics and public health, including a monograph issued by the National Research Council on the potential risk of lung cancer from diesel engine emissions. Dr. Harris received his A.B. degree from Harvard University and his Ph.D. and M.D. degrees from the University of Pennsylvania.

MAURICE R. HILLEMAN is director of the Merck Institute for Therapeutic Research and adjunct professor of pediatrics at the School of Medicine of the University of Pennsylvania, Philadelphia. From 1948 to 1958 he was chief of the Department of Respiratory Diseases, Walter Reed Army Institute of Research, Washington, D.C. He has published more than 400 original articles in the fields of virology, immunology, epidemiology, and infectious diseases. He has served on numerous advisory boards and committees, academic and governmental, and has been a member of the Expert Advisory Panel of the World Health Organization, Geneva, since 1952. He received the Lasker Medical Research Award in 1983 and is a member of the National Academy of Sciences. Dr. Hilleman received his B.S. degree from Montana State University in 1941 and a Ph.D. from the University of Chicago in 1944. He holds several honorary doctorate degrees.

RICHARD T. JOHNSON is Eisenhower Professor of Neurology and professor of microbiology and neuroscience at the Johns Hopkins University School of Medicine. He is a neurologist at the Johns Hopkins Hospital and holds a joint appointment in the Johns Hopkins School of Hygiene and Public Health. His research has been on the pathogenesis of acute and chronic viral infections of the nervous system. He has served on and chaired advisory boards for federal and voluntary agencies and has served on editorial boards of 15 scientific journals. He received his A.B. and M.D. degrees from the University of Colorado.

ARTHUR LIFSON is a vice president of the Equitable Life Assurance Society of the United States. He is responsible for government relations for Equitable Group and Health Insurance Company, which is a division of Equitable. Prior to joining Equitable in 1972, he was assistant director of the Northeast Ohio Regional Medical Program. Mr. Lifson is a gubernatorial appointee to the Health Care Financing Council of New York State and a member of the boards of directors of the National Health Council, Elderplan, Grantmakers in Health, and the Metropolitan Jewish Geriatric Center. He chairs and serves on a variety of committees of various health-related organizations and trade groups. He has written in the areas of long-term care, health education, and health economics. He received a B.S. degree from Hunter College and an M.S. from Case Western Reserve University.

FRANK LILLY is professor and chairman of the Department of Genetics, Albert Einstein College of Medicine, where most of his scientific work has been performed. His studies have been mainly in the areas of oncogenetics and immunovirology. He obtained his B.S. degree from

West Virginia University and, after a period of study at the University of Paris, received his Ph.D. degree from Cornell Medical College. He is a member of the National Academy of Sciences and of the Board of Directors of the Gay Men's Health Crisis, New York City.

ROBERT F. MURRAY, Jr., is professor of pediatrics and medicine, professor of oncology, and professor and chairman of genetics and human genetics at Howard University College of Medicine in Washington, D.C. His professional activities have included many appointments as chair or member of advisory bodies on bioethics, genetics, sickle-cell anemia, and the like for organizations including the National Research Council, the National Foundation-March of Dimes, and the National Institute for General Medical Sciences. A member of the Institute of Medicine, he has served on its governing council, has held a year-long appointment as its senior scholar-in-residence, has served on several of its study committees, and chaired the IOM study on health and performance of airline pilots related to age. He holds a baccalaureate degree from Union College, and an M.D. from the University of Rochester. He also holds a degree in genetics from the University of Washington and occupied a Rotary Foundation Fellowship in biochemistry at the University of Heidelberg.

DOROTHY NELKIN is a professor in the Program on Science, Technology, and Society and in the Department of Sociology of Cornell University. Her research focuses on the social and political implications of controversial areas in science, technology, and medicine and on the process of decision making in complex technical areas. She is on the Board of Directors of the American Association for the Advancement of Science (AAAS), Medicine in the Public Interest, and the Council for the Advancement of Science Writing. She is also a fellow of the Hastings Center and of the AAAS and was a Guggenheim Fellow in 1984. She has served as an adviser and consultant to several organizations, including the National Academy of Sciences, the Office of Technology Assessment, the National Council on Health Technology, and the Milbank Memorial Fund. Her books include *Controversy: The Politics of Technical Decisions, Science as Intellectual Property, The Creation Controversy, Workers at Risk,* and *Selling Science: How the Press Covers Science and Technology.*

JUNE E. OSBORN is dean of the University of Michigan School of Public Health and professor of epidemiology, pediatrics, and communicable diseases at the University of Michigan Medical School. From 1966 to 1984 she was on the faculty of the University of Wisconsin Medical School as professor of medical microbiology and pediatrics, and from 1975 she served as associate dean of the Graduate School for Biological Sciences at the University of Wisconsin, Madison. She has served in a number of advisory capacities to the Food and Drug Administration, the National Institutes of Health, the U.S. Public Health Service, and the World Health Organization and is a member of the Institute of Medicine. She received her M.D. degree from Case Western Reserve Medical School, did pediatric training at the Boston Children's and Massachusetts General hospitals, and trained in virology and infectious diseases at the Johns Hopkins University and the University of Pittsburgh.

SAMUEL W. PERRY is associate professor of psychiatry at Cornell University Medical Center and associate director of the consultation-liaison division of the New York Hospital. As a certified psychoanalyst and a federally funded principal investigator, he has been interested over the past 10 years in the interface between mind and body, especially in the areas of narcotic analgesics, psychoimmunology, and most recently HIV-related disorders. He has published more than 150 articles in these areas as well as two recent books on treatment selection in psychiatry. Dr. Perry received his A.B. degree from Princeton University and his M.D. degree and psychoanalytic training at Columbia University, where he continues to teach.

ROLAND K. ROBINS is a vice president of ICN Pharmaceuticals, Inc., and vice president and director of Molecular Research Institute, Costa Mesa, California. He is also an adjunct professor of microbiology and molecular genetics at the University of California, Irvine, an adjunct professor of chemistry at Brigham Young University, and a former director of the Cancer Research Center of Brigham Young University. Dr. Robins has published extensively in the field of heterocyclic compounds, nucleosides, and nucleotides as medicinal agents that selectively inhibit specific aspects of nucleic acid metabolism. His research has resulted in the synthesis of a number of drugs that are being used clinically or are under clinical evaluation in the United States or abroad. He received his Ph.D. from Oregon State University and is especially well known for his work in the fields of cancer chemotherapy and antiviral agents. From 1964 to 1969 he was a professor of chemistry and medicinal chemistry at the University of Utah, and from 1976 to 1985 he was professor of chemistry and biochemistry at Brigham Young University. He is an assistant editor of the *Journal of Heterocyclic Chemistry* and serves on the editorial board of the *Journal of Nucleosides and Nucleo-*

tides, the *Journal of Cyclic Nucleotide and Protein Phosphorylation*, and *Current Abstracts of Chemistry and Index Chemicus*. He is a member of the Board of Directors of Viratek, Inc.

MARGERY W. SHAW is professor and senior scholar in the Health Law Program at the University of Texas Health Science Center at Houston, and adjunct professor of health law at the University of Houston Law Center. She has served visiting professorships at Yale University, the University of North Carolina, and the University of Utah and is Andrew D. White Professor-at-Large at Cornell University. She is past president of the American Society of Human Genetics and the Genetics Society of America, is a fellow of the American College of Legal Medicine, and is on the American Board of Medical Genetics and the board of the American Society of Law and Medicine. She has served on the Director's Advisory Committee of the National Institutes of Health and on several National Research Council committees. She is on the editorial board of the *American Journal of Medical Genetics* and the *American Journal of Law and Medicine* and has edited three books. She has written more than 200 publications on chromosomal research and disorders and on health law issues concerning reproductive alternatives, privacy and confidentiality, wrongful life, and fetal abuse. She received an A.B. degree from the University of Alabama, an M.A. from Columbia University, an M.D. from the University of Michigan, and a J.D. from the University of Houston, and she has honorary D.Sc. degrees from the University of Evansville and the University of Southern Indiana.

P. FREDERICK SPARLING is J. Herbert Bate Professor and chairman of the Department of Microbiology and Immunology at the University of North Carolina School of Medicine, a position he has held since 1981. He is also professor of medicine and former chief of the Division of Infectious Disease in the Department of Medicine at the University of North Carolina at Chapel Hill. His research has focused on the molecular basis of antibiotic resistance and bacterial pathogenesis. He has had a long-standing interest in sexually transmitted diseases and is coeditor of a recent major textbook on this subject. He has served on a number of scientific advisory boards, was chairman of the Bacteriology and Mycology Study Section, and is a councillor of the Infectious Diseases Society of America. He received his M.D. degree from Harvard University and his B.A. from Princeton University.

CLADD E. STEVENS is a senior investigator and head of the Laboratory of Epidemiology at the New York Blood Center. She trained in pediatrics and in public health at the University of Washington, Seattle.

She began research in viral hepatitis as a consultant to the U.S. Navy Medical Research Unit No. 2 in Taiwan while a postdoctoral fellow at the University of Washington. In 1975 she joined the late Wolf Szmuness at the New York Blood Center, where she helped to run efficacy trials of hepatitis B vaccine. In addition to continued research on viral hepatitis and immunoprophylaxis, her recent research has focused on the epidemiology of AIDS. Dr. Stevens received a B.A. degree from Pomona College, an M.D. from Baylor College of Medicine, and an M.P.H. from the University of Washington.

HOWARD M. TEMIN is American Cancer Society Professor of Viral Oncology, Harold P. Rusch Professor of Cancer Research, and Steenbock Professor of Biological Sciences at the University of Wisconsin School of Medicine, Madison, where he has been since 1960. He has worked on retroviruses continuously since 1956, when he was a graduate student at the California Institute of Technology. In 1975 he received the Nobel Prize, along with David Baltimore and Renato Dulbecco, for some of this work. He is a member of the National Academy of Sciences and has served on the National Institutes of Health Virology Study Section and on the editorial boards of several virology journals.

PAUL VOLBERDING is associate professor of medicine at the University of California, San Francisco, and chief of the Medical Oncology Division and AIDS Activities Division at San Francisco General Hospital. During the past several years he has served on a variety of committees on AIDS for the city of San Francisco and the state of California, and he is a member of the National Institutes of Health Executive Committee. Dr. Volberding is actively involved in the provision of care to ARC and AIDS patients and undertakes clinical research in the treatment of HIV infection and Kaposi's sarcoma. He received an A.B. from the University of Chicago and an M.D. from the University of Minnesota.

LeROY WALTERS is director of the Center for Bioethics at the Kennedy Institute of Ethics and associate professor of philosophy at Georgetown University in Washington, D.C. He is coeditor of two books, the annual *Bibliography of Bioethics* and an anthology entitled *Contemporary Issues in Bioethics*. He is a member of the National Institutes of Health Recombinant DNA Advisory Committee and chairs the committee's Subcommittee on Human Gene Therapy. In 1976 and 1977 Dr. Walters chaired the Work Group on Informed Consent for the national immunization policy studies conducted by the Assistant Secretary for Health. From 1979 to 1981 he was a member of the National Council for Health Care Technology. He has served as a consultant to the National

Commission for the Protection of Human Subjects, the Department of Health, Education, and Welfare Ethics Advisory Board, and the President's Commission on Bioethics. Dr. Walters is an ethicist who received his Ph.D. degree from Yale University.

IRVING WEISSMAN is professor of pathology and biology at Stanford University. His research concerns the normal, pathologic, and neoplastic development and function of the central cells of the immune system—the T and B lymphocytes. He also studies the retroviruses that cause T- and B-cell malignancies. A member of the faculty at Stanford since 1968, Dr. Weissman is coauthor of two textbooks on immunology. He has served on several review committees and study sections for the National Institutes of Health, the American Cancer Society, and the Howard Hughes Medical Institute. He is on the editorial board of several journals in the fields of immunology, developmental biology, and cellular biology and is currently a member of the directorate of the Stanford Center for Molecular and Genetic Medicine. He received a B.S. from Montana State University and an M.D. from Stanford University.

SHELDON M. WOLFF is Endicott Professor and chairman of the Department of Medicine, Tufts University School of Medicine, and physician-in-chief at the New England Medical Center Hospital. Dr. Wolff received his B.S. degree from the University of Georgia, his M.D. degree from Vanderbilt University School of Medicine, and an honorary doctorate from the Federal University, Rio de Janeiro, Brazil. From 1960 through 1977 Dr. Wolff worked at the National Institute of Allergy and Infectious Diseases (NIAID), and for the last 10 years of his stay there he was clinical director of NIAID and chief of the Laboratory of Clinical Investigation. Dr. Wolff's research has dealt with the biological properties of bacterial endotoxins and, in particular, with the pathogenesis of fever. In addition, he has published widely on host defenses and responses to infectious diseases. He is a member of the Institute of Medicine, past president of the Infectious Diseases Society of America, past chairman of the Subspecialty Board of Infectious Diseases, and a member of the Board of Governors of the American Board of Internal Medicine. Dr. Wolff is a member of the advisory council of NIAID and was chairman of the Institute of Medicine-National Academy of Sciences Committee on the Toxic Shock Syndrome.

Glossary

Acquired immune deficiency syndrome (AIDS). A severe manifestation of infection with human immunodeficiency virus (HIV).

Active surveillance. The process of actively seeking out and identifying health problems within a population. (*See also* Passive surveillance.)

AIDS-related complex (ARC). A variety of chronic symptoms and physical findings that occur in some persons who are infected with HIV but do not meet the Centers for Disease Control's definition of AIDS. Symptoms may include chronic swollen glands, recurrent fevers, unintentional weight loss, chronic diarrhea, lethargy, minor alterations of the immune system (less severe than those that occur in AIDS), and oral thrush. ARC may or may not develop into AIDS.

Antibody. A protein in the blood produced in response to exposure to specific foreign molecules. Antibodies neutralize toxins and interact with other components of the immune system to eliminate infectious microorganisms from the body.

Antigen. A substance that stimulates the production of antibodies.

ARV (AIDS-associated retrovirus). Name given by researchers at the University of California at San Francisco to isolates of the retrovirus that causes AIDS.

Autologous transfusion. A blood transfusion in which the patient receives his or her own blood, donated several weeks before elective surgery.

353

B lymphocyte (or B cell). A type of white blood cell that produces antibody in response to stimulation by an antigen.

Candida albicans. A yeastlike fungus that causes whitish sores in the mouth. The infection is called candidiasis or, more commonly, thrush. In AIDS patients, candidiasis often extends into the esophagus.

Case-control study. A design for epidemiologic studies that matches individuals with a disease or health problem (cases) with others who do not have that condition (controls). Frequently, individuals included in the study are matched for factors such as age, race, socioeconomic status, occupation, and area of residence. Comparisons are then made between the two groups.

Casual contact. Refers to day-to-day interactions between HIV-infected individuals and others in the home, at school, or in the workplace. It does not include intimate contact, such as sexual or drug use interactions, and it implies closer contact than chance passing on a street or sharing a subway car.

CD4 lymphocyte or CD4 T cell. A T lymphocyte that expresses the cell surface marker molecule CD4. The majority of these cells are thought to consist of helper/inducer lymphocytes, which play important regulatory roles in the human immune system. These cells appear to be the primary targets for infection by HIV.

CD8 lymphocyte or CD8 T cell. A T lymphocyte that expresses the cell surface marker molecule CD8. The majority of these cells are thought to consist of suppressor/cytotoxic lymphocytes, which play important regulatory and functional roles in the human immune system.

Cell-mediated immunity. A defense mechanism involving the coordinated activity of two subpopulations of T lymphocytes, helper T cells and killer T cells. Helper T cells produce a variety of substances that stimulate and regulate other participants in the immune response. Killer T lymphocytes destroy cells in the body that bear foreign antigens (e.g., cells that are infected with viruses or other microorganisms).

Cofactor. A factor other than the basic causative agent of a disease that increases the likelihood of developing that disease. Cofactors may include the presence of other microorganisms or psychosocial factors, such as stress.

Cryptosporidium. A protozoan parasite that causes severe, protracted diarrhea. In persons with a normal immune system, the diarrhea is self-limited and lasts one to two weeks. In AIDS patients, the diarrhea often becomes chronic and may lead to severe malnutrition.

Cytomegalovirus (CMV). A virus that belongs to the herpesvirus group.

Prior to the appearance of AIDS, it was most commonly associated with a severe congenital infection of infants and with life-threatening infections in patients who had undergone bone marrow transplants and other procedures requiring suppression of the immune system. It rarely causes disease in healthy adults. In AIDS patients, CMV may produce pneumonia, as well as inflammation of the retina, liver, kidneys, and colon.

Cytopathic. Disease-induced or disease-inducing changes to cells.

DNA (deoxyribonucleic acid). A nucleic acid found chiefly in the nucleus of living cells that is responsible for transmitting hereditary characteristics.

ELISA. An acronym for "enzyme-linked immunosorbent assay," a test used to detect antibodies against HIV in blood samples.

Encephalitis. Inflammation of the brain.

Encephalopathy. Any degenerative disease of the brain.

End-stage renal disease (ESRD). A collection of diseases affecting the kidney and resulting in the failure of that organ, necessitating hemodialysis or transplantation to sustain life.

Epstein-Barr virus. A member of the herpes group of viruses and the principal cause of infectious mononucleosis in young adults. It also has been implicated as a causal factor in the development of Burkitt's lymphoma in Africa.

False negative. A negative test result for a condition that in fact is present.

False positive. A positive test result for a condition that in fact is not present.

Frank AIDS. Those cases of infection with HIV meeting the Centers for Disease Control's definition of AIDS.

Genome. The genetic endowment of an organism.

Gold standard. In medical testing, an independent means of unequivocally verifying the presence or absence of the condition being tested for.

Hemophilia. A rare, hereditary bleeding disorder of males, inherited through the mother, caused by a deficiency in the ability to make one or more blood-clotting proteins.

Herpes simplex. An acute disease caused by herpes simplex viruses types 1 and 2. Groups of watery blisters, often painful, form on the skin and mucous membranes, especially the borders of the lips (cold sores) or the mucous surface of the genitals.

Herpesvirus group. A group of viruses that includes the herpes simplex viruses, the varicella-zoster virus (the cause of chicken pox and shingles), cytomegalovirus, and Epstein-Barr virus.

HIV (human immunodeficiency virus). The name proposed for the causative agent of AIDS by a subcommittee of the International Committee on the Taxonomy of Viruses. (*See also* ARV, HTLV-III, and LAV.)

HTLV-III (human T-cell lymphotropic virus type III). The name given by researchers at the National Cancer Institute to isolates of the retrovirus that causes AIDS.

Humoral immunity. The human defense mechanism that involves the production of antibodies and associated molecules present in body fluids such as serum and lymph.

Immune system. The natural system of defense mechanisms, in which specialized cells and proteins in the blood and other body fluids work together to eliminate disease-producing microorganisms and other foreign substances.

Interferons. A class of proteins important in immune function and known to inhibit certain viral infections.

Interleukin-2. A substance produced by T lymphocytes that stimulates activated T lymphocytes and some activated B lymphocytes to proliferate. Also known as T-cell growth factor.

In vitro. Literally, within glass. The term refers to those experiments conducted in tissue culture or another artificial environment.

In vivo. Literally, within a living body. The term refers to those experiments conducted in animals or humans.

Interstitial pneumonitis. Localized acute inflammation of the lung. Interstitial pneumonitis persisting for more than two months in a child (under 13 years of age) is indicative of AIDS unless another cause is identified or tests for HIV are negative.

Intravenous. Injected into or delivered through a needle in a vein.

Kaposi's sarcoma. A cancer or tumor of the blood and/or lymphatic vessel walls. It usually appears as blue-violet to brownish skin blotches or bumps. Before the appearance of AIDS, it was rare in the United States and Europe, where it occurred primarily in men over age 50 or 60, usually of Mediterranean origin. AIDS-associated Kaposi's sarcoma is much more aggressive than the earlier form of the disease.

LAV (lymphadenopathy-associated virus). The name given by French researchers to the first reported isolate of the retrovirus now known to cause AIDS. This retrovirus was recovered from a person with lymphadenopathy (enlarged lymph nodes) who also was in a group at high risk for AIDS.

Lentiviruses. A subfamily of retroviruses that includes the visna viruses of sheep, the equine infectious anemia virus of horses, and the caprine arthritis-encephalitis virus of goats. Most researchers believe that HIV, the cause of AIDS, also belongs to this subfamily. The animal lentiviruses produce diverse chronic diseases in their natural hosts, but all cause encephalitis. The diseases are characterized by erratic relapses and remissions. The visna viruses cause a chronic interstitial pneumonitis similar to that seen in AIDS virus infections in infants. Lentiviruses persist in the body by evading natural defense mechanisms; the chronic carrier state—in which infected animals do not get sick themselves but can transmit the virus to other animals—is common.

Macrophage. A type of white blood cell that has the capacity to ingest or phagocytize foreign particulate matter, such as bacteria.

Mitogen. A substance that induces cell division.

Monocyte. A phagocytic white blood cell that engulfs and destroys bacteria and other disease-producing microorganisms. It produces interleukin-1, a substance that activates T lymphocytes in the presence of antigen.

Mycobacterium avium-intracellulare. A bacterium related to the organism that causes tuberculosis in humans, rarely seen by physicians prior to the appearance of AIDS. In AIDS patients it may cause a disseminated disease that responds poorly to therapy.

Oncoviruses. A subfamily of retroviruses that includes tumor-causing agents such as the Rous sarcoma virus and the bovine leukemia virus.

Opportunistic infection. An infection caused by a microorganism that rarely causes disease in persons with normal defense mechanisms.

Parenteral. Involving introduction into the bloodstream.

Passive surveillance. The process of monitoring health problems through the receipt of reports on those problems. (*See also* Active surveillance.)

Persistent generalized lymphadenopathy (PGL). A condition characterized by persistent, generalized swollen glands in the absence of any current illness or drug use known to cause such symptoms.

Phagocyte. A cell in blood or tissues that binds to, engulfs, and destroys microorganisms, damaged cells, and foreign particles.

Pneumocystis carinii ***pneumonia.*** The most common life-threatening opportunistic infection diagnosed in AIDS patients. It is caused by the parasite *Pneumocystis carinii.*

Prospective cohort study. A design for epidemiologic studies that follows a group of similar individuals over time, noting who develops the health problem of interest and who does not and comparing these two groups at the end of the study.

Provirus. A copy of the genetic information of an animal virus that is integrated into the DNA of an infected cell. Copies of the provirus are passed on to each of the infected cell's daughter cells.

Retrovirus. A class of viruses that contain the genetic material RNA and that have the capability to copy this RNA into DNA inside an infected cell. The resulting DNA is incorporated into the genetic structure of the cell in the form of a provirus.

Reverse transcriptase. An enzyme produced by retroviruses that allows them to produce a DNA copy of their RNA. This is the first step in the virus's natural cycle of reproduction.

RNA (ribonucleic acid). A nucleic acid associated with the control of chemical activities inside a cell. One type of RNA transfers information from the cell's DNA to the protein-forming system of a cell outside the nucleus. Some viruses carry RNA instead of the more familiar genetic material DNA.

Sensitivity. In serologic testing, the percentage of people who test positive who in fact do have the condition being tested for. (*See also* Specificity.)

Seroconversion. The initial development of antibodies specific to a particular antigen.

Serologic study. A study that compares the characteristics of the serum of individuals, especially those markers in blood that indicate exposure to a particular agent of disease.

Seropositive. In the context of HIV, the condition in which antibodies to the virus are found in the blood.

Shooting galleries. Locations where drug addicts gather for the administration of illicit drugs, often with sharing of injection equipment.

Specificity. In serologic testing, the percentage of people who test negative who in fact do not have the condition being tested for. (*See also* Sensitivity.)

Subunit vaccine. A vaccine that contains only portions of a surface molecule of a disease-producing microorganism.

Syndrome. A pattern of symptoms and signs, appearing one by one or simultaneously, that together characterize a particular disease or disorder.

T lymphocyte (or T cell). A cell that matures in the thymus gland. T lymphocytes are found primarily in the blood, lymph, and lymphoid organs. Subsets of T cells have a variety of specialized functions within the immune system.

T4 lymphocyte (or T4 cell). A synonym for CD4 T cell.

T8 lymphocyte (or T8 cell). A synonym for CD8 T cell.

Toxoplasma gondii. A protozoan parasite that is one of the most common causes of inflammation of the brain in AIDS patients. The infection is called toxoplasmosis.

Viremia. The presence of virus in circulating blood, which implies active viral replication.

Virion. A complete virus particle.

Western blot technique. A test that involves the identification of antibodies against specific protein molecules. This test is believed to be more specific than the ELISA test in detecting antibodies to HIV in blood samples; it is also more difficult to perform and considerably more expensive. Western blot analysis is used by some laboratories as a confirmatory test on samples found to be repeatedly reactive on ELISA tests.

Index

A

Acquired immune deficiency syndrome
(AIDS)
age, race, and sex trends, 72
cases by risk group, 70
causes of, 38-42, 60
clinical manifestations, 38, 47, 74-75
coordination of public resources against,
93-94
definition/defining, 7, 37, 46, 48, 63-64,
117, 316-319
diagnosis of, 49, 64, 72
disease presentation, 72-73
doubling time for cases, 70, 71
enteropathic, 75
epidemiologic and natural history studies
of, 66-67
geographic differences in clinical
manifestations, 46, 273
geographic distribution, 71-72
impediments to national involvement
with, 92-93; see also Fear of AIDS
incubation time for, 70
infections associated with, see
Opportunistic infections
international scope of, 29, 73-77; see
also specific countries/regions
involvement of disseminated sites, 45
malignancies associated with, 48, 292

media treatment of, 99
mortality, 72-73
National Commission on AIDS, 32-33,
94
natural history of, 44-46, 87
number of cases in U.S., 5, 7
pathogenesis of, 5-6, 141, 188
pattern of spread, 39
PHS plan for prevention and control of,
8-9, 85-86, 88, 91, 93-94, 326-333
projected cases and deaths, 5, 86
psychiatric/psychological problems
posed by, 148-149
remission of, 7, 46
reporting of, see Reporting of AIDS/HIV
infection
resources for dealing with, 92-94; see
also International resources for
fighting AIDS; Private resources for
fighting AIDS; Public resources for
fighting AIDS
risk population trends, 57-63; see also
High-risk groups; and specific
populations
sex education in schools, 11, 102; see
also Public education about AIDS
underreporting of, 14, 64, 88, 118, 159;
see also Epidemiologic surveillance
see also HIV infection; Human
immunodeficiency virus; Pediatric AIDS

Africa
AIDS cofactors in, 45, 52, 75, 190, 273
clinical manifestations of AIDS in, 74-75
heterosexual transmission of HIV in, 75, 90, 202, 269
Kaposi's sarcoma in, 75
onset of AIDS in, 74
maternal-infant transmission of HIV in, 56, 272
parenteral transmission of HIV in, 76, 269-271
prevalence of infection in, 8, 29, 74-76, 269, 272
Agency for International Development, 29, 267-268, 274, 276
AIDS Foundation, 144
AIDS patients
ability to mount antibody reactions to new antigens, 44
causes of death in, 47
CD4-to-CD8 ratio in, 43
costs of care for, 156-158
denial, 149
depression, 148
drug toxicity, 47, 211-218
equitable access to clinical trials, 100, 220
health care needs of specific populations, 146-149
immunodeficiency in, 42-43
isolation of retroviruses from, 39
loss of employment by, 168
measure of immunologic impairment in, 43, 213
nervous system diseases, 49
nursing requirements, 144, 160
other infections commonly found in, 39
psychiatric/psychosocial support of, 148-149
T-lymphocyte characteristics, 44
AIDS Project/LA, 144
AIDS-associated retrovirus (ARV), *see* Human immunodeficiency virus (HIV)
AIDS-related complex (ARC)
cases in U.S., 7, 70
course of disease, 38
definition/defining, 65
longitudinal studies, 149
national reporting of, 65
progression to AIDS, 7, 46
psychiatric/psychosocial support for patients, 149-150

symptomatology, 38, 149
see also Human immunodeficiency virus
Albumin, destruction of HIV infectivity in, 53
Alternative testing sites, 17, 68, 115-116, 131-132
American Red Cross
AIDS education efforts, 102
"Look Back" program, 117
Amyl and butyl nitrites
association with AIDS, 38, 45-46, 51
association with Kaposi's sarcoma, 48, 73
Anal intercourse
receptive, 51-52, 66, 75, 89, 190
risk to insertive partner in, 51
use of condoms in, 97-98
Animal models
chimpanzees, 25, 205, 207-208, 221, 226
in experimental transmission studies, 50
HIV-related viruses in Old World primates, 205-206
importance in HIV research, 25, 186, 204
lentiviruses of ungulates, 206-207
recommendations regarding, 25, 207-209
strategies for determining experimental counterparts of human diseases, 204
supplies of test animals, 25, 35, 207-208, 221
Antibodies to HIV
infectiousness of persons having, 40
neutralizing capabilities, 225
in sera from AIDS and ARC patients, 40
time to appearance of, 115
Antibody tests for HIV
availability of, 64
in children, 50
confidentiality of results, 15, 68, 115, 125
controversy over, 113
cutoff points in, 114, 116
false negatives, 115-117
false positives, 114, 116
as insurance screening device, 169
level of use, 13
number in U.S. annually, 116
private development of, 61, 113
reduction of risk to blood recipients through, 54, 113-117
sensitivity and specificity of, 13, 114
techniques, 113
see also Screening for HIV

Antigens, response of CD4 cells to, 44, 197
Antiviral agents
  alpha interferon, 218
  azidothymidine (AZT), 26, 215-216,
    219-220
  currently being studied, 213-218
  development strategies, 181, 188, 211,
    218-219
  foscarnet, 217
  HPA-23, 214-215
  ideal characteristics of, 25, 219
  mechanism of viral escape from, 194
  research recommendations on, 25-26,
    219-221
  ribavirin, 216-217
  suramin, 214, 219
  targets for, 184, 186, 211-212, 214
  see also Drugs; Vaccines against HIV
Autoimmune reactions due to repeated
  exposure to sperm, 39

B

B lymphocytes, function of, 43, 198
Bacterial infections, *see* Opportunistic
  infections
Bathhouses, 59, 128-129
Behavior modification
  content of education directed at, 97, 234;
    see also Public education about AIDS
  by homosexual men, 89, 101, 104
  of IV drug users, 89-90, 100, 105-112,
    232
  ways for inducing, 231-234
Bisexuals, *see* Homosexual men
Blacks
  IV drug use among, 60
  pediatric AIDS in, 61
  prevalence of AIDS among, 72, 102
Blood donation
  autologous transfusion, 117
  directed, 117
  during preantibody phase of HIV
    infection, 54
  lack of risk in, 98, 115
  limiting use of blood to research
    (self-deferral), 14, 115
  Red Cross "Look Back" program, 117
Blood donors
  alternative testing sites, 17, 68, 115-116,
    131-132
  risk to hemophiliacs from, 60
  screening of, 61
  self-exclusion of, 53, 61, 115, 270

Blood products
  AIDS cases attributable to, 70
  clotting factors, 54, 60
  HIV transmission through, 53
  packed red blood cells, 53-54
  risk factors in HIV transmission
    through, 6, 53-54, 115
  screening of, 53
Blood transfusion recipients
  number of AIDS cases in, 60-61, 70-71
  reduction of risk to, 6, 54
Blood transfusions
  heterosexual transmission and, 90
  HIV transmission through, 30, 40, 53, 62
  risks of HIV transmission through, 76,
    269-270, 309-313
Bovine leukemia virus, 223

C

California
  —expenditures for AIDS prevention, 18,
    131-132
  pediatric AIDS in, 61
  seropositivity among homosexuals in, 69
Cancers occurring in HIV-infected
  persons, 48, 292, 318
Candidiasis (oral and esophageal), 73, 150,
  284
Caprine arthritis-encephalitis virus, 206,
  223-224
Casual contact, evidence against
  transmission by, 6, 50-51, 98, 271
CD4 cells
  depletion by HIV, 43-44, 195-196
  function of, 43
CD8 cells, correction of defective
  cytotoxic activities of, 197
Central nervous system (CNS)
  cellular localization of HIV, 211, 295-296
  drug penetration of, 215
  infections and malignancies related to
    AIDS, 49
  unanswered questions on HIV infection
    of, 49
Children, *see* Infants and children
Cofactors in AIDS
  in Africa, 45, 52, 75, 190, 273
  correlates with disease development, 193
  forms of, 45
  in Haitians, 66
  history of sexually transmitted diseases,
    51, 66, 70, 75
  in IV drug users, 69, 89, 106-107

nitrites, 38, 45-46, 51
recommended studies of, 201, 273
tissue trauma, 52, 66, 75, 190-191
Colorado, HIV reporting requirements, 65
Condoms
    education about, 10, 101, 202
    effectiveness in inhibiting HIV
        transmission, 97-98, 101, 202
Confidentiality
    in outpatient settings, 143
    protection of, 125, 129-130
    in reporting of ARC, 65
    of results of HIV antibody tests, 15, 68,
        119, 125
Contact tracing and notification, 13, 119-120
Costs, *see* Health care costs
Cryptococcal disease, 49, 73, 285
Cryptosporidiosis, 73, 283-284
Cytomegalovirus (CMV)
    association with incidence of Kaposi's
        sarcoma, 48
    condoms to inhibit transmission, 97
    role in AIDS, 39, 46, 73, 287-288
    treatment, 288

D

Deaths
    causes of, in AIDS patients, 7, 47
    cumulative, projections of, 86
    from pediatric AIDS, 61
    underreporting of, 73
Dementia
    care for AIDS patients with, 147, 148
    severity in HIV-infected persons, 49
Developing countries
    health improvement assistance to,
        265-266
    immunization problems in, 262-262
    pediatric AIDS in, 56, 262
    scope of HIV infection in, 8
Diagnosis of AIDS
    change in methods, 72
    difficulties in, 49, 64
    international development of tools and
        training for, 267-268
    reliability of, internationally, 262
Discrimination
    against homosexuals, 59, 133-134
    countermeasures, 19, 134-135
    due to misinformation, 19, 98
    in employment, housing, and social
        services access, 19, 133-134
    laws against, 134

refusal to bury victims, 118
    see also Social stigma
DNA
    flow of genetic information from RNA
        to, in retroviruses, 41
    unintegrated, in HIV, 185, 195
Drug abuse education in schools, 102
Drug abuse treatment programs
    financing for, 171
    focus of, 108
    methadone maintenance, 107-109, 232
    planning for, 103
Drugs
    access to, by AIDS patients, 100
    design of, 182, 210
    evaluation in humans, 26, 212-213
    evaluation *in vitro*, 212, 214
    gamma interferon, 197
    hope offered by, 8, 95, 214-219
    interleukin-2, 197
    research recommendations, 23-25,
        219-221
    toxicity during treatment of AIDS
        patients, 47
    see also Antiviral agents

E

Education, *see* Public education about
    AIDS
Encephalitis, subacute, in AIDS patients,
    49, 293-294
Enzyme-linked immunosorbent assays
    (ELISA), 113-114
Epidemic
    dimensions of, 7, 8, 57-77
    future course of, 8-9, 85-92
    long-term prospects, 91-92
    projections by U.S. Public Health
        Service, 85-92
    spread of, within and outside high-risk
        groups, 89-91
    status of, 5-8
    ways to alter course of, 9-19, 95-135
Epidemiologic research
    approaches to, 24
    case-control studies, 66-67
    centers for, 66
    costs of, 66
    on improved serologic and virologic
        tests, 203-204
    on natural history of HIV infection, 24,
        200-202
    populations selected for, 65-68

prospective cohort studies, 15, 24, 67, 105, 124, 201
serologic surveys, 67-68
on transmission of HIV, 202-203
value of, 66, 105
Epidemiologic surveillance
of blood donors, 86
of clinical manifestations of HIV infection, 67
definition of AIDS for, 7, 37-38, 63-64, 316-319
difficulties in, 68, 87
for evidence of association between immune globulins and AIDS cases, 55
functions of, 117
of general population, 86
of high-risk groups, 24
of military applicants, 87
recommended approaches to, 14, 199-200, 273
serologic, 67-68
success of, 63, 96
see also Reporting of AIDS/HIV infection; Screening for HIV
Epstein-Barr virus, role in AIDS, 39, 198
Equine infectious anemia virus, 224
Ethical issues
clinical trials of drugs, 213, 220
in drug abuse treatment to reduce HIV transmission, 109
durable power of attorney, 154
in health care financing, 153
obligation to care for HIV-infected persons, 20, 153-155
obligations of at-risk individuals, 20, 153
terminal care decisions, 20-21, 154-155
Europe
pattern of AIDS in, 76-77
Western, concerted action by, 263, 269
Expenditures, state, for AIDS prevention, 17, 131

F

Fear of AIDS
effects of, 12, 59, 108, 148
reducing, 99, 100, 234-236
Feline leukemia virus (FeLV), 222
Female circumcision, 75, 271
Financing
see Funding; Health care financing
Florida, pediatric AIDS in, 61
Funding
for AIDS/HIV research, 28, 238-249

for alternative testing sites, 116
for CDC, 130, 239-240
current levels, 103, 130, 239, 241
determining appropriate levels of, 131, 244-248
distribution of, 244
for drug research, 218
for epidemiologic studies, 67
for federal and state agencies, 131-132, 240
of home-, community-, and hospice-based care, 163
mechanisms for, 16-17, 130, 239-244
needs, 131-132, 247-248
private sources of, 132, 240-241
for public health measures, 16-19, 112, 130-133; *see also* Public education about AIDS
recommendations for, 15-19, 28, 31, 33-34, 133, 162, 208, 248-249, 276-277
for social science research, 231
for treatment of IV drug users, 171
U.S. contributions internationally, 274-275
see also Health care financing

G

Gamma globulin, risk of HIV transmission from, 53
Gay Men's Health Crisis, 134, 144, 149
Genital mutilation, *see* Female circumcision
Genital ulcers, relation between HIV infection and, 45, 52, 76

H

Haiti
pattern of AIDS in, 76
transmission of HIV in, 261
Haitians
factors associated with AIDS in, 66
heterosexual transmission of HIV by, 66-67, 70, 261
pediatric AIDS in, 62
proportion of AIDS cases among, 70-71
Health care
AIDS units/teams, 20
bed needs, 160-161
community-based, 20, 143-145
coordination of, 19, 145
dedicated AIDS clinics, 142
demonstration projects, 17, 162

ethical issues in, 153-155
facilities needed for AIDS patient
    hospitalization, 160-161
home hospice care, 143, 144, 163
home nursing services, 143-144
in hospitals, 19, 141-142
infection control precautions, 157
length of inpatient stay, 156
needs of specific patient populations, 20,
    146-148
outpatient, 20, 142-143, 171
planning of patients' discharges from
    hospital, 142
recommendations for, 19-20, 34, 145-146
staff requirements, 20, 157
strains on, 19, 21-22, 49, 139
terminal, 20, 154-155
voluntary agencies providing, 20, 144,
    149
see also Psychiatric/psychosocial
    support
Health care costs
for ARC patients, 158-159
average lifetime cost per AIDS case, 12,
    109
direct, for AIDS patients, 21, 156-158
equity in sharing, 172
factors contributing to, 21-22
for HIV-related conditions, 21-22,
    155-162
hospital, 156-158
implications of projected AIDS cases,
    159-160
indirect, of HIV-related conditions,
    20-21, 159
prevalence-based estimates, 156
recommended research on, 22
reduction of, 142
for seropositive individuals, 158-159
type-of-patient factor in, 157
Health care financing
analogies, end-stage renal disease
    (ESRD), 166-167, 170-171
for drug abuse treatment, 171
eligibility for, 163, 171
ethical issues in, 153
for individuals with HIV-associated
    conditions, 22-23, 162-173
issues and problems, 161-162
Medi-Cal reimbursements, 164
Medicaid, 22, 144, 162-164, 172
Medicare, 22, 165
recommendations for, 22-23, 34, 172-173
reduction of, 142

reimbursement for hospice care, 144
Social Security Disability program, 163,
    165
sources of, 162-165
see also Funding; Health insurance
Health care personnel
AIDS specialists, 140
burnout of, 141
HIV exposure through accidental
    needlesticks, 54, 62, 271
labor force in U.S., 62
nursing staff and nurse practitioners, 142
prospective studies of, 62
psychological stress in, 147
risk of infection among, 62-63, 153
seropositivity in, 62
training of, 20, 141
Health care planning, major problems, 85,
    87
Health insurance
antidiscrimination laws governing, 169
costs of, 168
ethical issues relating to, 166-171
inadequate coverage, 22, 165-166
incentives to seek care, 171
last-resort coverage, 170
limitations on coverage, 144
misperceptions about coverage, 170
policy issues, 171-172
public versus private, 171-172
recommendations regarding, 172-173
screening devices for, 169
Health Resources and Services
    Administration, 145
Helper/inducer cells, *see* CD4 cells
Hemodialysis units, transmission of HIV
    through, 55, 203
Hemophiliacs
first cases of AIDS in, 60
heterosexual contacts of, 61
HIV transmission to, 54, 57, 60
life expectancy of, 60
number of AIDS cases in, 70
seropositivity rate in, 60
Hepatitis B virus
similarities between HIV and, 39, 55, 62,
    91, 97
Herpes simplex, 49, 73, 287
Herpes zoster, 287
Heterosexual contacts
anal intercourse in Africa, 52
populations at risk, 61
projections of AIDS cases from, 86
proportion of AIDS cases from, 71

Heterosexual transmission
in Africa, 30, 75
from men to women, 57
risk outside U.S., 70
sources of, 90, 105
from women to men, 52, 57
see also Sexual transmission
Heterosexuals
education of, about AIDS, 101
number of AIDS cases in, 70
High-risk groups
current, 6, 37, 57
disease trends by, 70-71
factors in HIV transmission, 57
largest, in U.S., 57-58
nondiagnostic infections in, 288-289
projections concerning, 86-87
psychiatric/psychosocial support,
151-152
self-exclusion of blood donors, 53, 61
spread of epidemic within and outside,
89-91
see also specific populations
Hispanics
pediatric AIDS in, 61
prevalence of AIDS among, 72, 102
HIV infection
antibody appearance after, 115
asymptomatic period, 6, 7, 15, 65, 92,
126, 150-151
cancers associated with, 48
cellular route to, 191-192
of chimpanzees, 191, 205
classification system for, 64-65, 320-324
clinical manifestations of, 7, 46-50, 65,
281-299
clinical staging system for, 64
earliest events in, 45, 191
geographical differences in epidemiology
of, 73-77
groups at high risk, *see* High-risk
groups; and specific populations
immune system response to, 42-44,
191-193
immunologic consequences of, 42,
193-198
international scope of, 8, 28-29, 73-77,
261-263; *see also* specific countries/
regions
interruption of, 183-187
national resources for dealing with, 92-94
natural history of, 23-24, 189-204
neurologic complications associated
with, 49, 147-148, 210-211, 292-297

number of viral particles needed to
initiate, 45
pathogenesis of, 74
persistence of, 92, 113, 192, 194, 209,
211
preantibody phase of, 54
prevalence of, 69-70, 74-76, 89-90, 105,
107
progression to AIDS or ARC, 7, 57, 87,
95
receptor for, 43-44
recommendations for research on, 23-27,
198-203
reduction of risk of, 53-54
risk factors in, 6; *see also* Cofactors in
AIDS
similarities to hepatitis B virus, 39, 55,
62, 91
spread of, 62, 66-68, 75, 90-91, 107
symptoms of, 42, 49
treatment for, 8, 140, 198-199, 209-211
in women, 10, 57
see also Human immunodeficiency virus
(HIV)
Hodgkin's disease, 48, 291-292
Homosexual men
attitudes about testing, 124
behavior modification, 89, 101, 104
discrimination against, 59
education of, about AIDS, 10-11, 101
estimated U.S. population, 58
Hodgkin's disease in, 291-292
incidence of Kaposi's sarcoma in, 47
Kinsey report regarding, 58
number of AIDS cases in, 70
progression from seropositivity to
clinical AIDS in, 45
projections of HIV infection among, 7,
89
prospective cohort studies of, 67, 69,
149-150
recruiting of, for studies, 67
risk factors for HIV infection in, 51, 66
serologic surveys of, 67
seropositivity among, 69, 104
spread of epidemic through, 30, 89, 269
Human immunodeficiency virus (HIV)
antibodies to, 40, 115, 192
antibody testing of donated blood, *see*
Antibody tests for HIV
cytopathic effects of, 43-44, 195-197, 210
depletion of CD4 cells by, 43-44,
195-196, 210
discovery, 188

earliest indicators of transmission, 44
entry into body, 45, 50-57
entry into cell, 184
envelope glycoprotein, 183, 196, 210,
    225, 227
etiologic role in AIDS, 40
evolution of, 92
genes involved in replication, 178-180,
    184-186
genomic variation, 225
host cells for, 45, 191, 193-194, 210-211
infectiousness of, 153
interaction between CD4 molecule and,
    44-45, 195-196
isolation from body fluids, 40, 51, 189
life cycle, 180, 183
mutation of, 183, 186, 226
nervous system involvement, 49, 211,
    295-296
organ damage by, 194
origin, 74
propagation of, 40
receptor for initiation of viral infection,
    43, 179, 183, 199
replication of, 179-181, 185, 210, 216
replication sites, 45
research recommendations on, 23, 26-28,
    188-189
serologic reactivity with, 40
structural and functional constituents,
    181-182
syncytia formation by, 195
transmission modes, 6, 50-57; *see also*
    Casual contact; Maternal-infant
    transmission; Parenteral transmission;
    Sexual transmission
unintegrated DNA in, 185, 195
variation in shedding of, 51
viral classification of, 41
virion structure, 182
Human T-cell lymphotropic virus type I
    (HTLV-I), 41, 223
Human T-cell lymphotropic virus type II
    (HTLV-II), 41
Human T-cell lymphotropic virus type III
    (HTLV-III), *see* Human
    immunodeficiency virus
Human T-cell lymphotropic virus type IV
    (HTLV-IV), 42, 224

I

Immune globulins, HIV transmission from,
    55
Immune overload from repeated infections,
    39
Immune system
    cellular, 192-193, 226
    composition and function of, 42-43
    response to HIV, 191-193
Immunocompromised state
    in AIDS patients with Kaposi's sarcoma,
        47
    causes of, 37
    results, 42
    susceptibility to live-virus vaccines, 122,
        226-227
Immunodeficiency, 196, 197, 210
Immunofluorescent assays, 114
Infants and children
    foster care for, 147
    health care needs of, 146
    of IV drug users, 62
    projections of HIV infection in, 91
    schooling of infected individuals, 16, 130
    time to development of AIDS in, 56
    see also Pediatric AIDS
Infection, *see* HIV infection; Opportunistic
    infections
Infectious diseases, 50, 96, 266
Insect vectors, lack of evidence for, 6, 30,
    271
Institutionalized populations
    compulsory testing among, 16, 128, 130
    health care for, 16, 147-148
International efforts, U.S. contribution to,
    30-31, 35, 274-276
International issues
    development of tools and training for
        diagnosis, 267-268
    diagnostic reliability, 262
    prevalence of AIDS, 28-29, 261-263
    rationale for U.S. involvement to control
        AIDS, 29, 264-268
    risk of HIV infection, 29-30, 268-272
    risks of exposure through blood
        transfusions, 269-270
    scope of HIV infection, 28-29, 261-263
International research
    cofactor investigations, 273
    of perinatal and heterosexual
        transmission, 272
    opportunities for, 30-31, 266-267, 272-273

International resources for fighting AIDS
organizations, 29-31, 35, 263-264,
267-270
recommendations, 30-31, 276-277
U.S. contribution to, 274-276
Intravenous drug users
AIDS occurrence in, 59, 70
behavior modification in, 100, 102,
105-112
biases in studies of, 69
demographic data on, 59-60
distribution of sterile needles and
syringes for, 13, 34, 108-110
factors related to HIV infection of, 69,
89, 106-107
health care needs of, 146
HIV transmission mode in, 52-53
international risks of HIV transmission,
270
prevalence of HIV infection, 69, 89-90,
105, 107
prevention of HIV infection, 12-13, 100,
102, 105-112
projections of HIV infection, 7, 89-90
recruiting for studies, 69
representation in prison populations, 60
risk to offspring of, 62
sharing of injection equipment, 30,
52-53, 100, 107, 270
spread of HIV through, 107
stereotypes of, 107-108
viral dose factor in risk to, 55
see also Drug abuse treatment programs
Isospori belli, 284
Italy, seropositivity among drug users in,
77

K

Kaposi's sarcoma
AIDS-associated outbreaks, 37
of central nervous system, 49
cofactors, 73
death from, 47, 73, 75
definition, 47
diagnosis, 48, 64
health care costs, 157
in homosexual men, 47, 66, 198, 273
in non-AIDS populations, 189-190
reporting of, 73
role in AIDS, 198, 273, 289

L

Legal issues
closing and regulation of facilities,
128-129
compulsory public health measures,
126-129
Consolidated Omnibus Budget
Reconciliation Act of 1985, 160
criminal sanctions for transmitting
AIDS, 127
health-insurance-related, 169
Rehabilitation Act of 1973, 134-135
reporting of seropositivity, 127-128
requests for assistance with, 134
restrictions on sale of sterile drug
paraphernalia, 100
sex education in schools, 102
sodomy laws, 59, 129
vaccine liability, 222, 229-230
see also Discrimination
Lentiviruses
disorders caused by, 41-42, 224
HIV similarities to, 41, 207
of ungulates, 206-207, 223
visna virus, 185, 206, 224
Lymphadenopathy, *see* Persistent
generalized lymphadenopathy
Lymphadenopathy-associated virus (LAV)
disorders associated with, 42
see Human immunodeficiency virus
Lymphoid interstitial pneumonitis,
chronic, 318

M

Macrophages, function of, 43
Malignancies occurring in AIDS patients,
196, 198, 289-292
Maternal-infant transmission
in Africa, 272
breast-feeding/breast milk, 56, 125, 203
populations at risk for, 62, 90
rate of, 56-57
research needs on, 203
routes of, 56, 62
Meningitis, aseptic, 293
Mitogens, effect of HIV on, 44
Models/modeling
biological, limitations in constructing, 87
of care, 145
of incidence of AIDS, 86-87
uncertainties in, 8-9, 87-88
of vaccine delivery, 226-228

Monitoring, *see* Epidemiologic surveillance
Monkeys, immunodeficiency resembling
    AIDS in, 42; *see also* Simian
    immunodeficiency virus (SIV)
Murine leukemia virus, 222-223
Myelopathy in AIDS patients, 49, 294

N

National Commission on AIDS, 32-34, 94
National Institute of Allergy and Infectious
    Diseases, 240
National Institutes of Health, funding by
    and of, 67, 240-244
Natural killer cells, 43
Needles and other unsterile implements,
    HIV infection from, 76, 270-271
Needlesticks, accidental, HIV infection
    from, 30, 54-55, 62, 202-203, 271
Netherlands, distribution of sterile
    injection equipment in, 110
Neurologic complications
    associated with HIV infection, 49
    care needs of patients with, 147
    clinical and pathologic features of,
        292-295
    dementia, 49, 147, 148
    unsolved problems of, 211, 296-297
New Jersey
    pediatric AIDS in, 61, 146
    proportion of AIDS cases in IV drug
        users, 72
New York City
    AIDS case trends in, 71-72, 89, 164
    closing and regulation of facilities in, 128
    expenditures for AIDS prevention, 131
    hospital facility needs, 21-22, 160
    pediatric AIDS, 61, 146
    public education efforts in, 102
    seropositivity rates among IV drug
        users, 107
    study of Kaposi's sarcoma in
        homosexual AIDS patients in, 66
Non-Hodgkin's lymphomas, 48, 291,
    318-319

O

Ohio public education efforts, 102
Oncoviruses, 41, 222-223
Opportunistic infections
    associated with Hodgkin's disease, 48
    associated with non-Hodgkin's
        lymphomas, 48

bacterial, 285-287, 317
causes, 46-47, 196, 198
of central nervous system, 49
characteristics in AIDS patients, 47
fungal, 284-285, 317
helminthic, 317
with major role in AIDS epidemic, 37
protozoal, 281-284, 317
relation to mortality in AIDS patients,
    73
treatment, 212
trends in, 72-73
viral, 287-288, 317-318
Oral transmission of AIDS, 56
Oregon public education efforts, 102

P

Pan American Health Organization, 263
Parenteral transmission
    accidental needlesticks, 30, 54-55, 62,
        202-203
    blood transfusions, 53; *see also* Blood
        transfusions; Hemophiliacs
    from bloody fecal material, 56
    from child to mother, 56
    through hemodialysis units, 55
    risk outside U.S., 76, 269-270
    shared IV injection paraphernalia, 30,
        52-53, 100, 107, 270; *see also*
        Intravenous drug users
    through unsterile needles and syringes,
        76, 270-271
    viral dose factor in, 55
Pediatric AIDS
    clinical manifestations, 49-50, 61,
        297-298
    definition, 64-65, 318
    demographic data, 61-62
    diagnosis, 297-299
    immunization problems in developing
        countries, 265
    international prevalence, 262, 272
    number of reported cases, 61
    projected cases, 86
    time to development in infants, 56
    transmission routes, 62
Perinatal transmission, *see* Maternal-infant
    transmission
Peripheral neuropathies, 294-295
Persistent generalized lymphadenopathy
    (PGL), 38, 197
Plasma-derived hepatitis B vaccines, 55-56

Pneumocystis carinii pneumonia
AIDS-associated outbreaks of, 37
death from, 7
diagnosis, 64
health care costs for, 157
prevalence, 72
symptoms, 281-282
treatment, 47, 216, 282
Poppers, *see* Amyl and butyl nitrites
Prevention strategies
closing and regulation of facilities,
128-129
condoms, 10, 97-98, 101
isolation and quarantine, 126-128
for IV drug users, their sexual partners,
and offspring, 12-13, 34, 105-110, 112
monitoring effectiveness of, 68
personal hygiene, 98
PHS plan, 326-333
recommendations for, 12-13, 34, 110-112
state expenditures for, 131
viricidal lubricants for vaginal and anal
use, 202
WHO guidelines on blood transfusions,
269-270
see also Public education about AIDS;
Vaccines against AIDS
Private resources for fighting AIDS, list of,
315
Projections
of AIDS cases, 5, 85-92
bases for, 88, 90
empirical models of incidence of, 86-87
international, 261-263; *see also* specific
countries/regions
problems in making, 86-89
Prostitutes, transmission of AIDS by, 65,
75-77, 90, 269
Psychiatric/psychosocial support
for AIDS patients, 20, 148-149
for ARC patients, 20, 149-150
for asymptomatic seropositive patients,
150-151
for denial, 149
for depression, 148
for seronegative individuals in high-risk
groups, 151-152
Psychosocial effects
of knowledge of antibody status,
122-123, 149
ostracism, 149
recommendations regarding, 152-153,
234-236
Public education about AIDS
aims of, 71, 98, 100

assessing efficacy of, 68, 104-105
communication of scientific results, 189
content of, 10, 97-100, 102, 233
"dirty words" issue, 99
funding for, 11, 15-19, 101, 103, 112
media costs for, 17-18
recommendations for, 9-12, 18, 33,
110-112
responsibility for, 102-104
sex education in schools, 11, 102
success of, 101
targets of, 10-11, 100-103, 233
for youth, 101-102, 108
Public health measures
blood banking, 115-117
closing and regulation of facilities, 128-129
compulsory, 15-16, 126-129
contact tracing and notification, 13,
119-120
factors complicating, 112-113
among institutionalized populations, 128,
130, 147-148
isolation or quarantine, 15, 126-128, 130
mandatory screening, 120-122; *see also*
Screening for HIV
recommendations on, 13-16, 33, 124,
129-130
reporting schemes, 118-119; *see also*
Reporting of AIDS/HIV infection
surveillance, 117-118; *see also*
Epidemiologic surveillance
tests for HIV infection, 113-114; *see also*
Antibody tests for HIV
voluntary testing, 122-126; *see also*
Testing/tests for HIV
Public resources for fighting AIDS
coordination of, 93-94
extent of, 92
list of, 314-315
noninvolvement, 92-93
Pyogenic infections, 287

Q

Quarantine, 126-128

R

Reporting of AIDS/HIV infection
asymptomatic, 65
Colorado program for, 65, 118
delays in, 88
mandatory, 65, 117

passive, 63
recommendations on, 24, 199-200
responsibility for, 63
schemes for, 117-119
state laws and regulations for, 14, 63-64
Reporting of ARC, 65
Research, *see* Epidemiologic research;
International research
Research needs, 177-249; *see also* specific
subject areas
Retroviruses
diseases caused by, 41
features of, 40-41
human, 39; *see also* Human
immunodeficiency virus
isolation of, 39, 209
from nonhuman primates, *see* Simian
immunodeficiency virus
replication by, 179-181
species harboring, 39
structure of, 178-179
subfamilies of, 41-42; *see also*
Lentiviruses; Oncoviruses;
Spumiviruses
transmission of genetic information by,
41
type D primate, 223
Reverse transcriptase
in cultures of T lymphocytes from AIDS
patients, 39
inhibition of, 213-217
role in HIV, 41, 180, 184, 212
RNA, transmission of genetic information
by retroviruses, 41
Robert Wood Johnson Foundation, 145

S

Saliva, HIV virus isolated from, 51
Salmonella infections, 286
San Francisco
AIDS case trends in, 71-72, 164
Bay Area Lawyers for Individual
Freedom, 134
closing and regulation of facilities, 128
community-based AIDS care, 143
expenditures for AIDS prevention, 131
homosexual population, 58
hospital facility needs in, 160
seropositivity among homosexuals in,
69, 104
Scarification, 75, 271
Scotland, seropositivity among drug users
in, 77

Screening for HIV
of asymptomatic persons, 44
of blood, 13, 53
of blood donors, 68
compared with genetic screening, 121
confidentiality in, 15, 68, 119, 125
mandatory, 14-15, 112, 120-122
of military inductees, 68, 121-122
premarital, 121
sites for, 68
of subgroups, 14-15, 120-121
of women in high-risk categories, 57,
125-126
Semen, HIV isolated from, 51
Seroconversion
time between transmission and, 44-45
see also HIV infection
Serologic testing, *see* Antibody tests for
HIV; Screening for HIV; Testing/tests
for HIV
Seronegativity in infected individuals, 191
Seropositive individuals
anxiety and depression in, 150
costs of care for, 158-159
psychiatric/psychosocial support for,
150-151
Seropositivity
among African men and women, 52
in health care personnel, 62
in hemophiliacs, 60
in homosexuals, 69, 89, 104
in husbands of women with
transfusion-associated AIDS, 52
in military recruit applicants, 68
in recipients of HIV-infected blood, 53
Sexual behavior, *see* Behavior
modification
Sexual transmission of HIV
age distributions indicative of, 52
artificial insemination, 190
case-control studies of, 51
condoms to prevent, 10, 97-98, 101, 202
contact with partners from areas with
high prevalence of AIDS, 51
drug use and, 51, 90
female circumcision and, 75
female to male, 6, 52, 75, 191
genital ulcers and, 45, 52, 76
heterosexual intercourse, 51-52
history of sexually transmitted disease
and, 51, 66, 70, 75, 190
kissing, 51
male to female, 62, 52, 75, 90, 191
manual-rectal intercourse (fisting), 51

mutual masturbation, 51
nitrites and, 51
oral intercourse, 51
oral-genital sex, 51
oral-rectal sex, 51
by prostitutes, 66, 75-77, 90
receptive anal intercourse, 6, 51-52, 66, 75, 89, 190
rectal douching and, 51-52
repeated exposure to infected partners, 52
risk outside U.S., 202, 268-269
scarification and, 75, 271
socioeconomic class and, 75
tissue trauma and, 52, 66, 75
vaginal inoculation, 190-191
vaginal intercourse, 6, 52, 75, 202
see also Heterosexual contacts; Homosexual men; Prevention strategies
Shanti Project, 143, 144
Shooting galleries, 53, 107
Simian immunodeficiency virus (SIV), 74, 202, 206, 209, 224
Skin abrasions, HIV infection through, 62
Slim disease, characteristics of, 75
Social science research
approaches to, 233
breaking train of transmission, 231-234; *see also* Behavior modification
funding, 231
needs, 27, 34, 230-238
organizing health and social services, 237-238
recommendations for, 27, 34, 238
reducing public fear of AIDS, 234-236
role in AIDS challenge, 231
Social stigma
attached to being tested/test results, 114, 119, 123
complication of public health measures by, 112
effects of, 19
see also Discrimination
Southeast Asia, pattern of AIDS in, 77, 272
Spain, seropositivity among drug users in, 77
Sperm, autoimmune reactions due to repeated exposure to, 39
Spumiviruses, disorders caused by, 42
Squamous cell cancers, association with HIV infection, 48

Suppressor/cytotoxic cells, *see* CD8 cells
Surveillance, *see* Epidemiologic surveillance

T

T lymphocytes
CD4 molecule, 43, 183-184, 191, 196, 199
CD4-to-CD8 ratio in AIDS patients, 43
CD8 molecule, 43
characteristics of, in AIDS patients, 44
culturability of HIV in, 39-40
cytopathic effect of HIV envelope protein on, 183, 210
functions of, 197
reduction of, in AIDS patients, 43
see also CD4 cells; CD8 cells
T-cell leukemia, 40-41
Tears, HIV isolation from, 51
Testing/tests for HIV
anonymous, 119-120, 124-125
antigen assays, 24
confirmatory, 114, 116
costs of, 17
counseling with, 15, 17
current methods, 304
improvements needed in, 30, 203-204
insurance-related, 169
performance characteristics of, 306-307
recommendations for, 30, 34, 124-125, 129
surrogate blood tests, 169
virologic, 203, 204, 213
voluntary, 15, 122-126
without subject's knowledge, 15, 125
see also Antibody tests for HIV; Screening for HIV
Thrush, *see* Candidiasis
Toxoplasma gondii, 49, 73, 282-283
Transmission of AIDS/HIV
breaking train of, 231-234
cellular route, 192
dose factor in, 190
efficiencies of, 190-191
epidemiologic approaches to research, 202-203
erroneous beliefs about, 98
outside the U.S., 29-30
sources of, 190
see also Casual contact; Cofactors in AIDS; Maternal-infant transmission; Parenteral transmission; Sexual transmission

Treatment strategies, *see* Antiviral agents;
    Drugs; Vaccines against HIV
Tuberculosis, 273, 285-286

U

United States
    agencies and organizations with
        international responsibilities, 267-268
    contribution to international efforts,
        30-31, 35, 274-276
    foreign policy considerations, 264
    health improvement assistance to
        developing countries, 264-265
    infection risks outside, 268-272
    rationale for international involvement to
        control AIDS, 264-268
U.S. Public Health Service
    AIDS Task Force, 93
    funding for, 17, 130-131
    plan for prevention and control of AIDS,
        8-9, 85-86, 88, 91, 93-94, 326-333
    projections for incidence and prevalence
        of AIDS, 85-92
    use of information related to antibody
        tests, 68

V

Vaccines, animal retrovirus, 222-225
Vaccines against HIV
    availability, 26, 92, 95, 113, 229
    development approaches, 23, 26-27,
        183-184, 192, 221-222, 225-226, 228-229
    difficulties in developing, 221, 223, 225
    liability and, 222, 229-230
    models for delivery of, 226-228
    private sector role, 27, 222, 230
    research recommendations for, 27,
        229-230
    testing in humans, 222, 228-229
Viral shedding, variability in, 51

W

Washington, D.C., seropositivity among
    homosexuals in, 69
Western blot analysis, use with ELISA
    test, 114, 116
World Health Organization, AIDS-related
    activities of, 29, 30-31, 35, 263,
    269-270, 273-277